IARC Handbooks of Cancer Prevention (Programme Head: Harri Vainio, M.D., Ph.D.)

Volume 5: Sunscreens

Editors:	Harri Vainio, M.D., Ph.D. Franca Bianchini, Ph.D.
Technical Editor:	Elisabeth Heseltine
Bibliographic assistance:	Agnès Meneghel
Layout:	Josephine Thévenoux
Photographic assistance:	Georges Mollon
Printed by:	Imprimerie Darantiere, BP 8, 21801 Quétigny, France Dépôt légal : janvier 2001 - N° d'impression : 20-1353
Publisher:	International Agency for Research on Cancer 150 cours Albert Thomas, 69372, Lyon, France Tel. +33 4 72 73 84 85 Fax. +33 4 72 73 83 19

WORLD HEALTH ORGANIZATION

INTERNATIONAL AGENCY FOR RESEARCH ON CANCER

IARC Handbooks of Cancer Prevention

Volume 5

Sunscreens

This publication represents the views and expert opinions
of an IARC Working Group on the
Evaluation of Cancer-preventive Agents,
which met in Lyon,

11–18 April 2000

2001

Published by the International Agency for Research on Cancer,
150 cours Albert Thomas, F-69372 Lyon cedex 08, France

Distributed by Oxford University Press, Walton Street, Oxford, OX2 6DP, UK (Fax: +44 1865 267782) and in the USA by
Oxford University Press, 2001 Evans Road, Carey, NC 27513, USA (Fax: +1 919 677 1303).
All IARC publications can also be ordered directly from IARC*Press*
(Fax: +33 4 72 73 83 02; E-mail: press@iarc.fr).

The International Agency for Research on Cancer welcomes requests for permission to
reproduce or translate its publications, in part or in full. Applications and enquiries should be addressed
to the Editorial & Publications Service, International Agency for Research on Cancer,
which will be glad to provide the latest information on any changes made to the text, plans for new
editions, and reprints and translations already available.

IARC Library Cataloguing in Publication Data

Sunscreens/
    IARC Working Group on the Evaluation of
    Cancer Preventive Agents (2001 : Lyon, France)

(IARC handbooks of cancer prevention ; 5)

1. Sunscreening agents – congresses. I. IARC Working Group on the Evaluation of Cancer
    Preventive Agents II Series

ISBN 92 832 3005 1   (NLM Classification: W1)
ISSN 1027-5622

Printed in France

International Agency For Research On Cancer

The International Agency for Research on Cancer (IARC) was established in 1965 by the World Health Assembly, as an independently financed organization within the framework of the World Health Organization. The headquarters of the Agency are in Lyon, France.

The Agency conducts a programme of research concentrating particularly on the epidemiology of cancer and the study of potential carcinogens in the human environment. Its field studies are supplemented by biological and chemical research carried out in the Agency's laboratories in Lyon and, through collaborative research agreements, in national research institutions in many countries. The Agency also conducts a programme for the education and training of personnel for cancer research.

The publications of the Agency contribute to the dissemination of authoritative information on different aspects of cancer research. A complete list is printed at the back of this book. Information about IARC publications, and how to order them, is also available via the Internet at: **http://www.iarc.fr/**

Note to the Reader

Anyone who is aware of published data that may influence any consideration in these *Handbooks* is encouraged to make the information available to the Unit of Chemoprevention, International Agency for Research on Cancer, 150 Cours Albert Thomas, 69372 Lyon Cedex 08, France

Although all efforts are made to prepare the *Handbooks* as accurately as possible, mistakes may occur. Readers are requested to communicate any errors to the Unit of Chemoprevention, so that corrections can be reported in future volumes.

Acknowledgements

The Foundation for Promotion of Cancer Research, Japan, is gratefully acknowledged for its generous support to the meeting of the Working Group and the production of this volume of the *IARC Handbooks of Cancer Prevention.*

List of Participants

H.N. Ananthaswamy
Department of Immunology
The University of Texas
M.D. Anderson Cancer Center
1515 Holcombe Boulevard
Box 178
Houston, TX 77030
USA

C. Arlett
MRC Cell Mutation Unit
University of Sussex
Falmer
Brighton, BN1 9RR
United Kingdom

B.K. Armstrong *(Chairman)*
Cancer Research and Registers
Division
New South Wales Cancer Council
PO Box 572
Kings Cross
1340 Sydney
Australia

P. Autier
European Institute of Oncology
Division of Epidemiology &
Biostatistics
Via Ripamonti 435
20141 Milan
Italy

J.A. Crowell
Chemoprevention Branch
Division of Cancer Prevention and
Control
National Institutes of Health
National Cancer Institute
Bethesda, MD 20892
USA

F.R. de Gruijl
Dermatology
University Hospital Utrecht
G02 124
PO Box 85500
3508 GA Utrecht
The Netherlands

B.L. Diffey
Regional Medical Physics Department
Newcastle General Hospital
Newcastle NE4 6BE
UK

J.-F. Doré *(Vice-Chairman)*
INSERM U453
Biologie des Gènes Suppresseurs de
Tumeurs
Bâtiment Le Cheney
Centre Léon Bérard
28, rue Laënnec
69373 Lyon Cedex 08
France

P.D. Forbes
Argus Research Laboratories, Inc.
905 Sheehy Drive
Horsham, PA 19044
USA

A. Fourtanier
Department of Dermato-Biology
L'Oréal-Advanced Research-Life
Sciences Research
Centre Charles Zviak
90 rue du Général Roguet
92583 Clichy Cedex
France

R.P. Gallagher
Cancer Control Research Program
British Columbia Cancer Agency
600 West 10th Avenue
Vancouver, BC, V5Z 4E6
Canada

G.M. Halliday
Department of Medicine (Dermatology)
Royal Prince Alfred Hospital
University of Sydney
Sydney, NSW
Australia

K. Hemminki
Centre for Nutrition and Toxicology
Karolinska Institute
Novum
141 52 Huddinge
Sweden

D.J. Hill
Centre for Behavioural Research in
Cancer
Anti-Cancer Council of Australia
100 Drummond Street
Carlton Victoria 3053
Australia

C. Jansén
Department of Dermatology
Turku University Central Hospital
Kiinamyllynkatu 4-8
20520 Turku
Finland

A. Kawada
Department of Dermatology
Kinki University School of Medicine
377-2 Ohno-Higashi,
Osaka-Sayama
Osaka 589 8511
Japan

A.M. Mommaas
Department of Dermatology and
Center for Electron Microscopy
Leiden University Medical Center
PO Box 9503
2300 RA Leiden
The Netherlands

M.F. Naylor
Department of Dermatology
University of Oklahoma Health
Sciences Center
Oklahoma City,
OK 73190
USA

V.E. Reeve
Department of Veterinary Anatomy
and Pathology
University of Sydney
B14 - McMaster Building, Room 225
Sydney NSW 2006
Australia

J.K. Robinson
Loyola University Chicago
2160 South First Avenue
Room 341
Cardinal Bernardin Cancer Center
Maywood, IL 60153
USA

B.W. Stewart
Cancer Control Program
South Eastern Sydney Area Health
Service
PO Box 88
Randwick NSW 2031
Australia

R.M. Tyrrell
Department of Pharmacy and
Pharmacology
University of Bath (5 West – 2.27)
Claverton Down
Bath, BA2 7AY
United Kingdom

A.R. Young
Department of Photobiology
St. John's Institute of Dermatology
Guy's, King's and St Thomas' School
of Medicine
University of London
London SE1 7EH
United Kingdom

Observer
Dr Romano Mascotto
L'Oréal
6 rue Bertrand Sincholle
92585 Clichy Cedex
France

Secretariat
R. Baan
F. Bianchini
M. Friesen
J. Hall
E. Heseltine
V. Krutovskikh
B. Pignatelli
A.B. Miller
H. Ohshima
C. Partensky
A. Sasco
H. Vainio
J. Wilbourn

Technical assistance
S. Egraz
A. Meneghel
D. Mietton
J. Mitchell
S. Reynaud
J. Thévenoux

Contents

Chapter 1

Sun, Skin and Cancer Prevention

Skin cancer is more common than any other type of cancer. The estimated age-standardized incidence rates of cutaneous melanoma in several countries are reported in Figure 1. It has been estimated with reasonable certainty that 106 000 melanomas of the skin were diagnosed worldwide in 1990 (Parkin *et al.*, 1999) (Table 1). Less certainly, it was estimated that at least 2 750 000 non-melanocytic cancers (basal- and squamous-cell carcinomas) of the skin were diagnosed in 1985, representing more than 30% of all newly diagnosed cancers (Armstrong & Kricker, 1995). While non-melanocytic skin cancers are usually considered to be of little concern, they are the reason for many hospital admissions each year in white populations and for higher direct health care costs than any other cancer in Australia (Mathers *et al.*, 1998). The incidence rates of melanoma and non-melanocytic skin cancers have been rising steadily for some decades in many white populations (Armstrong & Kricker, 1994; Gray *et al.*, 1997; Staples *et al.*, 1998).

While the contribution of sunlight is difficult to estimate with any certainty, it probably causes the majority of melanomas of the skin worldwide. In predominantly white populations, it is estimated to cause approximately 80–90% of such cancers (Armstrong & Kricker, 1993). The proportion of non-melanocytic skin cancers caused by sunlight has not been estimated but

is probably about the same as that of melanoma. Given the apparently overwhelming importance of solar radiation as a cause of skin cancer (IARC, 1992), public health programmes aimed at preventing skin cancer focus almost totally on protection from sunlight. These programmes usually incorporate a range of strategies, including dissemination of knowledge about the intensity of sunlight in the local environment (as measured, for example, by the solar ultraviolet index (WHO *et al.*, 1995), staying out of direct sunlight during times when the ambient intensity is high, wearing a hat and clothing on unprotected skin when in direct sunlight, and using broad-spectrum, water-resistant sunscreens that protect uncovered skin from direct sunlight.

The first use of sunscreens was reported in 1928 (Shaath, 1997a). While sunscreens have been portrayed as a 'last resort' in sun protection (Marks, 1996), they have become increasingly popular, particularly during outdoor recreation in which as little clothing is worn as possible, such as at the seaside (Koh *et al.*, 1997; Robinson *et al.*, 1997a). Sunscreens were first developed to protect against sunburn and were designed to filter out the burning rays of sunlight (ultraviolet B, UVB; 280–315 nm). More recently, because of evidence that longer wavelengths of sunlight (ultraviolet A, UVA; 315–400 nm) participate in the sunburn reaction and can cause skin cancer in animals, and

concern that staying in the sun longer with protection against UVB increases exposure to UVA, UVA absorbers have been added to most sunscreens to widen their absorption spectra (Gasparro *et al.*, 1998).

Sunscreens undoubtedly protect against sunburn, because they are routinely tested in humans and can be assigned a sun protection factor (SPF) which reflects their ability to prevent sunburn. Whether they can prevent skin cancer is the subject of this volume of handbooks.

Sun and skin cancer in humans

An association between non-melanocytic skin cancer and exposure to the sun appears to have first been suggested in 1894; it was not until about 1952 that it was argued that exposure to the sun also causes melanoma (Armstrong *et al.*, 1997). Exposure to the sun causes the three major types of skin cancer: basal-cell carcinoma, squamous-cell carcinoma and melanoma, although the evidence does not permit identification of the causative part of the solar spectrum. Lip cancer may also be caused by solar exposure (IARC, 1992). Exposure to the sun may also cause some other, rarer skin cancers and, possibly, an internal cancer, non-Hodgkin lymphoma (IARC, 1992; English *et al.*, 1997; Iscovich *et al.*, 1998; McGregor *et al.*, 1999; Miller & Rabkin, 1999).

What is the evidence that skin cancer is caused by exposure to the sun?

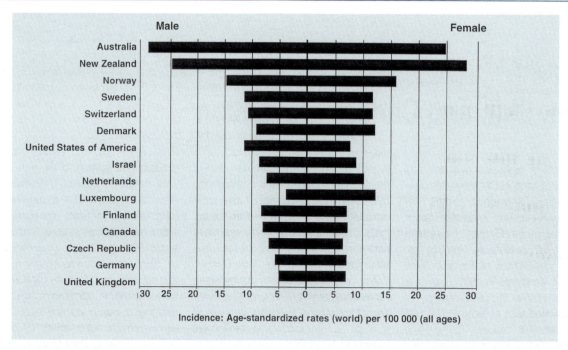

Figure 1 Estimated age-standardized incidence rates of malignant melanoma of the skin around 1990 in the 15 countries with the highest rates

Table 1. Proportional distribution of new cases of malignant cutaneous melanoma of the skin by region for persons of all ages, 1990		
Region	Distribution of cases (%)	
	Males	Females
Africa	6	7
Asia	8	10
Central and South America	7	9
Europe	47	34
North America	25	33
Oceania	7	7

The risk for skin cancers at all sites increases with proximity to the equator in people with white skin in Australia and the USA, countries that cover a wide range of latitudes. At the individual level, the risk is greater for people who have lived much of their lives at low latitudes or in sunnier climates than people who have lived in such areas little or not at all. Migrants to countries where there is heavy solar exposure, such as Australia and Israel, from countries were there is little solar exposure, such as northern and western Europe, have lower risks for skin cancer than people born in the countries with heavy exposure. Furthermore, the risk is greater the younger a person is when he or she migrates to a country with heavy solar exposure. People with black skin, which is comparatively insensitive to sunburn, have a much lower risk for skin cancer than do people with white skin, and among white-skinned people the risk of those with fairer skin is higher than that of people with darker skin (Fig. 2). Few studies have been conducted of patterns among people with other skin types, such as Asians. People who tan easily and rarely burn are less likely to get skin cancer than people who sunburn easily and tan with difficulty. The highest density of occurrence, per unit of surface area, of the common types of skin cancer is on skin that is usually exposed to the sun (the head and neck), and the lowest density is on skin that is rarely if ever exposed (the buttocks) (English et al., 1997).

These lines of evidence are all indirect, in that they do not relate

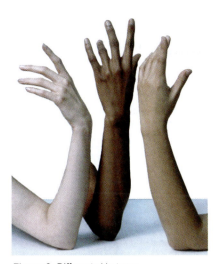

Figure 2 Different skin types

people's actual exposure to the sun to their risk for skin cancer. Studies that have attempted to do this have generally had less persuasive results. Such studies are not easy to perform, because people have difficulty in recalling details of their exposure to the sun accurately. Nevertheless, a number of studies have shown relationships between recalled exposure to the sun and the occurrence of skin cancer at the time or subsequently. A particularly consistent relationship has been found between heavy recreational exposure to the sun and individual risk for melanoma (IARC, 1992; Elwood & Jopson 1997). Establishment of a relationship between total exposure to the sun and melanoma has been more elusive, and some studies have suggested that people with heavy occupational exposure to the sun have a lower risk for melanoma than people with little such exposure (Elwood & Jopson, 1997). A high frequency of sunburn has been shown to increase the risks for all major types of skin cancer, and people who have benign conditions associated with heavy exposure to the sun, such as solar keratoses ('sun

spots'), also have a high risk for skin cancer (English *et al.*, 1997).

The paradoxical findings that melanoma is more common among people working indoors than those working outdoors and, more recently, that heavy occupational exposure to the sun is associated with a lower risk for melanoma than light exposure led to the suggestion that the pattern as well as the intensity of exposure to the sun influences the risk for melanoma (Holman *et al.*, 1980). It was also suggested that the risk increases with increasing intermittency of exposure. This suggestion is strongly supported by evidence that increasing recreational exposure to the sun increases the risk for melanoma. The relationship may also be true for basal-cell carcinoma (Kricker *et al.*, 1995) but probably not for squamous-cell carcinoma, the risk for which appears to depend only on the total accumulated amount of exposure to the sun (English *et al.*, 1998a).

Does reducing exposure to the sun reduce the risk for skin cancer? Evidence that it does is quite limited. A number of white populations are now experiencing falling incidence and mortality rates of melanoma, particularly among young people, and it has been argued that these trends are due to greater protection from the sun over the past 20 years or so (Giles & Thursfield, 1996). In addition, at least one population has shown a similar trend for basal-cell carcinoma, but not squamous-cell carcinoma (Staples *et al.*, 1998). There have also been reports of downward trends in the incidence of melanoma in areas where local initiatives have been made to reduce the population's exposure to the sun (Cristofolini *et al.*, 1993; MacKie *et al.*, 1997). In a randomized, controlled trial of the effects of isotretinoin on the risk for further basal-cell carcinomas over 36

months, the risk of people who had reduced their solar exposure was lower than that of those who had not (Robinson & Rademaker, 1992). Reduction of recent exposure to the sun may also reduce the risk for squamous-cell carcinoma, as shown in a randomized, controlled trial of four to five years' use of sunscreens (Green *et al.*, 1999a,b).

It may be difficult to demonstrate that reducing exposure to the sun reduces the risk for skin cancer, since studies of migrant populations suggest that the lifetime risk is strongly determined by exposure to the sun during the first 15 or so years of life (English *et al.*, 1997; 1998b). There is some evidence, however, that exposure to the sun later in life also influences the risk for skin cancer (Robinson, 1987; Zanetti *et al.*, 1996; Armstrong, 1997; English *et al.*, 1998a).

What evidence do we have that ultraviolet radiation (UVR), the component of the sun's rays that is attenuated by sunscreens, is that which causes skin cancer? In humans, exposure to UVB produces a range of chemical changes in DNA, consisting most commonly of intra-strand cross-links between adjacent pyrimidine bases (IARC, 1992). These cross-links, if not repaired, can produce mutations, which might in turn lead to cancer development. This form of DNA damage can also produce 'signature mutations' in DNA, CC to TT transitions (in which two adjacent cytidine bases are mutated to two adjacent thymidine bases) or C to T transitions at dipyrimidine sites — the definitive indicator of carcinogenesis by UVR. These signature mutations have been found in the tumour suppressor *p53* gene in normal skin cells (and are probably present in other genes as well), and their presence has been correlated with the extent of exposure of the body site from which the skin was taken (Ouhtit *et al.*, 1997). They have also been found quite frequently in the *p53* gene in basal- and squamous-cell carcinomas of the skin, whereas they are rare in *p53* gene mutation patterns of other types of cancer (IARC, 1992). Mutation of the *p53* gene is probably an important step in the development of these skin cancers (Ziegler *et al.*, 1996). The estimated density of CC to TT transitions in the *p53* gene in normal skin was shown to predict the risk for basal-cell carcinoma in one study, although the density did not correlate with estimates of individual exposure to the sun (Ouhtit *et al.*, 1998). Signature UVR-associated mutations have also been found in cyclin-dependent kinase (*p16*) genes in a primary melanoma cell line. While these signature mutations have been found in melanoma cell lines, only one was found in 26 samples from human tumours (Pollock *et al.*, 1995; Healy *et al.*, 1996; Pollock *et al.*, 1996; Xu *et al.*, 2000).

Additional evidence that UVR, specifically, causes skin cancer is provided by the observation that people with the rare genetic syndrome xeroderma pigmentosum have a very high risk for skin cancer (IARC, 1992). With regard to the general population, there is conflicting evidence about the relationship between the capacity for excision repair of DNA and the risk for basal-cell carcinoma (Hall *et al.*, 1994; Wei *et al.*, 1995; D'Errico *et al.*, 1999; Xu *et al.*, 2000).

Solar radiation of concern and its attenuation

Solar ultraviolet radiation

The spectrum of extraterrestrial solar radiation approximates to a black body at a temperature of about 5800 K. Of this, about 9% is UVR ($\lambda < 400$ nm). Sunlight consists of visible light in the spectrum from 400 nm (violet) to 700 nm (red), infrared radiation (> 700 nm) and UVR. UVR has been subdivided by the International Commission for Illumination into UVA (315–400 nm), which is sometimes called 'black light', UVB (280–315 nm) and UVC (100–280 nm). The quality (spectrum) and quantity (intensity) of sunlight are modified during its passage through the atmosphere. The principal interactions in the stratosphere (~10–50 km above sea level) are absorption by ozone and scattering by interaction with molecules such as N_2 and O_2 (Fig. 3). In the troposphere (~0–10 km above sea level), absorption by pollutants such as ozone, NO_2 and SO_2 and scattering by particulates such as soot and clouds are the main attenuating processes. At ground level, UVR comprises about 5% of solar energy (Madronich, 1993).

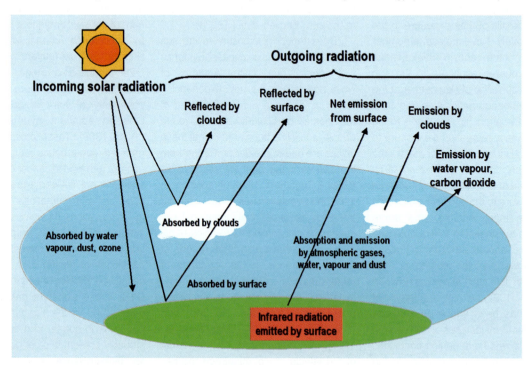

Figure 3 Interactions of solar radiation in the atmosphere

Both the quality and quantity of terrestrial UVR vary with the elevation of the sun above the horizon, or solar altitude. (The complementary angle between the sun and the local vertical is termed the 'solar zenith angle'.)
The solar altitude depends on the time of day, the day of the year and geographical location (latitude and longitude). On a summer's day, UVB comprises approximately 3.5% of terrestrial UVR, and UVA the remaining 96.5%; UVC is blocked by the stratospheric ozone layer and does not reach the earth's surface. Since UVB is much more effective than UVA at causing biological damage (Figure 4), solar UVB contributes about 80% towards sunburn, and solar UVA contributes the remaining 20% (Figure 5). The spectrum of terrestrial sunlight measured at Melbourne, Australia (latitude 38°S) at noon in midsummer (solar altitude, 75°) is shown in Figure 4.

Normally, less than 10% of sunlight is reflected from most ground surfaces. The main exceptions are gypsum sand, which reflects about 15–30%, and snow, which can reflect up to 90%. Contrary to popular belief, calm water reflects only about 5% of incident UVR, although up to 20% is reflected from choppy water (Diffey, 1998). Since UVR passes easily through water, swimming in either the sea or open-air pools offers little protection against sunburn. Furthermore, if sunscreens that are not water-resistant have been applied, they will wash off rapidly (Stokes & Diffey, 1999a) and increase the risk for sunburn if users believe they are protected and extend their time in the water accordingly.

Several artificial sources of UVR have been developed, including incandescent sources, gas discharge lamps, arc lamps, fluorescent lamps, metal halide lamps and electrodeless lamps (IARC, 1992; WHO, 1994). These sources differ in the power consumption, rare gas and phosphor used, type of metal or metal halide incorporated, composition of the housing and pressure within the lamp (Council on Scientific Affairs, 1989). Depending on the filters used, they can provide either unfiltered UVR or simulated sunlight.

Sunscreens

Absorption by sunscreens

Topical sunscreens applied to the skin act by absorbing and/or scattering incident UVR. The shape of the absorption spectrum is the fundamental attribute of a topical sunscreen. It is expressed as the extinction coefficient, which is a measure of the degree to which the sunscreen absorbs individual wavelengths across the terrestrial UVR spectrum (290–400 nm). Absorbance is the product of the extinction coefficient, the concentration of the active ingredient and the effective thickness of application. The monochromatic protection factor, $mPF(\lambda)$, at wavelength λ is related to the absorbance $[A(\lambda)]$ as follows:

$$mPF(\lambda) = 10^{A(\lambda)}.$$

The monochromatic protection factors of a typical, modern, broad-spectrum sunscreen product are shown in Figure 6.

Sun protection factor

The concept of a sunscreen effectiveness index (ratio) is attributed to Schulze (1956a,b). The specific term 'sun protection factor' (SPF) and the associated method were proposed by Greiter (1974, 1981). Use of the SPF was subsequently adopted by many regulatory authorities and by the cosmetics and pharmaceutical industries. The SPF is defined as the ratio of the least amount of ultraviolet energy required to produce minimal

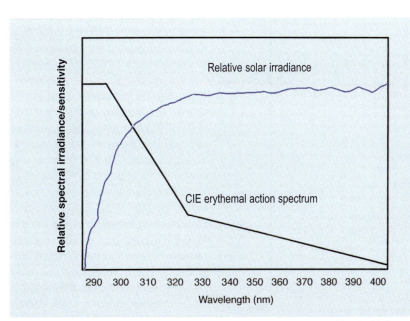

Figure 4 Relative spectral irradiance of ambient midday summer sunshine in Melbourne, Australia (38°S) and the action spectrum of the International Commission for Illumination (CIE) for minimal erythema in human skin

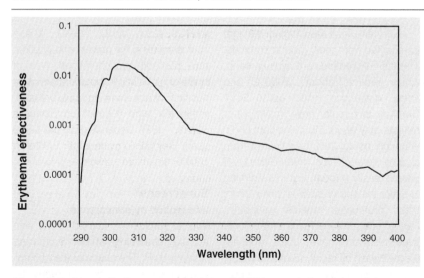

Figure 5 Erythemal effectiveness spectrum of sunlight. This curve is the product of the relative solar irradiance and the erythemal action spectrum of the International Commission for Illumination (see Figure 4) at each wavelength.

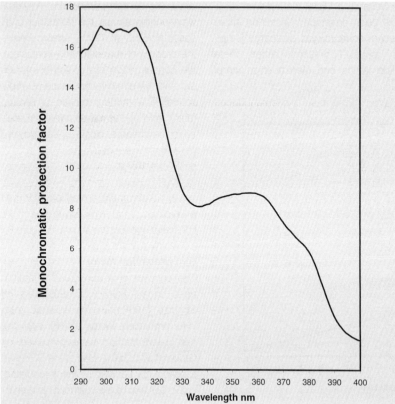

Figure 6 Monochromatic protection factors of a broad-spectrum sunscreen (SPF 15) with butyl methoxydibenzoylmethane, methylbenzylidine camphor, octyl salicylate and titanium dioxide as active ingredients

erythema (reddening of the skin) on sunscreen-protected skin to the amount of energy required to produce the same erythema on unprotected skin (Food & Drug Administration, 1978, 1993, 1998, 1999). It is popularly interpreted as how much longer skin covered with sunscreen takes to burn compared with unprotected skin (Health Education Authority, 1996). Internationally agreed procedures (Food & Drug Administration, 1978; COLIPA, 1994) define protected skin as that to which a 2 mg/cm² layer of sunscreen has been applied.

The SPF of sunscreens applies strictly to human skin exposed *in vivo* to a simulated source of sunlight achieved by defined optical filtering of xenon arc lamps. Determination of SPFs by phototesting *in vivo* is subject to increasing variability with increasing SPF. This is illustrated in Table 2, which shows the results of a series of inter-laboratory tests performed by seven major European sunscreen manufacturers (Ferguson, 1997). It can be seen that even under the same laboratory conditions there is a threefold variation in the measured SPF for the high-factor (SPF 20–25) sunscreen.

The numerical value of the SPF appearing on sunscreen products is usually not identical to the measured mean SPF, since other factors, such as regulatory requirements and commercial considerations, also influence the choice of the declared SPF. The measured protection factor depends strongly on the topology of the surface to which the sunscreen is applied. Determinations *in vivo* in experimental animals, such as hairless mice, or *in vitro* in artificial substrates, such as Transpore tape, may result in protection factors different from those obtained in human skin (Diffey, 1989a). Furthermore, the strong dependence of the efficacy of sunscreens on wavelength means that the spectral

Table 2. Measured SPFs of four products tested in seven laboratories by the COLIPA SPF test method

Nominal SPF	Measured SPF	
	Mean	Range
4	4.2	3.9–4.6
15	12.7	11–14
15	15.5	14–18
20–25	22.4	11–34

From Ferguson (1997)
SPF, sun protection factor; COLIPA, European Cosmetic Toiletry and Perfumery Association

emission of the UVR source will influence the measured protection factor (Wilkinson, 1998). This is particularly important when fluorescent UVB sun-lamps (e.g. Philips TL12) are used as the source (Farr & Diffey, 1985). For high-SPF products (> 30), the SPFs determined with a solar simulator will be higher than those expected in sunlight because of the relatively small amount of UVA in xenon arc solar simulators (Stokes & Diffey, 1997a; Wilkinson, 1998).

In 1990, the labelled SPFs on most commercially available sunscreen products were < 10, but by 2000 there was a trend for higher factors, most manufacturers offering products with factors of 15–20 and, not uncommonly, products claiming a factor of 50 or higher.

It is important to know if protection from erythema results in comparable levels of protection from photobiological end-points that are thought to be important in photocarcinogenesis. These include epidermal DNA photodamage and mutation as well as immune suppression. In theory, an agent that gives protection from erythema without giving comparable levels of protection from these end-points could enhance the risk for skin cancer.

As the SPF of a sunscreen is a measure of protection from erythema in human skin that is determined with solar-simulated UVR (see above), valid comparisons of the SPF with the degree of protection against other biological end-points, such as immune suppression, can be made only when these have been determined in human skin with a solar-simulated UVR source and the standard sunscreen application density of 2 mg/cm^2. Comparison of SPFs with protection from important end-points other than erythema induced by other sources of UVR (such as UVB fluorescent lamps) is not valid, because protection factors depend on the spectral emission of the UVR source.

Although ideally all studies of sunscreens should be done with solar-simulated UVR, there may be situations in which this is not feasible or appropriate, for example, in studies in animals that require the use of selected wavebands. Furthermore, studies of dose-response relationships for the same biological end-points should be done with and without sunscreen. When studies are conducted with sources that do not simulate sunlight, it is important to compare the level of protection from the end-point in question with protection from erythema or other markers of inflammation, such as mouse skin oedema.

Interaction of solar radiation with biomolecules

Chromophores

Since solar UVC does not reach the earth's surface, the radiation wavelengths of interest are in the UVA and UVB regions. Changes following the excitation induced by absorption of solar energy in molecules known as chromophores may generate a biological effect either directly or by secondary reactions. Chromophores are endogenous biomolecules, such as DNA, or exogenous molecules, such as the active molecules of sunscreens. They absorb energy from the different wavelengths with differing efficiencies, and this pattern of response is defined as the absorption spectrum characteristic of the particular chromophore. Genetic effects such as mutation (Brash et al., 1991) implicate DNA as a major chromophore. In particular, induction of skin cancer by UVB involves damage to DNA, which then leads to a cascade of events including cell cycle arrest, DNA repair, mutation and transformation (Fig. 7). Both UVB and UVA have been reported (Morlière et al., 1991; Punnonen et al., 1991; Vile et al., 1994) to cause lipid peroxidation at biologically relevant fluences in the membranes of human fibroblasts and keratinocytes.

As the wavelength increases through the UVB and UVA regions, damage to proteins becomes increasingly important because of the absorptive properties of aromatic amino acids relative to nucleic acids. In addition, many proteins (which include the antioxidant enzymes catalases and peroxidases) contain haem groups, thus making the proteins UVA chromophores and potentially photosensitizers.

Photoimmunological effects implicate trans-urocanic acid, DNA photodamage

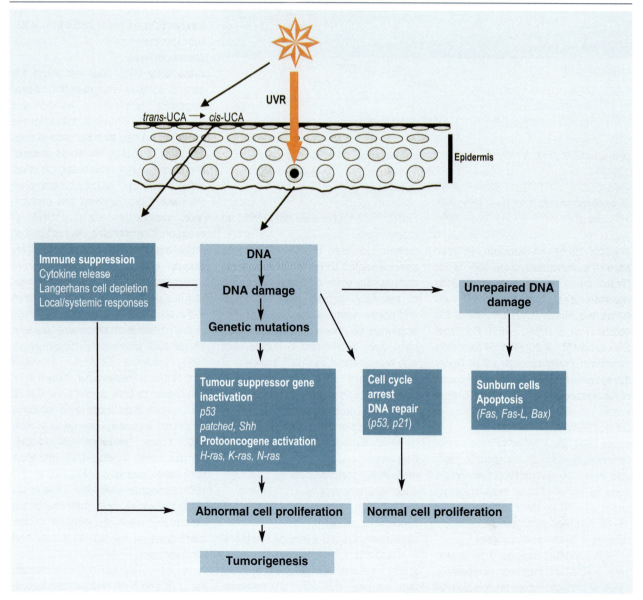

Figure 7 DNA and *trans*-urocanic acid (UCA) are chromophores implicated in the induction of non-melanoma skin cancer by ultraviolet radiation (UVR). Absorption of UVR by the chromophores DNA and *trans*-UCA initiates the process of non-melanoma skin carcinogenesis, involving at least two distinct pathways. One is the action of UVR on keratinocyte (neoplastic) transformation; the other is the action on the host's immune system. These two pathways interact or converge to cause skin cancer.

and cytokines (Kripke *et al.*, 1992; Noonan & De Fabo, 1992; Ullrich, 1995; Nishigori *et al.*, 1996; Kibitel *et al.*, 1998; Petit-Frère *et al.,* 1998). Melanin, the major pigment in the skin, is also considered important in human photoprotection.

As solar radiation is composed of many wavelengths, their effects may interact.

The skin is a complex, many-layered organ, and the radiation spectrum that impinges on its surface is not the same as that which reaches the lower layers

(Fig. 8). The consequence of this interaction is that the action spectrum or wavelength dependence of a specific biological end-point, as measured in the skin, is unlikely to match exactly the absorption spectrum of a chromophore.

The lesions

The major photoproducts formed in DNA by direct absorption can be detected in human skin *in vivo* (Freeman *et al.*, 1986; Young *et al.*, 1998a,b; Bykov *et al.*, 1999). These include cyclobutane pyrimidine dimers (TT > TC > CT >> CC) and pyrimidine (6–4) pyrimidone photoproducts (Fig. 9) (Cadet & Vigny, 1990; Cadet *et al.*, 1997). Specific lesions such as TT and TC dimers and 6–4 photoproducts have been described in humans *in vivo* (Bykov *et al.*, 1998), and such lesions constitute 70–80% and 20–30% of the total UVC-induced damage, respectively (Mitchell, 1988; Sage, 1993). The thymine-containing pyrimidine dimer is also the commonest lesion induced by UVB (Mitchell *et al.*, 1992). Thymine glycols (Hariharan & Cerutti, 1977; Mitchell *et al.*, 1991), pyrimidine hydrates (Fisher & Johns, 1976), purine or purine–pyrimidine moieties (Gallagher & Duker, 1989),

DNA single-strand breaks and DNA–protein cross-links are all present but at much lower frequencies than pyrimidine dimers.

UVA induces direct damage, but less efficiently than it does indirect damage (Tyrrell, 1973; Freeman *et al.*, 1989). Techniques have been developed to measure specific types of oxidative damage, in particular 8-hydroxy-2'-deoxyguanosine (8-OHdG), which is one of many such lesions. UVA induces significant levels of 8-OHdG in mammalian cells (Kvam & Tyrrell, 1997a; Zhang *et al.*, 1997), although the action spectra demonstrate that there are various wavelength dependences for this induction (Kielbassa *et al.*, 1997; Kvam & Tyrrell, 1997b). Although the measurements were not made in the same way, the difference between a response peaking with UVA (Kvam & Tyrrell, 1997b) and one peaking with near-visible radiation (Kielbassa *et al.*,

1997) may be due to a difference in the chromophore profile of the two cell types—human skin fibroblasts and Chinese hamster cells—used in these studies. In an investigation of oxidative DNA damage induced by several types of broad-spectrum sources, Douki *et al.* (1999) concluded that 8-OHdG-induced damage was not involved in cell death and was unlikely to be involved in mutagenesis. This conclusion was based on the spectrum of UVA-induced mutations, which proved to be characteristic of changes at dipyrimidine sites rather than oxidized guanines. Analysis of UVA-induced damage in mouse skin tumours led to a similar conclusion (van Kranen *et al.*, 1997). Until a more detailed picture of the spectrum of oxidative DNA damage emerges, however, no final conclusion can be drawn.

Modulation of gene expression

Alterations in gene expression at both the transcriptional and the translational levels occur in response to UVR, the effect being dependent on cell type and the intensity and wavelength of radiation used (Tyrrell, 1996a,b). Cell signalling pathways activated after exposure to UVR include those involving jun and p38MAP kinases and, in some cases, ERK kinases. The activation states of various transcription factors (AP-1, NFκβ) and *p53* stability change specifically in response to short-wavelength UVR. Increased production of stress proteins is seen after exposure of epidermal and dermal cells to UVR.

Many of the studies of changes in gene expression have involved use of high, usually lethal levels of irradiation, although physiologically relevant doses were used in some studies in cells and human skin (e.g. Fisher *et al.*, 1996). Low levels of UVA and UVB can activate cytokine production in strains

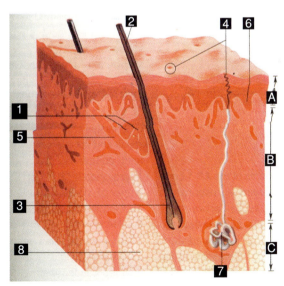

Figure 8 Section of the skin showing the three different layers:
(A) epidermis (B) dermis and (C) hypodermis.
(1) sebaceous gland; (2) hair; (3) hair root; (4) sudoriparous gland pore; (5) hair erector muscle; (6) papillae dermis; (7) sudoriparous gland and its excretor channel;(8) adipose tissue

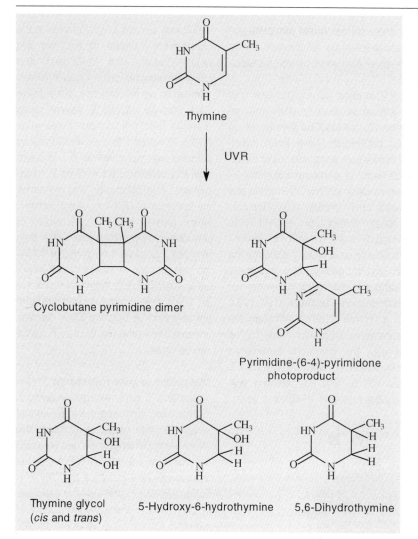

Figure 9 Chemical structures of major thymine photoproducts

cultured from primary fibroblasts and certain established lines (Ullrich, 1995). Physiological doses of solar-simulated UVR and UVB induce cytokines in human skin *in vivo* (Skov *et al.*, 1998; Barr *et al.*, 1999).

Exposure to UVA at physiologically relevant doses increases the expression of collagenase, intercellular adhesion molecule 1, CL100 phosphatase and haem oxygenase 1 in cultured human skin fibroblasts. Up-regulation of c-*fos*

and c-*jun* (components of the AP-1 complex) is also observed in response to UVA (Bose *et al.*, 1999; Soriani *et al.*, 2000). A growth stimulatory response may be detected after UVB irradiation, specifically including alterations in the status of STAT 1 and related kinases (Aragane *et al.*, 1997). Both UVA and UVB can activate nitric oxide synthase in a human cell strain cultured from primary keratinocytes (Romero-Graillet *et al.*, 1997). Formylated indolocarba-

zoles may act as Ah-receptor agonists, and UVB may activate CYP 1A (a cytochrome P450 subtype) in various human cell types (Wei *et al.*, 1999).

Certain patterns of gene expression elucidated in cultured cells, such as increases in p53, collagenase and ornithine decarboxylase, may be demonstrated in irradiated skin in both human and rodent models (Tyrrell, 1996a,b). Expression of the AP-1 components is increased in biopsy samples of human skin after irradiation *in vivo* (Fisher *et al.*, 1996).

Endogenous cellular defence mechanisms
Repair of DNA damage
One way in which the incidence of photolesions can be reduced is by repair of cellular DNA damage. The major mechanism for reducing the incidence of photolesions is excision repair (Lindahl & Wood, 1999). The importance of these mechanisms for the repair of UVB-induced damage is demonstrated most elegantly by the increased susceptibility of patients with xeroderma pigmentosum to solar-induced skin cancer (Arlett & Lehmann, 1996; Bootsma *et al.*, 1998). The majority of these patients have defects in the progressive steps of nucleotide excision repair and fall into seven genetically distinct complementation groups, A–G. Approximately 20% of these patients (variants) do not have defects in the excision repair genes but have defects in DNA polymerase η (Masutani *et al.*, 1999), which is responsible for translesion synthesis, a component of post-replication repair.

Antioxidant defence
Small antioxidant molecules are crucial in protecting human skin against UVR, particularly at the longer wavelengths

(Tyrrell *et al.*, 1991; Fuchs & Packer, 1999). In cultured human skin fibroblasts, glutathione depletion leads to strong sensitization to mutations caused by UVB (302–313 nm), UVA (334–365 nm) and near-visible (405 nm) radiation (Tyrrell & Pidoux, 1986, 1988), and there is a direct correlation between cellular glutathione content and the degree of photosensitization. Glutathione is depleted by exposure of human skin to UVA (Connor & Wheeler, 1987).

All the major antioxidant enzymes are present in skin, but their role in protecting the cells against oxidative damage induced by UVA has not been fully elucidated. Likewise the role of other endogenous antioxidant molecules such as ascorbate, carotenoids and α-tocopherol in protection against UVR-induced damage in humans requires further investigation.

Effects of solar radiation other than cancer

Erythema (sunburn)
Erythema is the most readily clinically apparent reaction to exposure to the sun (Fig. 10). It appears after 3–4 h and intensifies for 12–24 h, resulting in vasodilatation and an increased volume of blood in the dermis. UVB, particularly the shorter wavelengths, is most efficient in causing erythema. UVA can also cause erythema but at much higher doses (Gange & Parrish, 1983); however, as UVA represents the majority of sunlight, it contributes to about 15–20% of sunburn.

The clinically observed minimal erythemal dose (MED) is defined as the minimal amount of energy required to produce a qualifying erythemal response, usually after 24 h. The erythemal responses that qualify can be either just perceptible reddening or uniform redness with clearly demarcated borders, depending on the criterion adopted by

the observer. The former end-point (just perceptible) is more reliable than the latter (Quinn *et al.*, 1994; Lock-Anderson & Wulf, 1996). The MED depends on factors such as phenotype (e.g. skin complexion and hair colour), anatomical site and previous exposure, the amount of melanin in the epidermis at the time of irradiation and the intensity of the radiation. Individuals who burn easily and tan slightly reach their MED value after about 20 min of unprotected exposure to midday sun in midsummer in temperate latitudes. Five MEDs (100 min for such an individual) produce a painful burn. Ten MEDs lead to oedema, vesciculationand the formation of bullae.

Individual susceptibility to solar radiation depends on skin complexion (pigmentation of unexposed skin), hair colour and eye colour, which define the phenotype of the individual. The population can be grouped broadly into three levels of risk for burning in response to solar exposure: very sensitive, moderately sensitive and less sensitive. Very sensitive individuals burn easily and have difficulty tanning. Moderately sensitive individuals burn initially but then tan. Less sensitive individuals rarely or never burn and always tan. The Fitzpatrick six-point scale for human skin type defined the burning and tanning response of individuals to UVR. Generally, individuals with skin types I and II are very sensitive, types III and IV are moderately sensitive, and V and VI are less sensitive to UVR (Weinstock, 1992). The predisposition to burn correlates with the risk for developing skin cancer (IARC, 1992).

The typical histological changes associated with sunburn include slight epidermal spongiosis, increased nuclear diameter and nucleolar size of keratinocytes, alterations of Langerhans cells, induction of sunburn cells, hyperkeratosis,

acanthosis and migration of inflammatory cells in the exposed areas. Depending on the amount of the skin surface involved, severe sunburn can cause systemic symptoms including fever, nausea, vomiting, severe headache and even shock.

Pigmentation (suntanning)
Individuals have varying degrees of basic melanization of the skin. Fair-skinned individuals have limited melanin, which may be nested predominantly in freckles. Those with deeply pigmented skin tend to have a uniform distribution of melanin over the surface. The tanning response depends on the biological distribution of melanocytes. Tanning is the facultative increase in epidermal melanin pigmentation above the constitutional baseline level in response to UVR. Immediate pigment darkening, a transient greyish-brown change in skin colour due to oxidation of existing melanin, is induced by UVA and some visible wavelengths. It begins during exposure and persists, depending on the duration and intensity of exposure, but does not involve the production of new melanin. Tanning, the production of melanin, begins 48–72 h after UVR exposure, peaks at 7–10 days, may persist for several weeks to months, and is the result of increased production of melanin. Tanning

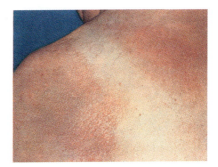

Figure 10 Shoulder of a man overexposed to the sun

may follow exposure to either UVB or UVA, but larger doses of UVA are required to give the same degree of tan as can be obtained with UVB.

Immune suppression

Studies on UVR-induced suppression of the immune system have been reviewed (Ullrich *et al.*, 1999). UVR induces local immune suppression, defined as an inability to induce contact hypersensitivity through locally UVR-irradiated skin, or systemic immune suppression at a skin site distant from that which was irradiated. The effects of UVR that contribute to such immune suppression include depletion from the skin of Langerhans cells, epidermal dendritic antigen-presenting cells which pick up antigen and transport it to local lymph nodes where they activate specific T lymphocytes. UVR also disrupts production of cytokines by various cells in the skin, creating an environment which is not conducive to activation of immunity. Upon exposure to UVR, urocanic acid is isomerized from the *trans* to the *cis* form (see Fig. 7), which is immune suppressive. Application of antigen to the skin under these conditions activates suppressive rather than protective immunity.

Photoageing

The changes seen in human skin with age are really due to a combination of ageing of the skin *per se* and ageing of the skin due to exposure to sunlight (photoageing). Ageing skin in doubly covered areas such as the buttocks is characterized primarily by atrophy (Gilchrest, 1996). This results in a thinner, more transparent skin, increasing prominence of the underlying vasculature and loss of elasticity. While there are relatively few changes in the stratum corneum, the epidermis thins and the rete ridges are effaced, reflected histologically by flattening of the undulations of the dermo-epidermal junction. The dermis also thins with age, resulting in more fragile skin (Fig. 11).

Changes considered to be signs of photoageing include wrinkling, mottled pigmentation, telangiectasia and epidermal thickening (Pearse *et al.*, 1987; Montagna *et al.*, 1989; Gilchrest & Yaar, 1992; Gilchrest, 1996). The dermal changes include the deposition of large quantities of abnormal, thickened, elastic fibres, a decrease in mature collagen, changed production of proteoglycan, chronic inflammation and damage to the microcirculation (Kligman, 1969, 1979; Mera *et al.*, 1987).

Photodermatoses

Up to 20% of the fair-skinned adult populations in Sweden and the USA has been reported to experience symptoms of polymorphic light eruption, a sun-sensitivity disorder that manifests as itching papules on sun-exposed skin. (Morison & Stern, 1982; Ros & Wennersten, 1986). Even though some sufferers from this condition may require medical care, most cases are mild and tend to resolve with further exposure to the sun, in a so-called 'hardening' phenomenon. Other, less common but more severe photodermatoses include solar urticaria and chronic actinic dermatitis. There are no indications that sufferers from photodermatoses are more prone to skin cancers than the general population.

Melanocytic naevi

Naevi (moles) are focal collections of non-dendritic melanocytes (naevocytes), usually found at the junction of the epidermis and dermis (junctional naevi) or at various depths in the dermis (compound or dermal naevi) (Fig. 12). Some naevi show a clinical resemblance to melanoma and may in addition be histologically atypical (Piepkorn *et al.*, 1994). Common acquired naevi arise after birth, and their ultimate density is related to a family history of naevi and increases with exposure to the sun (Harrison *et al.*, 1994). Acute exposure to the sun is implicated in the development of naevi in children. The number of naevi increases with age through adolescence and with a history of exposure to the sun and sunburn (Gallagher *et al.*, 1990; Harrison *et al.*, 1994). Naevi occur more frequently on sun-exposed areas, and there is strong evidence that the number of naevi on exposed areas increases with total cumulative exposure to the sun during childhood and adolescence (Holman & Armstrong, 1984; Kelly *et al.*, 1994). Children with

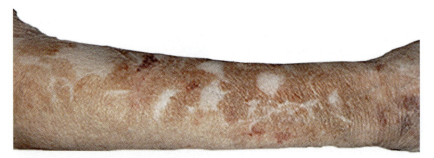

Figure 11 Severe signs of photoageing with mottled pigmentation and stellate pseudoscars indicating epidermal and dermal damage

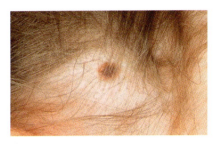

Figure 12 Intradermal naevus on scalp

light skin who tend to burn rather than tan have more naevi at all ages. Many cutaneous melanomas arise in acquired naevi (Sagebiel, 1993; Skender-Kalnenas *et al.*, 1995). Most acquired naevi are clonal, while most melanocytes in areas without naevi are not (Robinson *et al.*, 1998a). The number of common naevi or the number of atypical naevi in any given individual constitutes the best predictor of individual risk for melanoma (Holman & Armstrong, 1984; Holly *et al.*, 1987; Grob *et al.*, 1990; see Boyle *et al.*, 1995, for review).

Actinic (solar) keratosis
Actinic keratoses are proliferations of epidermal keratinocytes. They are associated with total and occupational exposure to the sun (Marks *et al.*, 1983; Goodman *et al.*, 1984; Vitasa *et al.*, 1990), with phenotypic indicators of cutaneous sensitivity to the sun (Vitasa *et al.,* 1990) and with other indicators of solar damage (Holman *et al.*, 1984; Green, 1991). Some of these lesions develop into squamous-cell carcinomas (Marks *et al.*, 1988).

Carcinogenicity of ultraviolet radiation in animals
The carcinogenicity of UVR in experimental animals (including studies on solar-simulated UVR, UVB and UVA) were reviewed in detail (IARC, 1992).

The first proof of the carcinogenicity of UVR was provided by Findlay (1928) in experiments in which he induced skin tumours in mice by repeated daily exposure. Subsequently, Roffo (1934) showed that sunlight induced skin cancer in rats and that this carcinogenic action was blocked by glass, which filters out UVB. The finding of the carcinogenic effectiveness of UVB concords with its genotoxicity, which is considerably greater than that of UVA (IARC, 1992).

Studies in experimental animals conducted in the course of the twentieth century have yielded much information on the induction by UVR of skin tumours. Most of these studies investigated fibrosarcomas and squamous-cell carcinomas in mice and melanomas in opossum and fish (hybrids of the genus *Xiphophorus*). The commonest sun-related skin cancer in humans, basal-cell carcinoma, is, however, hardly ever observed in such experiments, underlining the need for a suitable animal model for each type of human skin tumour. The suitability of an animal model depends on the fidelity with which it reproduces the biology and pathology of the human tumour and on the genes that are involved in its development. The mouse model for the induction of squamous-cell carcinoma with long-term exposure to UVR is now well established: UVR-induced mutations in the *p53* tumour suppressor gene appear to play a role in both human (Brash *et al.*, 1991) and murine tumours (Kress *et al.,* 1992; Kanjilal *et al.*, 1993; Dumaz *et al.,* 1997). The validity of the opossum and fish models for melanoma is still being debated, but the genes and oncogenic pathways involved in hereditary melanoma in fish resemble those in humans (Kazianis *et al.*, 1998; Wittbrodt *et al.*, 1989), notably the *INK4a/p16* locus and the *RTK-RAS* pathway.

Species differences such as the absence of photolyase activity in human melanocytes will, however, complicate attempts to extrapolate the results of carcinogenicity studies in these animal models to humans. In humans, mutations in the *PTCH* gene (part of the *sonic hedgehog* pathway) were found to be involved in basal-cell carcinomas, and in heterozygous *Ptch* knock-out mice the development of basal-cell carcinomas was enhanced by UVR (Aszterbaum *et al.*, 1999). Thus, there is a robust model for the induction of squamous-cell carcinoma by UVR, and transgenic mouse models for basal-cell carcinoma and melanoma are emerging, which will facilitate further investigation of relevant genetic changes and an assessment of the protective effect of sunscreens against these tumour types.

Protection by a sunscreen depends on dose, time and wavelength
Although experiments with animals may elucidate and allow quantification of the role of some of these factors, the number of variables in such experiments must be limited, and they must be standardized in certain well-controlled ways in order to provide reproducible, comparable data. Specification of the animals, the UVR sources, the exposure regimen, the UVR dosimetry and tumour evaluation are of the utmost importance. Unfortunately, many studies on the carcinogenicity of UVR do not fullfil these requirements and are, therefore, of limited use, especially for quantitative analyses such as are needed for the evaluation of protective effects of sunscreens.

Three physical dimensions are of the essence to UVR carcinogenesis: the spectrum (wavelength) of UV irradiation, the radiant energy (dose), the exposure scheduling and the latency of the tumour (time). Knowledge about the relationship between these physical aspects and tumour induction has been advanced greatly by experiments in animals. In the 1940s, Blum et al. (1941) conducted an elaborate series of experiments on skin tumours induced by long-term exposure to UVR in which they carefully determined the quantitative relationships between tumour induction and the schedule of exposure (Blum et al., 1941; Blum, 1959). The quantitative relationships they found were very similar to those reported by Druckrey (1967) after long-term application of chemical carcinogens to the skin and to those found by Raabe et al. (1980) for induction of bone cancer by radium. They all found that $D^r.t_m =$ constant, where t_m is the median tumour latency period, r is a power constant which depends on the carcinogen ($0 < r < 1$), and D is the average daily (monthly or yearly) dose. Thus, a two-fold higher daily dose does not shorten the tumour induction time by a factor of 1 but by a factor < 2 , i.e. there is no direct reciprocity between dose fraction and induction time. This lack of reciprocity is fully understandable if tumour development is envisaged as a process of multiple rate-limiting steps (e.g. mutations), of which only some are directly dependent on the carcinogen. The lack of reciprocity may be further attributed to protective mechanisms that become more active as the daily dose is increased. The nature of the dose–response relationship must be taken into consideration carefully in assuming a protective effect of a sunscreen (see page 91): a reduction of the dose by a factor of 10 will delay tumour development by a factor of 2–4, and, because of the steep increase in the incidence over time, the lifetime risk may decrease by a factor of up to 10 000.

Protection from carcinogenesis must be determined from dose–response

relationships with and without sunscreen: the degree of protection should be assessed from the ratios of the UVR doses required to evoke identical tumour responses. As this has been done in only a few studies, the level of protection from carcinogenesis by sunscreens is generally unknown.

In these early experiments, exposure to UVR induced fibrosarcomas and carcinomas on the ears of haired animals (see page 91). In the 1960s, immune-competent hairless mice became available, which respond consistently to UVR with induction of squamous-cell carcinoma, with actinic keratoses or sessile-based papillomas as precursor lesions, similar to the lesions observed in chronically exposed human skin. This model was studied extensively at the former Skin and Cancer Hospital in Philadelphia, USA (from which the hairless strain 'SKH' originates), and at

the department of Dermatology of the University Hospital in Utrecht, the Netherlands (for a review, see de Gruijl & Forbes, 1995). The earlier results of Blum et al. (1941) were refined, and the dependence of the induction of squamous-cell carcinoma on wavelength (the 'action spectrum') was derived mathematically from accumulated data obtained with UVR sources of various spectral compositions (de Gruijl et al., 1993). The result was called the 'SCUP-m' action spectrum (SCUP stands for Skin Cancer Utrecht–Philadelphia, and the '-m' for murine). From the SCUP-m, a SCUP-h action spectrum ('-h' for human) could be estimated by correcting for differences in UVR transmission between human and murine epidermis (de Gruijl & van der Leuw, 1994), the differences being largest below 300 nm. The result is depicted in Figure 13, with the directly measured action spectrum

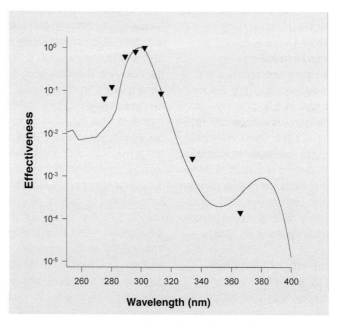

Figure 13 Comparison of the SCUP-h action spectrum (line; de Gruijl & van der Leuw, 1994) with the wavelength dependence of the dimers in induction of cyclobutane pyrimidine dimers in human skin (inverted triangles; Freeman *et al.*, 1989)

of UVR-induced DNA damage in human skin (Freeman *et al.*, 1989). The similarity of these two action spectra clearly indicates the importance of UVB-induced pyrimidine dimers in the formation of squamous-cell carcinoma. This in turn is fully in line with the nature of the mutations found in the *p53* gene (see previous section).

In view of the dominance of pyrimidine dimers in the genotoxicity of sunlight, one would expect the SCUP action spectrum to be generally valid for all types of UVR-induced skin cancer. This appears to be confirmed by the finding of gene point mutations (*p53* and *Ptch*) in murine (genetically modified) and human basal-cell carcinoma (Aszterbaum *et al.*, 1999). Surprisingly, the action spectrum for the induction of melanoma in certain hybrid fish (Setlow *et al.*, 1993) appears to be quite different from the SCUP-m action spectrum. The data on melanoma induction in opossum do not appear to confirm those in fish. UVB induces melanoma in opossum, and although UVA induces precursor lesions it does not appear to cause a conversion to malignancy (Ley, 1997).

The protective effect of sunscreens can be tested in the robust model of UVR-induced squamous-cell carcinomas. The action spectrum indicates that most protection would be provided by passive shielding from UVB; however, as a significant portion of the carcinogenic dose of sunlight stems from the UVA band, good protection can be achieved only if a substantial amount of UVA is filtered out. Any deviation from the expected results of UVR filtering would be suspect and would need further investigation (see section 6.2 of the handbook on sunscreens). Because the available data refer to squamous-cell carcinoma, any protective effect of suncreens against melanoma, or even basal-cell carcinoma, would differ importantly. A proper assessment of such protection must await good animal models for derivation of relevant action spectra for these types of skin cancer.

Experiments in transgenic mice and human skin

As described earlier, great advances are being made in basic research on skin cancer by the use of transgenic mice. The natural proneness of mice to develop primarily squamous-cell carcinomas after exposure to UVR may be overcome by activation of the *Hedgehog* pathway (e.g. by introducing a defect in the *Ptch* gene), which will enhance the induction of basal-cell carcinomas (Aszterbaum *et al.*, 1999). Transgenic mice can also be used to introduce human proteins (such as H-ras) into the murine system and thus test their specific responses (Chin *et al.*, 1997). Moreover, mice can be manipulated to accept human skin, which can then be tested freely. For example, immune-deficient RAG-1 mice have been used to host human skin grafts in which skin tumours were subsequently induced by long-term exposure to UVB in combination with application of a known promoter of skin tumours. One of the lesions in one of 48 grafts was a melanoma (Atillasoy *et al.*, 1998). The latter experiment is, of course, not a true in-vivo experiment, since human skin grafts lack the normal interaction with the rest of the body.

Although animal models for basal-cell carcinomas and melanomas are emerging, they are not yet well established. The effects of sunscreens can be tested most reliably in the model for squamous-cell carcinomas. A proper model for assessment of the protective effect against the most frequently fatal skin cancer, melanoma, is not yet available but clearly deserves to be high on the research agenda.

- **Skin cancer is more common than any other type of cancer**
- **It has been estimated that 106 000 melanomas of the skin were diagnosed worldwide in 1990.**
- **At least 2 750 000 non-melanocytic cancers of the skin were diagnosed in 1985**
- **Exposure to sun causes the three major types of skin cancer, basal-cell carcinoma, squamous-cell carcinoma and cutaneous melanoma.**
- **Sunscreens protect against sunburn**

Chapter 2
Chemical and physical characteristics of sunscreen constituents

Active ingredients
The active ingredients of sunscreens may be classified as organic or inorganic chemical absorbers. Table 3 and Appendix 1 show those ingredients that are approved for use in Australia, Europe, Japan and the USA.

Organic chemical absorbers
The organic chemical absorbers are generally aromatic compounds conjugated with a carbonyl group. One classification of such UVR absorbers (Shaath, 1997b) is based on their chemical structure, as follows: cinnamates, *para*-aminobenzoate (PABA) derivatives, salicylates, benzophenones, camphor derivatives, dibenzoyl methanes, anthranilates (Fig. 14) and miscellaneous compounds. Cinnamates, PABA derivatives, salicylates and camphor derivatives are all principally UVB absorbers, while benzophenone derivatives, dibenzoyl methanes and anthranilates are principally UVA absorbers. In most organic chemical absorbers, an electron-releasing group (an amine or a methoxyl) is substituted in the *ortho* or *para* position of the aromatic ring. UVA absorbers are all *ortho*-substituted, allowing easier electron delocalization of the internal hydrogen bonding.

Inorganic chemical absorbers
Inorganic chemical absorbers, such as titanium dioxide (TiO_2) and zinc oxide (ZnO), absorb and scatter UVR, unlike organic chemicals which only absorb.

ZnO and TiO_2 were used relatively little in commercial sunscreens until microfine forms became available, providing formulators with the opportunity to produce an effective product that was cosmetically acceptable (Anderson *et al.*, 1997; Fairhurst & Mitchnick, 1997). Inorganic absorbers are generally used in conjunction with organic absorbers to achieve high SPFs.

Historical perspective
Sunscreens appeared in commerce in the 1920s in the USA and in the 1930s in Europe. During the Second World War, red petrolatum was used by US armed forces. The varieties and uses of sunscreens proliferated after that time with changes in fashions, increased leisure time and greater awareness of health issues (Shaath, 1997a). PABA was a popular sunscreen in the 1950s and 1960s. It presents two extremely polar groups (amino and carboxylic acid moieties) with a *para* orientation on the benzene nucleus, which gives it certain characteristics that make its use difficult. These groups induce some hydrogen bonds either intermolecularly (giving rise to a crystalline physical state, unsuitable for cosmetic formulations) or with solvents (resulting in high water solubility and a dramatic solvent effect on absorption spectra). As doubts were raised about the safety of PABA with regard to the induction of contact sensitization (Kligman, 1966; Funk *et al.*, 1997), derivatives have been prepared, and

the two functional groups are now protected in several sunscreens, diminishing many of the problems associated with PABA itself, namely its physical aspect and water solubility. One of these compounds, ethylhexyldimethyl PABA, is one of the best UVB absorbers, with one of the highest extinction coefficients.

Salicylates were the first UVR filters used in sunscreen preparations. They are *ortho*-disubstituted compounds, which allows the formation of internal hydrogen bonds and thus decreases the ability of electrons to interact with other ingredients or solvent or biological substrates. Although they are relatively weak UVR absorbers, they have excellent safety records and, because they are easily incorporated into cosmetic formulations, some are used to solubilize other usually insoluble cosmetic ingredients, such as benzophenones. Of the salicylates on the market today, homosalate and ethylhexyl salicylate are the most widely used in sunscreen preparations.

Cinnamates have an extra unsaturation conjugated to both the aromatic ring and the carbonyl group portion of the carboxylic acid, thus allowing electron delocalization throughout the molecule. Cinnamates have been improved over the years. Ethylhexyl methoxycinnamate is currently the most popular sunscreen chemical, with good UVR absorption, safety, solubility in oils and insolubility in water, so that it is suitable for use in most waterproof sunscreen formulations.

Table 3. Chemical UVR absorbers approved for use in Australia, Europe, Japan and the USA

INCI nomenclature	CAS No.	COLIPA No.	Approved for use in			
			EU[a]	Japan[b]	USA[c]	Australia[d]
ORGANIC CHEMICAL ABSORBERS						
UVB absorbers						
Cinnamates						
– Cinoxate	104-28-9	S-29		Y	Y	Y
– DEA-methoxycinnamate	56265-46-4	S-24				Y
– Diisopropyl methyl cinnamate	32580-71-5	S-23		Y		
– Ethylhexyl methoxycinnamate	5466-77-3	S-28	Y	Y	Y	Y
– Ethyl methoxycinnamate	99880-64-5	–				Y
– Glyceryl ethylhexanoate dimethoxycinnamate	–			Y		
– Isoamyl-*para*-methoxycinnamate	71617-10-2	S-27	Y			Y
– Isopropyl-*para*-methoxycinnamate and diisopropylcinnamate mixture	–	–		Y		
para-Aminobenzoic acids (PABAs)						
– Amyl dimethyl PABA	14779-78-3	S-5		Y		Y
– Ethyl dihydroxypropyl PABA	58882-17-0	S-2				Y
– Ethylhexyl dimethyl PABA	21245-02-3	S-8	Y	Y	Y	Y
– Ethyl PABA	94-09-7	–		Y		
– Glyceryl PABA	136-44-7	S-6		Y		Y
– PABA	150-13-0	S-1	Y	Y	Y	Y
– PEG-25 PABA	116242-27-4	S-3	Y			
Salicylates						
– Dipropylene glycol salicylate	7491-14-7	–		Y		Y
– Ethylene glycol salicylate	87-28-5	–		Y		
– Ethylhexyl salicylate	118-60-5	S-13	Y	Y	Y	Y
– Homosalate	118-56-9	S-12	Y	Y	Y	Y
– Isopropylbenzyl salicylate	94134-93-7	S-16				Y
– Methyl salicylate	119-36-8	–		Y		
– Phenyl salicylate	118-55-8	S-14		Y		
– TEA salicylate	2174-16-5	S-9			Y	Y
Camphor derivatives						
– 3-Benzylidene camphor	15087-24-8	S-61	Y			
– Benzylidene camphor sulfonic acid	56039-58-8	S-59	Y			
– Camphor benzalkonium methosulfate	52793-97-2	S-57	Y			
– 4-Methylbenzylidene camphor	38102-62-4	S-60	Y			Y
– Polyacrylamidomethyl benzylidene camphor	113783-61-2	S-72	Y			
Miscellaneous						
– Diethylhexylbutamido triazone	154702-15-5	S-78	Y			
– Digalloyl trioleate	17048-39-4	S-55				Y
– Ethylhexyl triazone	88122-99-0	S-69	Y			Y
– 5-Methyl-2-phenylbenzoxazole	7420-86-2	S-47		Y		
– Octocrylene	6197-30-4	S-32	Y		Y	Y

Table 3. (contd)						
INCI nomenclature	**CAS No.**	**COLIPA No.**	**Approved for use in**			
			EU[a]	**Japan**[b]	**USA**[c]	**Australia**[d]
– Phenylbenzimidazole sulfonic acid	27503-81-7	S-45	Y		Y	Y
– Urocanic acid	104-98-3	S-46				Y
UVA absorbers						
Benzophenones						
– Benzophenone-1	131-56-6	S-33		Y		
– Benzophenone-2	131-55-5	S-34		Y		Y
– Benzophenone-3	131-57-7	S-38	Y	Y	Y	Y
– Benzophenone-4	4065-45-6	S-40	Y	Y	Y	Y
– Benzophenone-5	6628-37-1	S-40	Y	Y		
– Benzophenone-6	131-54-4	S-35		Y		
– Benzophenone-8	131-53-3	–			Y	Y
– Benzophenone-9	76656-36-5	S-36		Y		
– Benzophenone-10	1641-17-4	S-39				Y
Camphor derivative						
– Terephthalylidene dicamphor sulfonic acid	90457-82-2	S-71	Y			Y
Dibenzoylmethane						
– Butyl methoxydibenzoylmethane	70356-09-1	S-66	Y	Y	Y	Y
Anthranilate						
– Menthyl anthranilate	134-09-8	–			Y	Y
Miscellaneous						
– Bisymidazylate (proposed INCI name)	180898-37-7	S-80	Y			
UVA and UVB absorbers						
Miscellaneous						
– Anisotriazine (proposed INCI name)	187393-00-6	S-81	Y			
– Drometrizole trisiloxane	155633-54-8	S-73	Y			
– Methylene-bis-benzotriazolyl tetramethylbutylphenol	103597-45-1-P	S-79	Y			
INORGANIC CHEMICAL ABSORBERS						
– Titanium dioxide (CI 77891)	13463-67-7	S-75	Y[e]	Y[e]	Y	Y
– Zinc oxide (CI 77947)	1314-13-2	S-76	Y[e]	Y[e]	Y	Y

INCI, International Nomenclature of Cosmetic Ingredients; CAS, Chemical Abstracts Service; COLIPA, European Cosmetic, Toiletry and Perfumery Association; EU, European Union

[a] From European Commission (2000)

[b] From Ministry of Health and Welfare (1999)

[c] From Food and Drug Administration (1999)

[d] ' The chemical UVR absorbers approved by the FDA (USA) and European Commission (EU) would be acceptable in Australia ' (Commonwealth Department of Human Services and Health, 1995)

[e] Approved as a cosmetic colourant

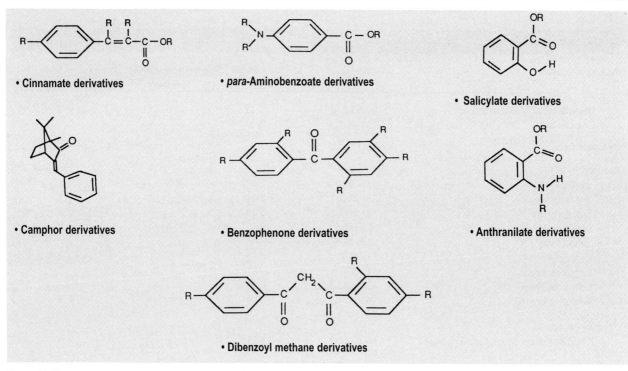

- Cinnamate derivatives
- *para*-Aminobenzoate derivatives
- Salicylate derivatives
- Camphor derivatives
- Benzophenone derivatives
- Anthranilate derivatives
- Dibenzoyl methane derivatives

Figure 14 The seven major groups of organic chemical sunscreen filters currently used in sunscreens

Benzophenones are dibenzoyl-methane derivatives that belong to the aromatic ketone category. They resonate easily, thus requiring a low quantum of energy; they therefore have a longer wavelength for electron transition. The main drawbacks to use of benzophenones as UVR filters are concern about their safety, as aromatic ketones are more difficult to detoxify than esters, and their solid state, which impairs their solubilization in cosmetic formulations. When high SPFs (20–30) are required, benzophenone-3 is usually used in combinations with solubilizers.

Camphor derivatives are bicyclic compounds with high extinction coefficients. With only one exception, they are solid. They are approved for use in Europe but not in the USA.

Anthranilates, such as menthyl anthranilate, are *ortho*-disubstituted aminobenzoates. This allows easy elec-tron delocalization and a shift in the maximum absorption. Anthranilates, like salicylates, are stable and safe and have no significant solvent effects in cosmetic formulations.

Dibenzoylmethanes are substituted diketones with a keto–enol tautomerism which confers the characteristics of UVA filters (enol form). The keto form is responsible for high photoisomerization, resulting in a significant loss of protective power. These compounds have exceptionally high molar extinction coefficients but low photostability.

Of the miscellaneous compounds, phenylbenzimidazole sulfonic acid is a water-soluble sunscreen with effective dose-response relationships with SPFs. It has limited use in the USA.

TiO_2 became more popular after the introduction of micronized grades, but this product is still difficult to formulate. ZnO is used largely as a UVA absorber.

Biological pigments

Melanin is the only natural pigment considered to be a sunscreen ingredient. It absorbs UVR and might provide both practical protection and the 'tanned' appearance desired by some people, but it is not available commercially (Chedekel & Zeise, 1997).

Vehicles and formulations

pH and various solvents can profoundly influence the effectiveness of a sunscreen chemical because of shifts in absorption characteristics (Shaath, 1997b). In addition, the final formulation strongly influences the suspension, distribution, stability and retention of the sunscreen on the skin (Klein, 1997).

Additional ingredients

At various times and under various circumstances, products containing sunscreening agents have also contained a wide variety of other ingredients, including urocanic acid, antioxidants, stabilizers, vitamins, hormones, animal and plant extracts and preservatives. Whether and how these ingredients interact with the sunscreen chemical during use is not well documented.

Topically applied psoralens are known to enhance the induction of melanogenesis in skin exposed to UVR. For this reason, some sunscreen formulations were marketed with bergamot oil containing 5-methoxypsoralen. Since psoralens are known to enhance photocarcinogenesis (see IARC, 1987), they are no longer permitted in sunscreen formulations in Europe or the USA (Autier et al., 1995, 1997a).

Stability, photostability and reactivity

Analysis and quality control measures indicate that sunscreens stored under standard conditions meet or exceed the requirements for stability (Shaath, 1997c). Ideally, sunscreen molecules should absorb UV photons and then dissipate the excess energy through such processes as radiative decay (fluorescence and phosphorescence), self-quenching or internal conversion and vibrational relaxation (heat). In short, they should undergo little or no photochemistry. The following examples show that not all sunscreens meet this ideal.

Butyl methoxydibenzoylmethane was introduced in 1978 in Europe as a sunscreen ingredient that absorbed principally in the UVA region. The first formulation containing this ingredient that was marketed in the USA lost a significant amount of its effectiveness during use, reportedly because of photoreactions (Sayre & Dowdy, 1999).

The use of several esters of PABA has been reduced or discontinued because of real or perceived cutaneous reactions, including irritation and contact sensitization (Funk et al., 1997). One such ester (ethylhexyl dimethyl PABA) is reported to induce phototoxicity and photomutagenicity in budding yeast cells (Knowland et al., 1993). Gulston and Knowland (1999) reported enhancement of DNA damage in human keratinocytes in vitro by a SPF-15 sunscreen formulation, and they attributed the effect to ethylhexyl dimethyl PABA.

Martincigh et al. (1997) catalogued the reported photochemical and photophysical characteristics of sunscreens, related compounds and their photoproducts. They also reviewed the evidence for photodimerization of DNA by sunscreens in vitro. They speculated that these events presage mutagenesis in vitro and, by extension, in vivo. They acknowledged that if such events occur only in the stratum corneum during use of sunscreens, little damage would be caused to viable cells.

Analysis, verification and quality control

Analytical techniques of particular use in sunscreen chemistry have been reviewed (Shaath et al., 1997a). The quality control procedures first involve physical and chemical analysis (Shaath, 1997c). The physical analysis includes tests for odour, colour, physical appearance, melting-point, refractive index, specific gravity, optical rotation, solubility, moisture, viscosity, pH and flash-point. The chemical analysis involves determination of saponification value, acid value, functional groups and metal content. Chromatographic and spectroscopic (UVR spectrum, infrared spectrum, nuclear magnetic resonance spectroscopy, mass spectrometry) analyses are also performed (Klein, 1992; Shaath et al., 1997b).

New chemical absorbers

Several patents have been assigned for modifications of chemical UVR absorbers, including benzophenones, derivatives of dibenzoylmethane, ferulic acid amides, polyvalent metal salts of PABA, para-dimethyl PABA and 4-methoxycinnamic acid (Shaath, 1997a). Other derivatives (indoline derivatives, chalcone derivatives, benzylidene camphor) appear to be useful as chemical absorbers.

Natural and biosynthesized raw materials have also been described in patents and articles, including DL-α-tocopherol, thiamine or thiamine esters and genetically produced melanin incorporated in a polymer-based delivery system.

Several forms (microparticles and ultrafine powder) of the inorganic chemical absorbers TiO_2 and ZnO and other metal oxides have been shown to be superior to those available on the market. In addition, plastics, resin emulsions and particles have been studied for use as reflectors to block UVR

Other properties of sunscreen ingredients

Sunlight generates active oxygen intermediates, including free radicals, in cells and tissues (Tyrrell, 1994), and these may damage cellular defence pathways. The free-radical scavenging antioxidant properties of the active components of sunscreens have not been investigated systematically. They will be relevant when sunscreens penetrate the cells and tissues in which active damaging intermediates are generated.

Chapter 3

Human use of sunscreens

Availability

Sunscreen products are available for general public use as a consumer product all over the world. There is thus no constraint on the availability of approved sunscreens, other than cost. Sunscreens are distributed in numerous ways, e.g. in many types of outlets and in pharmacies as over-the-counter products. They are also sold directly by physicians (e.g. in the USA), by hospitals (e.g. in Italy) and by cancer control organizations and cancer charities (e.g. in Australia). In Australia, the availability of sunscreens has been maximized through sales tax exemptions; sunscreens are also available in the work place as part of occupational health and safety programmes; they are widely available in schools, and their use by children is actively promoted. In contrast, in the USA, sunscreens are rarely promoted by schools, in part because of fear of litigation, as these products are classified as drugs.

Regulation

Regulatory control strongly influences the availability of specific sunscreen formulations in most countries. Sunscreens are currently regulated as cosmetics in the European Union (Janousek, 1997), in Japan (Fukuda & Naganuma, 1997), in South Africa, in South America and in Taiwan. Sunscreens are regulated as drugs in Australia, Canada, New Zealand and the USA through procedures specific to each country. Australia and New Zealand maintain a standard for the acceptable method of determining the effectiveness of sunscreens available in those countries (Australian/New Zealand Standards, 1998). Canada's regulation calls for independent evaluation of the safety and effectiveness of sunscreens (Health Canada, 1999). In the USA, several monographs of the Food and Drug Administration (1993, 1998, 1999) list previously approved sunscreens and their active ingredients with acceptable labelling information. The monographs also prescribe detailed methods for determining the effectiveness of each formulation to be marketed, whether or not the active ingredients were previously approved. Furthermore, any new sunscreen active ingredient must fulfil the testing requirements for safety associated with a 'new drug application' before it is approved for marketing in the USA. Of the sunscreen ingredients approved by the Food and Drug Administration, about 15 are still in use, and fewer than half of these account for the bulk of the US market (Murphy, 1997).

Whether they are regulated as cosmetics or drugs, sunscreens are tested toxicologically by the procedures mandated in each country and, in Europe, by the European Commission (1976). Panels of experts and regulatory staff reviewers judge the adequacy of the data on preclinical and clinical safety. The emphasis is usually placed on detecting cutaneous or ocular irritancy or contact sensitivity, but the respective agencies in Canada and the USA anticipate inclusion of data from photocarcinogenesis testing before approval of new sunscreen ingredients (Health Canada, 1999; Food & Drug Administration, 2000).

A directive of the European Commission (2000) mandated that a list of 'full ingredient labelling' in decreasing order of concentration be included on the label of the container of all cosmetics, including sunscreen formulations.

Production

Regrettably, there is no data collection system in place that would make it possible to estimate the total annual use of sunscreen products on a country-by-country basis. The world market for sunscreen formulations and related products was estimated as US$ 3.47 thousand million for the calendar year 1998, the most recent year for which trade journal figures were available. Eight countries accounted for 70% of the consumption in dollar terms: Canada, France, Germany, Italy, Japan, Spain, the United Kingdom and the USA. For the category of sunscreens alone, the European Union and the USA represent about 75% of the world wide market. Table 4 gives estimates of the numbers of units of sunscreen products and the volume of UVR filters sold in 1998.

In the European Union 55% of the market is for sunscreens with a 0–8 labelled SPF, 16% for SPF 9–14 or 15–24, and 13% for SPF > 25. In Germany there is a clear tendency to use of higher-SPF products.

Table 4. Amounts of sunscreen products and UVR filters sold annually worldwide

Area	Estimated number of units (thousands)	Estimated volume of UV filters (t)
USA[a]	163 000	2934
European Union[b]	227 775	4100
Rest of the world[c]	130 225	2164
World	521 000	9198

[a] According to Kline & Co. Inc., the estimated number of units of sunscreen products sold in the USA in 1998 was 163 million. If the average concentration of UV filters is 15%, and the volume/unit is 120 g, the volume sold is 2934 t.
[b] The volume of UV filters was estimated at 4100 t. This results in an estimated number of 227 775 thousand units.
[c] The volume for the rest of the world is estimated by assuming that it represents 25% of world sales.

Sun exposure and protection
Exposure to sunlight
The UVR to which an individual is exposed depends on :

- ambient sunlight,
- the fraction of ambient exposure received on different anatomical sites and
- behaviour and time spent outdoors.

The UVR dose absorbed by the skin is further modified by the use of photoprotective agents such as hats, clothing and sunscreens.

The maximum daily exposure to ambient sunlight under clear summer skies represents about 70 standard erythemal doses (SEDs) in the tropics (10–30°), 60 SED at latitudes approximating those of southern Europe (around 40°) and 45 SED at temperate latitudes (50–60°) (Roy et al., 1996). The SED is a measure of erythemal UVR (Commission Internationale de l'Éclairage, 1998). Just perceptible reddening (minimal erythema) of unacclimatized skin requires exposure to about 1.5 SED for individuals who burn easily and never tan (skin type I) (Lock-Andersen et al., 1998), about 2 SED for people who burn easily but tan minimally (skin type II) and 3 SED for those who burn but tan readily (skin

type III) (Weinstock, 1992). Clinical studies have shown no difference in the erythemal response to UVR between children (< 15 years) and adults (Cox et al., 1992).

Sun exposure of adults
Estimates of personal exposure can be obtained in two ways: by direct measurement with UVR-sensitive film badges (Diffey, 1989a) or by independent determination of ambient sunlight, the fraction of ambient exposure received on different anatomical sites and behaviour and time spent outdoors, either by measurement, modelling or a combination of the two (Parisi et al., 2000) (Fig. 15). The results obtained from a number of studies in northern Europe (Challoner et al., 1976; Leach et al., 1978; Larkö & Diffey, 1983; Schothorst et al., 1985; Webb, 1985; Slaper, 1987; Knuschke & Barth, 1996) indicate that indoor workers received an annual exposure of around 200 SED, mainly from exposure during weekends and holidays (Fig. 15) and principally on the hands, forearms and face. This value is approximately 5% of the total ambient sunlight available. It must be stressed, however, that there are large variations in the annual doses received by individuals within a given population group, depending on the propensity for outdoor activities.

Outdoor workers at the same latitudes receive two to three times these doses (Larkö & Diffey, 1983; Webb, 1985), while studies of three groups of outdoor workers on the Sunshine Coast in Queensland, Australia (27° S) wearing film badges suggested that the annual exposure would be considerably higher — certainly in excess of 1000 SED per year (Gies et al., 1995).

Sun exposure of children and adolescents
Few longitudinal studies have been conducted on children's exposure to the sun (Diffey et al., 1996; Gies et al., 1998; Kimlin et al., 1998a; Moise et al., 1999a,b,c; O'Riordan et al., 2000; Parisi et al., 2000), and differences in the methods used in those that were conducted make detailed comparisons problematic. Table 5 summarizes the findings from three of these studies (Diffey et al., 1996; Gies et al., 1998; Moise et al., 1999b). The median dose measured on the chest or shoulder as a percentage of the ambient sunlight is significantly lower for infants and small children than for older children and adolescents, even though the percentage of time spent outdoors between 8:00 and 18:00 is similar. There are two probable reasons for this. The infants were outside between 9:00 and

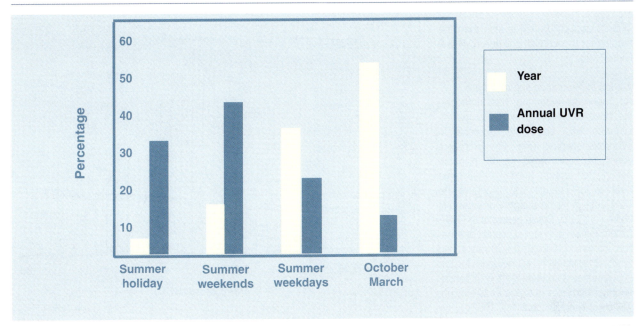

Figure 15 How adult indoor workers in northern Europe are exposed to sunlight (e.g. a 2-week summer holiday, 4% of the year, contributes 30% of the annual dose)

Table 5. Median exposure to UVR (expressed as per cent of ambient) and time spent outdoors between 8:00 and 18:00 for infants, children and adolescents in England and in Queensland, Australia

Age (years)	Location	Season	% ambient UVR	% time ourdoors	Reference
1	Queensland	Spring	0.7	17	Moise *et al.* (1999b)
2	Queensland	Autumn	1.6	25	Moise *et al.* (1999b)
9–10	England	Spring/Summer	6.6	24	Diffey *et al.* (1996)
12	Queensland	Summer	7.0	21	Gies *et al.* (1998)
14–15	England	Spring/Summer	4.5	17	Diffey *et al.* (1996)

16:00, when the UVR intensity is high, for only 5% of the time during weekdays and 9% at weekends; they were therefore exposed most of the time when the ambient UVR intensity was relatively low. Secondly, infants and small children are more likely to be under the supervision of adults than are older children, and such supervision may well involve the use of shade as a means of limiting exposure to UVR.

The annual ambient dose of UVR in England is typically 3000–4000 SED, which is considerably less than that in Queensland where it is 11 000–15 000 SED. Behaviour can be equally, or more, important than the ambient UVR dose in determining an individual's exposure (Diffey & Saunders, 1995; Diffey, 1996). Figure 16 shows the distribution of daily outdoor exposure of English children (1575 child-days) and children in

Queensland (568 child-days) to UVR in two of the studies summarized in Table 5 (Diffey *et al.*, 1996; Gies *et al.*, 1998). While the median daily personal exposure in Queensland was twice that received in England, there was a wide overlap between the two distributions: on any one day, the daily exposure of 17% of English children exceeded the median exposure of the children in Queensland, and the exposure of 26% of the

Queensland children was less than the median for the English children (Diffey & Gies, 1998).

Trends in population sun exposure

An important factor that has increased the dose of people living in temperate latitudes has been the increase in overseas holidays (Fig. 17). In recent years the most rapid trends in destinations for foreign holiday travel have been to low-latitude regions where the UVR dose is typically high. For example, holiday visits by British people to the USA (where Florida is the most popular destination) increased 15-fold in the 20 years up to 1997. Participation in outdoor leisure activities has also increased, with consequential increases in exposure to sunlight (Office of National Statistics, 1998).

Anatomical distribution of sunlight

Table 6 shows the mean percentages of ambient UVR relative to the top of the head received at various anatomical sites, as measured on rotating mannekins and living subjects pursuing outdoor activities such as tennis, sailing, swimming, walking, golf and gardening. The shoulders generally receive the greatest relative exposure in all activities (approximately two-thirds of that on the top of the head), with greater variation among the other sites, reflecting differences in posture for the different activities.

Facial exposure to sunlight

The face is particularly prone to solar damage (Fig. 18) because it receives significantly more exposure than other anatomical sites, which are usually covered when outside. A number of workers have used UVR-sensitive film badges to measure the exposure of the face relative to ambient exposure for both human subjects (Holman *et al.*, 1983; Rosenthal *et al.*, 1990; Melville *et al.*, 1991; Rosenthal *et al.*, 1991) and mannekins (Diffey *et al.*, 1977, 1979; Gies *et al.*, 1988; Diffey & Cheeseman,

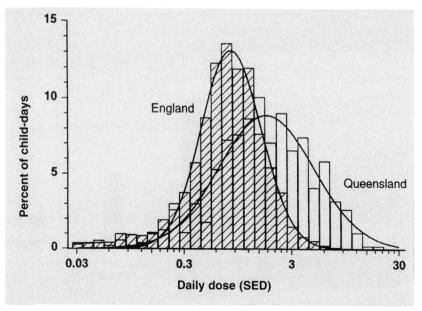

Figure 16 Distribution of daily personal outdoor exposure to UVR of English children and children in Queensland, Australia. Smooth curves are log-normal distributions obtained by regression analysis. SED, standard erythemal dose

1992; Gies *et al.*, 1992; Airey *et al.*, 1995; Kimlin *et al.*, 1998b). The data vary considerably, reflecting factors such as positioning of film badges on the face, behaviour of individuals, solar altitude and shade, but representative values for various sites on the face are given in Table 7. The variation is explained partly

by the posture or angle at which the head is held. In a study of the effect of head tilt on relative exposure over the face, Airey *et al.* (1995) showed that the exposure of the nose relative to the horizontal dropped from 59% to 11% as the head tilted from 0° to 60° to the normal. Wearing a hat can modify the exposure of

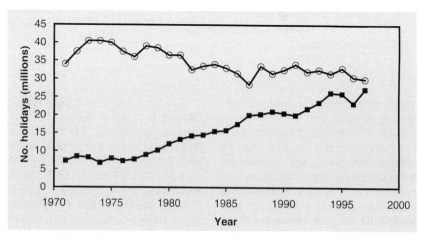

Figure 17 Domestic (open circles) and overseas (closed squares) holidays taken by British residents

Table 6. Exposure to sunlight (relative to 100% on the top of the head) of rotating mannekins and living subjects engaged in tennis, golf, gardening or walking

Site	Mannekin		Living subjects	
	Diffey *et al.* (1977)	Gies *et al.* (1992)	Holman *et al.* (1983)	Herlihy *et al.* (1994)ᵢ
Cheek	31	24	15	13
Hand	50	–	24	29
Shoulder	75	94	66	43
Back	43	36	58	40
Chest	68	50	44	23
Thigh	33	–	16	25

the face, especially if the hat has a wide brim (Diffey & Cheeseman, 1992; Wong *et al.,* 1996) (Fig. 19).

Influence of clothing on exposure

Most summer clothing provides protection factors against sunburn greater than 10; measurements of over 5000 fabrics submitted for testing to the Australian Radiation Laboratory revealed that 97% of fabrics fell into this category (Gies *et al.*, 1996). More than 85% of fabrics had protection factors of 20 or more. Studies on the spectral transmission of textiles (Robson & Diffey, 1990) showed that many materials absorb more or less uniformly over the solar UVR spectrum. In other words, most clothing, in common with other forms of shade such as trees, canopies and beach umbrellas, provides principally a quantitative rather than a qualitative change in cutaneous exposure to UVR. Factors that affect the protection offered by fabrics against sunlight include weave, colour, weight, stretch and wetness (Gies *et al.*, 1994).

Exposure to the sun and sunscreens

When sunscreens are used to prevent sunburn, how high should the SPF be to satisfy this requirement for the average person? The maximum daily ambient dose of UVR under clear summer skies is about 70 SED in the tropics (10–30°)

and about 45 SED in temperate latitudes (50–60°). These maximum ambient doses will not be received, simply because it would be unrealistic to lie in the sun all day without moving. An assiduous sunbather might spend half the time supine and half the time prone, resulting in a maximum exposure on much of the body surface of 50% of the ambient dose. For upright subjects engaging in outdoor pursuits such as gardening, walking or tennis, the exposure relative to ambient on commonly exposed sites such as the chest, shoulder, face, forearms and lower legs ranges from about 20% to 60% (Table 7). Thus, someone who is on holiday in southern Europe would receive a daily exposure of no more than 20 SED

over much of the body surface. Since a dose of 2–3 SED is necessary to induce minimal erythema on unacclimatized white skin, a photoprotective device (sunscreen or clothing) need have an SPF of only 10 to prevent sunburn. For exposure to the tropical sun, an SPF of 15 should be adequate for all-day exposure.

If sunscreens of SPF 15 are sufficient to protect against sunburn even with all-day exposure in tropical sunshine, why were people who usually or always used a high-factor (≥ 15) sunscreen more likely to report sunburn than those who rarely or never used sunscreens? Conversely, and not surprisingly, fewer people who usually or always sought shade, wore a hat or wore clothes

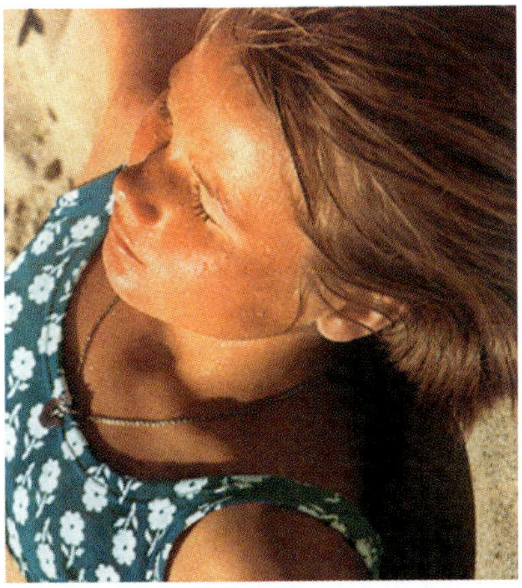

Figure 18 Intentional exposure to the sun for heavy suntanning effect

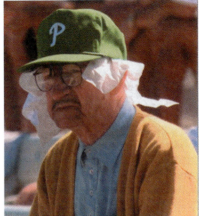

Figure 19 Head protection against the sun

Table 7. Exposure to sunlight on the head in studies on living subjects and mannekins

Site	Relative exposure
Top of head	100
Forehead	20–65
Nose	20–65
Cheek	15–40
Chin	20–35
Back of neck	20–35

got sunburnt than those who rarely or never did so (Dixon *et al.*, 1997). The protection against sunburn conferred by a sunscreen — defined by its SPF — is assessed by phototesting *in vivo* at an internationally agreed application thickness of 2 mg/cm² (Fig. 20). Approximately 35 ml of sunscreen would need to be applied to the total body surface of an adult to achieve the SPF quoted on the packaging. Yet, a number of studies have shown that consumers typically apply 0.5–1.5 mg/cm² (Stenberg & Larkö, 1985; Bech-Thomsen & Wulf, 1992; Diffey & Grice, 1997; Gottlieb *et al.*, 1997; Azurdia *et al.*, 1999). As application thickness has a significant effect on the degree of protection, most users probably achieve a mean value of 20–50% of that expected from the product label (Stokes & Diffey, 1997b). This problem is compounded by the likely variability of protection over the skin surface due to uneven application (Rhodes & Diffey, 1996). It is difficult to see which parts of the body have been missed when sunscreens are applied. Further, once a sunscreen has been applied to the skin, its adherence may be compromised by factors such as immersion in water (Stokes & Diffey, 1999a) and abrasion by beach sand (Stokes & Diffey, 2000). Therefore, people get sunburnt even when they use high-SPF sunscreens because inadequate amounts of sunscreen are applied, areas of the body are missed, and sunscreens are washed and/or rubbed off.

There is some evidence to suggest that the numerical measure of protection indicated on the product pack is generally higher than that achieved in practice (Diffey, 2000), and experience has led consumers to realize that if they want to spend several hours in the sun and avoid sunburn, they must use products labelled with factors of 20, 30 or higher.

Behavioural considerations in sunscreen use

Since 1950, an increasing number of white people have used sunscreens, principally in Australia, Europe and North America. Sunscreen use has also become common among several non-white populations, such as in Japan. In the USA, sunscreen use by adults increased from 35 to 53% between 1986 and 1996 (Robinson *et al.*, 1997a). Between 1989 and 1995, the average yearly increase in sunscreens sold was 17.6% in Japan (Fukuda & Takata, 1997) and 9.6% in the USA. In Germany during the 1990s, sunscreen sales increased by 16.7% per year (Sauermann *et al.*, 1997).

Sunscreen use is included in 'sun-related behaviour', i.e. any behaviour that increases or decreases the exposure of the skin or eyes to sunlight (Hill *et al.*, 1993). Sun-related behaviour other than sunscreen use includes wearing protective clothing, hats or sunglasses (Fig. 21), seeking or remaining in the shade, scheduling activity or work to be indoors around solar noon and minimizing the time spent outdoors at high and low latitudes and in sunny seasons. Since cloud cover reduces UVR intensity at ground level, modulating outdoor activity to take into account local prevailing weather conditions is also sun-related behaviour.

While the purpose of sunscreens is to reduce the amount of UVR that reaches the epidermis, the underlying reasons that people use them include: to reduce the risk for skin cancer, to prevent sunburn, to promote suntanning by avoiding burns that blister, to protect the skin from photoageing, to take part in outdoor activities or simply to comply with the expectations of others. The motivations of other populations may be quite different. For instance, in Japan, sunscreen use is often based on a desire to prevent 'disgraceful' pigmented spots, and sunscreens are used frequently during daily activities (Fukuda & Takata, 1997).

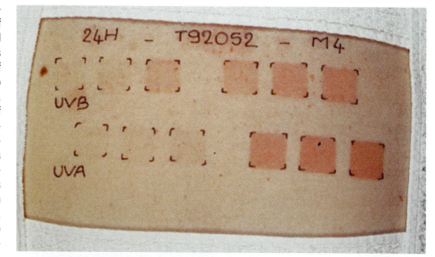

Figure 20 Both UVA and UVB induce erythema. The reactions, reproduced indoors by exposure of a volunteer to solar-simulated light attenuated by cut-off filters, are used to determine sun protection factors.

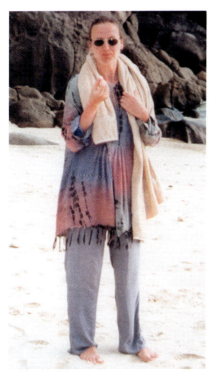

Figure 21 Sun-protective behaviour on the beach

Except for people who may use sunscreen routinely as a component of makeup, moisturizers and other anti-ageing products, sunscreen use (like other sun-related behaviour) is a contingent rather than a habitual behaviour. That is to say, it is contingent upon certain situations, such as a warm, sunny day. It therefore makes little sense to draw conclusions about an individual's predisposition to sun protection unless the prevailing conditions, in particular UVR intensity, can be estimated at the same time as the sun-related behaviour is recorded.

Another complication in the study of sun-related behaviour is that it is an alternative. It is false to conclude that people who do not use sunscreens are not interested in sun protection. Some of the studies considered in this section are open to the criticism that they assume that sunscreen use *per se* can be used

as an indicator of a predisposition to sun protection or that it is valid to add sunscreen use as an item in scales that include other sun-related behaviour. Someone who remains indoors needs neither a sunscreen, a hat, nor clothing to be protected from UVR, even if it is midday at the equator.

Two types of exposure to the sun can be distinguished, during which sunscreen may be applied on uncovered parts of the skin. The primary purpose of intentional exposure to the sun is to achieve a biological response, such as a tan. During intentional exposure, significant portions of the trunk and limbs are frequently uncovered. Sunbathing is the most typical such behaviour. Intentional exposure to sources of UVR other than the sun has become popular with the increasing availability of artificial tanning devices. The randomized trial of the effect of use of sunscreens with different SPFs on duration of exposure (Autier *et al.*, 1999), described on p. 61, was conducted in situations of intentional exposure. Unintentional exposure to the sun occurs during daily life, with no specific intention to acquire a tan or to stay in the sun. Unintentional exposure to UVR sources other than the sun may occur at the workplace. During unintentional exposure to the sun, the uncovered body parts are generally the face, ears, neck and hands. The forearms and legs (especially of women) may also be uncovered, but the trunk is usually covered. The randomized trials of the ability of sunscreens to prevent non-melanocytic sun-induced lesions (Thompson *et al.*, 1993; Naylor *et al.*, 1995; Green *et al.*, 1999a,b; Gallagher *et al.*, 2000) were conducted in situations of unintentional exposure, with sunscreens (or placebo lotion) applied essentially on the face, ears, neck and hands.

A serious concern is that use of sunscreens, which reduces the most immediate adverse effect of the sun (sunburn), may actually increase total exposure to sunlight and therefore the risk for harm

(Autier *et al.*, 1999). It is therefore important to understand both the behavioural consequences and the behavioural causes of sunscreen use.

It is difficult to assess actual sunscreen application from direct observation, and sunscreen use patterns have been assessed prospectively in few studies. Most of the data come from surveys in which people were asked directly whether they used a sunscreen when in the sun or about their knowledge about the properties of sunscreens. As sunscreen use has become a socially desirable behaviour which is widely promoted by cancer prevention campaigns and commercial advertising, it must be borne in mind that assessment of sunscreen use through questionnaires is subject to bias and over-reporting. There may be considerable discrepancy between knowledge about sun protection methods, self-reported sun protection and actual sun protection (von Schirnding *et al.*, 1991/92; Zinman *et al.*, 1995; Buller & Borland, 1999; Dixon *et al.*, 1999). The declared motives for using a sunscreen must be noted with caution, as they are likely to be influenced by the perception subjects have about the right answer (Buller & Borland, 1999). For these reasons, studies based only on knowledge of the properties of sunscreens have not been considered in this section.

What is known about the behavioural aspects of sunscreen use can be found in the answers to the following questions:

- Who uses sunscreens?
- Where and when do they use them?
- Why do they use them?
- How do they use them?
- What is their experience of using them?
- Which strategies to increase sunscreen use are effective?
- What effect does sunscreen use have on other sun-related behaviour, particularly the timing and scheduling of outdoor activities?

Who uses sunscreens and when and where they use them

There is great variation in the use of sunscreens by white-skinned populations, according to their natural susceptibility to the sun, socioeconomic status, attraction to sunlight, holiday habits, perception of skin cancer risk and background sun irradiation. Table 8 shows the sunscreen use reported by European subjects in two epidemiological studies conducted between 1988 and 1992, and the sunscreen use of European children as reported by parents in 1995–96. A South to North gradient in the proportion of children and adult sunscreen users is noticeable, paralleling the South to North gradient in natural susceptibility to sunlight prevailing in Europe. Sunscreen use is particularly high in Scandinavian countries, with use rates as high as 86–90% among Norwegian and Swedish adolescents (Wichstrom, 1994; Boldeman et al., 1996).

The prevalence of sunscreen use in various samples, including summer and winter/snow settings, was reported in 79 studies (see Tables 9 and 10). Unfortunately, no standard metric has been used to quantify use, and in a number of studies in which data on sunscreen use were collected they were not reported separately because the authors' focus was on indices of sun protection, into which prevalence of sunscreen use was merged. There is thus considerable variation in the way in which the data were reported. In some studies, a point prevalence of use is reported; for instance people interviewed on the beach were asked "Are you using a sunscreen now?" and people in a telephone survey were asked "Were you using a sunscreen between 11:00 and 15:00 yesterday?" A question about typical use is often asked, such as "In summer, how often do you use a sunscreen when out of doors?" For simplicity of presentation and ease of comparison, only the highest category of typical use, or the sum of the two highest categories, is taken to indicate 'use' (for instance, the sum of 'always' and 'frequently'). The few studies in which only 'ever used' was reported have been excluded.

The prevalence of sunscreen use has been reported for populations and subpopulations in 15 countries covering latitudes ranging from 60° to 18°, but for very few specific locations, except the beach. Women are far more likely to use sunscreens than men, regardless of age, country, location or whether use is reported as habitual or at a specific time. In all the studies in which sex differences were reported, use was greater among female than male subjects. In 16 of these, the difference was ≥ 10%, and in eight it was ≥ 20% . Another noteworthy feature is the consistency of reported use by age group within studies. In all studies in which use on young children and adults was compared, the children's use was higher. In three studies in which adolescents were compared with adults, use by adolescents was lower. The mean prevalence of regular use (in studies of the prevalence of use always/frequent/often) was 60% (18 estimates in 12 studies) on children up to the age of 13, 32% (19 estimates in 12 studies) for adolescents and 44% (37 estimates in 22 studies) for adults.

Sunscreens are most often used during intentional exposure to the sun (Fig. 22). The mean prevalence of usual use in studies in which precautions at the beach and/or sunbathing were recorded expressly was 65% in children (five studies), 68% in adolescents and young adults (three studies) and 48% in adults (six studies). Studies of the prevalence of sunscreen use conducted at the beach tended to give higher use rates than those in other or unspecified

Table 8. Latitude and sunscreen use by European children in 1995–96 and by European adults in 1988–92

Country (city)	Children aged 6–7 years (%)		Adults who ever used sunscreen (%)
	Often/always use sunscreen when in the sun[a]	% of sunscreens with SPF ≥ 15[a]	
Sweden (Lund)	–	–	71[b]
Germany (Bochum)	69	63	62[c]
Belgium (Brussels)	62	69	50[c]
France (Lyon)	42	74	48[c]
Italy (Rome)	45	51	–

[a] From Autier et al. (1998)
[b] From Westerdahl et al. (1995), control subjects ≥ 15 years old
[c] From Autier et al. (1995), control subjects ≥ 20 years old

Table 9. Prevalence of sunscreen use in summer (who uses them and where they use them)

Reference	PP or H	Location of study	Year	Location of use	Study population and prevalence of sunscreen use	Other comments
Australia						
Hill et al. (1984)	H	Australia, Victoria	1982		Adult volunteers, recruited in workplaces, average 37 years When on vacation 53% When at work 37% On weekends 43%	Self-report 'Very often/always' use sunscreen
Hill et al. (1992)	PP	Australia, Victoria	1987–88	When outdoors	Melbourne residents, 14–69 years All 21% Males 16% Females 25%	Self-report Had applied a sunscreen (55% of sunscreens used were SPF ≥ 15)
Baade et al. (1996)	PP	Australia, Queensland	1988–89 and 1991–92	Summer weekends on Sunday while outside between 11:00 and 15:00	Residents 14–69 years 1988–89 25% 1991–92 33%	Self-report Used sunscreen on Sunday
Hill et al. (1993)	PP	Australia, Victoria	1988–90 (only 1990 data reported here)	When outdoors on the previous summer weekend between 11:00 and 15:00	Melbourne residents, 14–69 years Males Females 14–29 years 16% 24% 30–39 years 18% 39% 40–69 years 9% 26% Skin type (sensitivity) High 24% 32% Medium 12% 30% None 11% 17%	Self-report Used sunscreen
Hill & Boulter (1996)	PP	Australia, Victoria	1988–95	11:00–15:00 on previous Sunday	Victorians 1988 1989 1990 1992 1995 19% 25% 24% 27% 34%	Self-report Used sunscreen
Pincus et al. (1991)	PP	Australia	1989 March	Queensland beach between 12:00 and and 14:30 (average temperature, 27 °C)	Beachgoers 2–78 years All 70% < 10 years (n = 8) 50% 10–19 years 57% 20–29 years 79% 30–39 years 62% ≥ 40 years 64%	Self-reports; parent proxy reports for children < 10 years 'Applied sunscreen on the day of survey'

Table 9. (Contd)

Reference	PP or H	Location of study	Year	Location of use	Study population and prevalence of sunscreen use		Other comments
Pincus et al. (1991) (contd)					Skin type: fair medium olive/dark	76% 68% 63%	
Bennetts et al. (1991)	PP	Australia	1989	Two Victorian beaches, temperature 30–37 °C	Children 8–12 years Observed to apply sunscreen 'when arrived at beach' Reported they had used 'a SPF ≥ 15 sunscreen'	75% 48%	Self-report and observation
Martin (1995)	H	Australia	1989 December	Adelaide	Patients ≥ 16 years	74%	Self-reports 'Used sunscreen'
Pratt & Borland (1994)	PP	Australia, Victoria	1990–91	On a surf beach between 11:30 and 16:00 on days > 25 °C	Adolescents, 15–20 years	74%	Self-report 'Wearing sunscreen on at least some parts of their body at time of interview'
Foot et al. (1993)	PP	Australia	1991	Beach	All Children < 15 years Adults 15–29 years Adults ≥ 30 years	69% ~85% ~55% ~60%	Parent proxy reports, self-reports 'SPF 15+ applied to at least one body region' (approximations from bar chart)
Green et al. (1999a)	H	Australia	1992	Nambour	Residents in sunscreen treatment group	75%	Self-reported compliance with 'Daily sunscreen application' at 12 months: head neck arms and hands 3–4 days per week
Whiteman et al. (1994)	PP	Australia, Northern Territories	1992 August–October	When sitting in the sun 11:00–13:00 at the Darwin markets	Non-Aboriginal people 3–76 years All Past history of skin cancer No history of skin cancer NT residents	 17% 44% 11% 14%	Self-report interview 'Had applied' sunscreen
Watts et al. (1993)	H	Australia	1992 Summer	Adelaide	Survey participants Males Females	83% 73% 92%	'Used' sunscreen to avoid sun-burn or getting too much sun

Table 9. (Contd)

Reference	PP or H	Location of study	Year	Location of use	Study population and prevalence of sunscreen use		Other comments
Segan et al. (1999)	H	Australia, Victoria	1993 November	When outside for > 15 min between 10:00 and 14:00 while on holiday in Queensland	Tourists, ≥ 17 years	90%	Self-report 'Always/usually or sometimes' used SPF ≥ 15 sunscreen
Whiteman et al. (1997)	H	Australia	1994		Queensland children 10–21 years at interview When on holiday Melanoma cases ≤ 15 years Controls ≤ 15 years When at school Melanoma cases ≤ 15 years Controls ≤ 15 years	64% 54% 21% 13%	Children's retrospective self-reports 'Often/always' use sunscreen
Broadstock et al. (1996)	H	Australia, Victoria	1994	When outside for ≥ 1 h in summer between 11:00 and 15:00	Secondary students 12–17 years	27%	'Always' use SPF ≥ 15 sunscreen
Dobbinson et al. (1999)	H	Australia, Victoria	1995–96		Lifesavers When sunny VIC lifesavers NSW lifesavers When no sun VIC lifesavers NSW lifesavers	97% 85% 76% 54%	'Regularly' use sunscreen on patrol
Pruim et al. (1999)	H	Australia, Nambour	1996	When in sun	Residents ≥ 29 years	36%	Self-report 'Usually' wore sunscreen in last 3 months (of those who used sunscreen, 61% reapplied it)
Dixon et al. (1999)	H	Australia, Victoria	1996–97 mid-spring	On sunny days when outside	Melbourne primary school-children 'Always/mostly/wear sunscreen on exposed areas (parent's report) Used sunscreen (children's report)	72% 86%	Parents' proxy and children's reports, observation

Table 9. (Contd)

Reference	PP or H	Location of study	Year	Location of use	Study population and prevalence of sunscreen use		Other comments
Canada							
Campbell & Birdsell (1994)	H	Canada, Alberta	1987	When exposed to sun	Adults 35–64 years Males 15% Females 35%		Self-report 'Usually use' sunscreen
Rivers & Gallagher (1995)	H	Canada	1991–93		General public attending screening programme 1991–93 Age group / Males / Females 0–19 — 70% / 94% 20–39 — 61% / 79% 40–64 — 61% / 78% ≥ 65 — 54% / 69% All — 60% / 78%		Self-report 'Usually use' sunscreen
Zinman et al. (1995)	PP H	Canada	1993	When child played outdoors in the sun for > 30 min	Children attending hospital emergency department Had 'used sunscreen at least once in previous 2 months' 84% Would apply an SPF ≥ 15 sunscreen 74%		Parents proxy reports
Lovato et al. (1998)	H	Canada	1996 June–August		Children 'Always/often' used sunscreen on body < 12 years 76% 6–12 years 68% ≤ 5 years 84% 'Always/often' used sunscreen on face < 12 years 76% 6–12 years 67% ≤ 5 years 84%		Parent proxy reports
Gooderham & Guenther (1999)	H	Canada, Ontario	1998 April and May	When outdoors in summer	Primary students Summer pre-test 'Always' use/plan to use/using sunscreen 41% When using sunscreen, 'always' use/plan to use/ using a SPF ≥ 15 sunscreen 69%		Self-report

Table 9. (Contd)

Reference	PP or H study	Location of	Year	Location of use	Study population and prevalence of sunscreen use	Other comments
Denmark						
Stender *et al.* (1996a)	PP	Denmark	1994 July	At a beach, park, swimming-pool in Copenhagen after bathing	Used sunscreen on day of interview Sunbathers Males 65% Females 52% 73% Reapplied sunscreen ≥ 10 years 43% ≤ 10 years 11%	Self-report interviews
Stender *et al.* (1996b)	PP	Denmark, eastern	1994	4 beaches, 1 park July (summer; *n* = 805) May (early spring; *n* = 100)	Sunbathers (average, 28 years) All 67% Males 52% Females 73%	Self-report; parent proxy report for children < 8 'Used sunscreen' on day of study
France						
Grob *et al.* (1993)	H	France, Marseilles	1989 April–May		Children 3 years 85% Adolescents 13–14 years 48%	Mothers' proxy reports for children aged 3 years; adolescents, self-reports Sunscreen 'used'
France & Switzerland						
Autier *et al.* (1999)	H	France & Switzerland	1997	Before study, during sunny holidays or leisure times in sun	Swiss & French participants in a sunscreen trial, 18–24 years SPF 10 57% SPF 30 55%	Self-report 'Always/often' use sunscreen
Greece						
Kakourou *et al.* (1995)	H	Greece	1993 September–November		Mothers & children ≤ 12 years attending outpatient department 'Used' sunscreen last summer Mothers 80% Children 84% 'Always' used sunscreen when at the beach Mothers 52% Children 64%	Mothers' reports of self and children

Table 9. (Contd)

Reference	PP or H	Location of study	Year	Location of use	Study population and prevalence of sunscreen use		Other comments
Israel							
Harth *et al.* (1995)	H	Israel	1993		Habitual use (at least 1 year after excision)		
					Patients treated for BCC	64%	
					Controls	36%	
					After swimming		
					Patients treated for BCC	48%	
					Controls	33%	
Japan							
Kawada *et al.* (1989)	H	Japan	1988		Outpatients 15–68 years		Self-report 'Sunscreen use'
					All	27%	
					Females	57%	
					Males	18%	
					< 30 years	39%	
					> 30 years	42%	
					Japanese skin type: 1	53%	
					Japanese skin type: 2	36%	
					Japanese skin type: 3	40%	
New Zealand							
McGee & Williams (1992)	H	New Zealand	1991		Students 13–15 years		Self reports 'Often/always' used sunscreen last summer
					All	54%	
					Males	49%	
					Females	59%	
McGee *et al.* (1995)	PP	New Zealand	1994	Summer weekends	Adults 15–65 years		Self reports 'Used a sunscreen when outside on the weekend (Of those who used sunscreen, 89% reported using SPF ≥ 15)
					Respondents outdoors	32%	
McGee *et al.* (1997)	PP	New Zealand	1994 January–March	Sunny summer weekend	Children ≤ 10 years 1 day on weekend:		Parents' proxy reports 'Were wearing' sunscreen
					Saturday	49%	
					Sunday	52%	
					Both days	37%	

Table 9. (Contd)

Reference	PP or H	Location of study	Year	Location of use	Study population and prevalence of sunscreen use		Other comments
Norway							
Wichstrom (1994)	H	Norway	1992		High-school students Very often/always' use sun-screen		Self-report
					Males	20%	
					Females	35%	
					Use SPF ≥ 6		
					Males	28%	
					Females	24%	
South Africa							
von Schirnding et al. (1991/92)	H & PP	South Africa	1989	At the beach	Whites, ≥ 1 years: 'Most/all' the time use sunscreens	72%	Self-reports
					At time of interview use sun-screen	50%	
					Using sunscreen lotion		
					Males	49%	
					Females	74%	
					Using SPF ≥ 15 on body	6%	
					Using SPF ≥ 7 on body	15%	
					Using SPF > 7 on face		
					Males	18%	
					Females	43%	
Sweden							
Jerkegren et al. (1999)	H	Sweden	1995	Habitual use	University students ~ 24 years When sunbathing		Self-report 'Always/very often' used sunscreen 70%
					Females	51%	
					Males	79%	
					When sunbathing in a southern country		
					When sunbathing 11–15 h	50%	
					When skin starts to turn red	50%	
					Every day	7%	

Table 9. (Contd)

Reference	PP or H	Location of study	Year	Location of use	Study population and prevalence of sunscreen use		Other comments
United Kingdom							
Hughes *et al.* (1993)	H	United Kingdom	1990	On holiday:	Children 12–16 years Warmer country United Kingdom Elsewhere	78% 41% 52%	Self-report Wearing a sunscreen 'when it was sunny'
Bourke *et al.* (1995)	H	United Kingdom	1992	On sunny days	People in city ≥ 15 years When at home Males Females People aware of melanoma People unaware When 'abroad' Males Females People aware of melanoma People unaware	12% 32% 27% 13% 73% 54% 71% 46%	Self-report 'often/always' use sunscreen
Bourke & Graham-Brown (1995)	H	United Kingdom	1993		Children ≤ 14 years Sunny day at home Abroad	53% 88%	Parents' proxy reports Frequently/always ensure children use sunblock (of these, 32% said they used SPF ≥ 15)
USA							
Michielutte *et al.* (1996)	H	USA, North Carolina	1994		Women > 20 years When sunbathing Spring/summer	48% 33%	Self-report interviews at health care clinic 'Always' use sunscreen
Putnam & Yanagisako (1982)	H	USA, Hawaii	1980–81 December– February	Before receiving educational package	Hawaii Kai residents ≥ 18 years 'Use' sunscreen 'Use' SPF 8–15	34% 19%	Self-reported changes

Table 9. (Contd)

Reference	PP or H	Location of study	Year	Location of use	Study population and prevalence of sunscreen use		Other comments
Robinson (1992)	H	USA	1983–87	At baseline 1 year after surgery	NMSC patients (average age, ~ 60 years)		Self-report (prior to education)
					Use SPF < 15	32%	
					Use SPF ≥ 15	1%	
					Use 'when sun exposure was expected	32%	
					Use 'daily'	0%	
Berwick et al. (1992)	H	USA, Connecticut	1988 May		Subjects attended community skin cancer screening		
					Used sunscreen at least once last summer	75%	
					'Almost always' used sunscreen	42%	
Ross & Sanchez (1990)	H & PP	USA, Puerto Rico	July 1988–January 1989		Beachgoers ≥ 18 years		Interviews
					Habitual use		
					Tourist group	82%	
					Peurto Rican residents	38%	
					While at the beach		
					Tourist group	77%	
					Puerto Rican residents	50%	
Banks et al. (1992)	H	USA	1989 April–June	In early part of sunny season before they acquire a tan	Paediatric patients 12–19 years	26%	Self-reports
							Used sunscreen on 'more than half the days of sun exposure'
Mermelstein & Riesenberg (1992)	H	USA, Chicago	1990		High-school students		Self-reports
					Used sunscreen 'at least most of the time'		
					Males	8%	
					Females	17%	
					High-risk skin type	17%	
					Low- risk skin type	7%	
					9th grade	12%	
					10th grade	14%	
					Usual sunscreen used was SPF ≥ 15		
					Males	14%	
					Females	20%	
					High-risk skin type	21%	
					Low-risk skin type	12%	

Table 9. (Contd)

Reference	PP or H	Location of study	Year	Location of use	Study population and prevalence of sunscreen use	Other comments
Vail-Smith & Felts (1993)	H	USA, Southeast	1990 autumn	When exposed to sun for ≥ 30 min	University students Use SPF ≥ 15 sunscreen 9% 'Usually' use SPF ≥ 15 sunscreen at beach All 17% Males 15% Females 16%	Self reports
Hourani & LaFleur (1995)	H	USA, southern California	1990 & 1992		Residents attending community screening, ≥ 17 years 50% Males Females 17–35 years 26% 41% 36–50 years 35% 31% ≥ 51 years 39% 29%	Self-reports 'Regularly' use sunscreen
Foltz (1993)	H	USA	1991		Parents at paediatric clinic aged 23–49 years 'Sometimes/always' wear sunscreen 67% 'Sometimes/always' ensure child has sunscreen on Beach 77% Garden 47%	Parent proxy reports
Mawn & Fleischer (1993)	H	USA, North Carolina	1991	Samples from cruise ship, shopping mall, social function	White adults ≥ 15 years 40%	Self-reports 'Almost always/very often' use sunscreen
Maducdoc et al. (1992)	PP	USA, Texas	1991 July 10:00–15:00	Galveston beach	Parents using sunscreen on children ≤ 12 years 51%	Had 'used' sunscreen on their children
Koh et al. (1997)	H	USA	1991 July–September	Aquatic recreational areas	Sunbathers > 16 years All 47% Males 36% Females 53% Low education 38% Middle education 53% High education 55%	Self-report 'Always/often' use sunscreen (55% of regular sunscreen users and 25% overall sunbathers used SPF ≥ 15 sunscreen)

Table 9. (Contd)

Reference	PP or H	Location of study	Year	Location of use	Study population and prevalence of sunscreen use		Other comments
Leary & Jones (1993)	H	USA	1991 September	When in the sun	White undergraduates 17–23 years	7%	'Used' sunscreen regularly
Rodriguez et al. (1993)	H	USA, Puerto Rico	November 1991–March 1992	San Juan beach	Adolescents (white Puerto Ricans) All 13–15 years 16–18 years High-risk skin type Low-risk skin type	68% 67% 71% 20% 11%	Self-report 'Always' used sunscreen
Rossi et al. (1994)	PP	USA, Rhode Island	1991–92 Summer	Beach	Beachgoers	81%	Individuals accepted free sunscreen
Nguyen et al. (1994)	PP	USA, New Jersey	1992	Beaches	Beachgoers All Males Females 13–18 years 19–25 years 26–40 years 41–87 years Skin type I & II Skin type III & IV Skin type V & V	78% 70% 84% 72% 78% 81% 82% 87% 78% 61%	'Number using sunscreen' (of those who used sunscreen, 87% provided detail on SPF used: 35% used SPF ≥ 16; 17% used ≥ 4)
Hall et al. (1997)	H	USA	1992	When outside on a sunny day for > 1 h	Whites ≥ 17 years All Males Females	32% 22% 41%	Self-reports 'Very likely" to use sunscreen
Friedman et al. (1995)	H	USA, Houston, Texas	1992 May	Worksite	Hospital employees (average, 44 years)	64%	Self-report 'Very/extremely likely to use sunscreen
Buller et al. (1995)	H	USA	1993		Children < 14 years Parents 19–56 years	76% 42%	Parents/proxy Use 'most or all of the time' in summer
Marlenga (1995)	H	USA	1993		Dairy farmers, average, 51 years 'Frequently/always' use sunscreen 'Never' use sunscreen	8% 54%	Self-reports

Table 9. (Contd)

Reference	PP or H	Location of study	Year	Location of use	Study population and prevalence of sunscreen use		Other comments
Hoegh et al. (1999)	H	USA, California	1993–95	When outside > 15 min	Non-Hispanic white residents ≥ 18 years:		Self-report on 'use of sunscreen'
					Males	13%	'Always' use sunscreen (regular use)
					Females	31%	
					High-school graduates	23%	
					Non-graduates	11%	
					Fair skin	27%	
					Medium/dark skin	18%	
Newman et al. (1996)	H	USA, San Diego	1994		Adults 18–65 years: When suntanning last summer		Self-report?
					'Always/sometimes' used sunscreens on face	39%	
					'Always/sometimes' used sunscreen on body	39%	
					While in the sun for recreation last summer		
					'Always/sometimes' used sunscreen on face	59%	
					'Always/sometimes' used sunscreen on body	51%	
Robinson et al. (1997b)	H	USA, Midwest	1994	When outside in summer	Adolescents		Self report
					'Every day'	26%	
					'About once a week'	23%	
					'A few times each summer'	49%	
					'Daily use'		
					11–13 years	23%	
					14–16 years	31%	
					17–19 years	23%	
					Males	17%	
					Females	35%	
					Skin type I, II	33%	
					Skin type III, IV	29%	
					Skin type V, VI	–	
Reynolds et al. (1996)	PP	USA, Southeastern states	1994		Average, 11 years		'Used sunscreen'
					On Saturday	29%	
					On Sunday	21%	
					On the weekend		
					Males	11%	
					Females	21%	

Table 9. (Contd)

Reference	PP or H	Location of study	Year	Location of use	Study population and prevalence of sunscreen use		Other comments
Miller et al. (1999)					Children < 13 years When outside		Proxy reports by parents 'Usually' wear sunscreen
					< 6 years	36%	
					6–13 years	33%	
					When at the beach		
					< 6 years	85%	
					6–13 years	65%	
					With continuous exposure for 6 h		
					< 6 years	47%	
					6–13 years	35%	
Rosenman et al. (1995)	H	USA	1995	When outside for more than 1 h	Farmers & spouses ≥ 40 years		Self-report 'Very likely to use a sunscreen'
					Males	13%	
					Females	42%	
Glanz et al. (1997)	H	USA, Hawaii	1995	When outdoors	General public	65%	Self-report questionnaire 'Always/usually' use sunscreen
Zitser et al. (1996)	PP	USA, Connecticut	1995	When at beach (three beaches) 9:30–15:30	Beachgoers Using sunscreen		Self-report interviews
					Males	56%	
					Females	48%	
					Using SPF > 14 sunscreen		
					< 6 years	60%	
					6–13 years	25%	
Glanz et al. (1998a)	H	USA, Hawaii	1995 Summer	Four summer programmes, one swimming-pool	Parents	61%	Self-report, proxy reports of parents 'Use' sunscreen (at baseline)
					Children	68%	
					Staff	51%	
Martin et al. (1999)	H	USA, Florida	1996	Subtropical climate	Students 9–13 years		'Often/very often used sunscreen in past month'
					Boys	17%	
					Girls	20%	
Robinson & Rademaker (1998)	PP	USA, Michigan	1996	Beach at Lake Michigan	Beachgoers:		Observation Applied sunscreen at the beach
					Males	46%	
					Females	71%	
					Children ≤ 10 years	76%	

Table 9. (Contd)

Reference	PP or H	Location of study	Year	Location of use	Study population and prevalence of sunscreen use		Other comments
Glanz et al. (1999)	H	USA, Hawaii	1996 mid-June	Summer recreation programmes	Children		Parents' proxy reports & self-report 'Usually or always'
					Use sunscreen	39%	
					Use before going to beach	81%	
					Parents		
					Use sunscreen	36%	
					Use before going outside	57%	
					Staff		
					Use sunscreen	29%	
					Use before going outside	59%	
Robinson et al. (1998b)	H	USA	1996		Parents magazine readers		
					Regularly apply sunscreen to their children when at beach	68%	
					Seventeen magazine readers 12–19 years		
					'Always/often' use sunscreen when outdoors		
					Males	30%	
					Females	40%	
Donavan & Singh (1999)	H	USA, Kansas	1997		Primary-school students		
					'Always use sunscreen'	29%	
					'Thought sunscreen only important in summer months'	51%	
McCarthy et al. (1999)	PP	USA, Texas	1997	Galveston Island beach	Beachgoers 16–59 years	76%	Self-report, observation Used sunscreen
Glanz et al. (1998b)	H	USA, Hawaii	1997	When in bright sun	Children 6–8 years, participating in prevention programme		
					'Usually used sunscreen (formative research)	62%	
					Parents		
					'Always' used sunscreen	~1/3	
					Staff		
					'Usually/always' used sunscreen	60%	

Year, the year data were collected, if reported, otherwise year of publication less 2 years
PP, point prevalence (i.e. at a specific time) or H, habitual (i.e averaged over many observations or what people say they typically do); BCC, basal-cell carcinoma; NMSC, non-melanoma skin cancer; VIC, Victoria State; NSW, New South Wales; NT, Northern Territories

Table 10. Prevalence of sunscreen use in winter or in the snow

Reference	PP or H	Location of study	Year	Location of use	Study population and prevalence of sunscreen use		Other comments
Gooderham & Guenther (1999)	H	Canada, Ontario	1998 April & May	During winter	Primary-school students Before test After test 1 After test 2	2% 14% 12%	Self-report 'Always' use/plan to use/using sunscreen when going outdoors in winter
Harth et al. (1995)	H	Israel	1993	Winter	BCC patients and controls average age, 54 years Patients Controls	51% 39%	Self-report after treatment Used sunscreen in winter
Jerkegren et al. (1999)	H	Sweden	1995	When skiing in sunny weather	University students ~ 24 years	50%	'Always/very often' used sunscreen
Buller et al. (1995)	H	USA	1993	In winter	Adults 19–56 (with children):	23%	Self-report 'At least some of the time' use sunscreen
Michielutte et al. (1996)	H	USA, North Carolina	1994	When outdoors	Women > 20 years Autumn Winter	10% 8%	Self-report (face-to-face interviews at a health care clinic) 'Always use'
Buller et al. (1998)	H	USA	1996–97	Winter	Skiers and boarders 'Wearing a sunscreen' Adults Children SPF ≥ 15 'Use of sunscreen lip balm' Adults Children	89% 13% 90% 64% 85%	Self-report

PP, point prevalence (i.e. at a specific time) or H, habitual (i.e averaged over many observations or what people say they typically do); BCC, basal-cell carcinoma
Year, the year data were collected, if reported, otherwise year of publication less 2 years

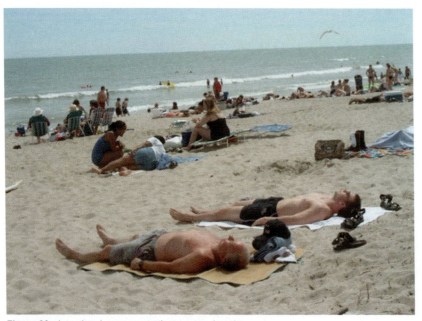

Figure 22 Intentional exposure to the sun on a beach

used sunscreens in the autumn, 8% in winter, 33% in spring and summer and 48% when sunbathing. Before a skin cancer education programme in Ontario, Canada (Gooderham & Guenther, 1999), 41% of primary-school students reported 'always' using, or planning to use, a sunscreen in summer, but only 2% did so in winter. In Sweden (Jerkegren *et al.*, 1999), 50% of a sample of university students 'always or very often' used sunscreens when skiing in sunny weather and 79% did so when sunbathing abroad. A study in Colorado, USA (Buller *et al.*, 1998), showed that 89% of adults used sunscreen on the snowfields.

How people use sunscreens

Few published data are available on how people use sunscreens, although cosmetics companies have probably collected much relevant information in the course of product development and testing. This lack of detailed published information, which would have to be based on unobtrusive observation and measurement, is a significant limitation. The literature on how people use sunscreens is thus heavily biased towards aspects of use that respondents can readily describe. The three main themes are application before exposure and re-application during exposure, SPF strengths used and the parts of the body to which sunscreens are applied.

In several studies, respondents were asked if they routinely applied sunscreen, as recommended, 30 min or so before going out into the sun. Among adolescents and adults, application before exposure was reported by 65% in Denmark (Stender *et al.*, 1996a), by 13% in Greece (Kakourou *et al.*, 1995), by 87% in New Zealand (McGee *et al.*, 1995) and by 2% in the USA (Robinson & Rademaker, 1998). Among parents, application on their children before exposure was reported by 20% in Greece (Kakourou *et al.*, 1995) and by 12% (Foltz, 1993) and 89% (Glanz *et al.*,

settings, probably because frequent beachgoers are more likely to use sunscreens and to be overrepresented in beach surveys. There is little doubt that the setting in which sunscreens are most commonly used is the beach and/or during sunbathing. The mean point prevalence of sunscreen use in 10 studies of beachgoers and one of sunbathers was 66%, and that in the studies in which sex differences were reported was about one-third times higher in women than in men. In five studies, the mean point prevalence of sunscreen use in people who were not beachgoers or sunbathers when out of doors in summer was 30%.

In two studies (Foltz, 1993; Jerkegren *et al.*, 1999) in which sunscreen use was compared in various settings, sunscreens were used more often at the beach than in any other setting. Four studies in northern Europe (Hughes *et al.*, 1993; Bourke & Graham-Brown, 1995; Bourke *et al.*, 1995; Jerkegren *et al.*, 1999) reported greater use of sunscreens when 'abroad' (presumably on summer vacations) than at home.

Some studies suggest that sunscreen use in sunny climates is more strongly associated with intentional than with unintentional exposure to the sun. In northern Australia, 71% of women and 68% of men on beaches applied a sunscreen (Pincus *et al.*, 1991). In contrast, less than 20% of fair-skinned adults at a market were found to have applied a sunscreen to uncovered areas of the skin (Whiteman *et al.*, 1994). In a case–control study of childhood melanoma in Queensland (the area of the world with highest incidence of melanoma), 83% of control children had used sunscreen when on holiday as compared with 44% when at school (Whiteman *et al.*, 1997).

The self-reported usual sunscreen use of the same respondents in seasons other than summer was contrasted in only five studies. In Arizona, USA (Buller *et al.*, 1995), 23% of 19–56-year-old parents used sunscreen 'at least some of the time' in winter, whereas 42% 'almost always' used sunscreen in summer. Of women in North Carolina, USA (Michielutte *et al.*, 1996), 10% 'always'

1999) in the USA. It cannot be determined whether this highly variable pattern reflects true differences among the population groups or artefacts of measurement.

Among adolescents and adults, reapplication was reported by 61% (Pincus et al., 1991) and 62% (Pruim et al., 1999) in Australia, by 43% in Denmark (Stender et al., 1996a), by 82% in France (Grob et al., 1993), by 9% in Greece (Kakourou et al., 1995), by 30% in Puerto Rico (Rodriguez et al., 1993) and by 8% in the USA (Banks et al., 1992). Among children, parents and/or children, the prevalence of sunscreen reapplication was 11% in Denmark (Stender et al., 1996a), 54% in France (Grob et al., 1993), 10% in Greece (Kakourou et al., 1995) and 45% in the USA (Foltz, 1993). Again, the high variability suggests that much of it is due to measurement artefact, and no generalization can be made about the prevalence of reapplication among sunscreen users from these data.

The choice of SPF level may vary according to the stage of tan acquired or desired (Vail-Smith & Felts, 1993; Wichstrom, 1994; Newman et al., 1996), skin sensitivity (Zitser et al., 1996), parental supervision (McGee et al., 1997) and regularity of use (Koh et al., 1997), but there are too few studies for conclusions to be drawn about common patterns of choice. Reported sunscreen use in the absence of details of SPF rating is likely to be highly ambiguous, and the reported numbers may include people using the most effective sunscreens as well as those who have deliberately chosen low-SPF formulations expressly to permit greater exposure to UVR. A number of studies do, however, indicate the proportion of sunscreen users using a high-SPF product on a specific occasion. The proportion reporting use of sunscreens with an SPF ≥ 15 was 48% (Bennetts et al., 1991), 47% (Pincus et al., 1991), 55% (Hill et al., 1992), 84% (Foot et al., 1993) and 27% (in adolescents; Broadstock et al., 1996) in

Australia; 89% in New Zealand (McGee et al., 1995); 6% in South Africa in 1989 (von Schirnding et al., 1991/92); and 48% (Nguyen et al., 1994), 45% (Zitser et al., 1996), 90% (in snow fields; Buller et al., 1998), 60% (Glanz et al., 1998a,b) and 47% (McCarthy et al., 1999) in the USA. The results of these studies indicate that a little over half of self-identified 'sunscreen users' use high-SPF products.

The SPF of sunscreens used on children appears to be higher than that of adults: in Europe in 1995–96, 50% of children who had ever received a sunscreen had a product of higher SPF than that used by their parents (Autier et al., 1998). Table 6 suggests that the South to North gradient observed in Europe for sunscreen use by children also exists for the SPF. In general, users were more likely to apply sunscreen to the face than to other parts of the body and to use a sunscreen with a higher SPF on the face.

The patterns of sunscreen use by families on an inland beach in the USA were measured by a combination of observational and interview methods (Robinson et al., 1998b). Women were most likely to provide and apply sunscreens to others, particularly children, and the median delay in application of sunscreen between arrival at the beach and application to the last family member was 51 min.

Why people use sunscreens
Table 11 lists the reasons why adults, adolescents and children use or do not use effective sunscreens (people deliberately using ineffective products were considered not to be using sunscreens). When significant associations between skin type and sunscreen use were found, it was assumed that knowledge about a propensity to burn was the reason for sunscreen use. In some studies, associations with sunscreen use were not sought, and people were simply asked why they used or did not use them. Reasons can be inferred from such studies

even if a link with behaviour was not demonstrated.

The commonest reason for using sunscreens among adults, adolescents and children was having a sensitive skin type. Self-perception of risk, previous experience of skin cancer and a family history of skin cancer were also frequently related to sunscreen use, particularly by adults. Two studies showed that sunscreen use was relatively more common among adults who knew people who had had skin cancer. Compliance with social norms was identified as another reason for using sunscreens.

A large majority of the studies of the role of knowledge about the dangers of exposure to the sun found that this predicted sunscreen use. Studies of adults and adolescents confirmed that sunscreens are used to prevent sunburn, and generally, positive attitudes to use of sunscreens and sun protection (measured variously) were related to sunscreen use.

Both positive and negative attitudes to suntanning have been found to be associated with sunscreen use by adults, and a positive attitude to a tan has been related to sunscreen use by adolescents, consistent with the results of behavioural studies, which show that sunscreen use increases with increasing exposure to UVR, and with those of epidemiological studies, in which skin cancer/melanoma was positively correlated with sunscreen use (see p. 69). Three studies of adolescents and two of adults have shown that sunscreen use is part of deliberate sunbathing, and other studies suggest that one motive for sunscreen use is to permit additional time in the sun. These conclusions raise concern that sunscreen use may result in unintended, additional, hazardous exposure to UVR.

Table 11 also presents reasons that people give for not using sunscreens, most of which are inferred, since often only non-users were asked their reasons. Those identified included finding them redundant (having skin that does not burn easily or is already tanned, not

Reason	Adults		Adolescents		Children	
	Yes	No	Yes	No	Yes	No
Reason to use						
Previously had skin cancer	Whiteman et al., 1994; Harth et al., 1995; Rademaker et al., 1996; Hall et al., 1997	Pruim et al., 1999				
Have skin that is fair/burns easily	Kawada et al., 1989; Miller et al. 1990; Ross & Sanchez, 1990; Berwick et al., 1992; Hill et al., 1992; Leary & Jones, 1993; Campbell & Birdsell, 1994; Newman et al., 1996; Stender et al., 1996b; Zitser et al., 1996; Hall et al., 1997; Glanz et al., 1999; Hoegh et al., 1999; Pruim et al., 1999		Fritschi et al., 1992; Mermelstein & Riesenberg, 1992; Wichstrom, 1994; Broadstock et al., 1996; Reynolds et al., 1996	Banks et al., 1992 Boldeman et al., 1996	Zinman et al., 1995; Robinson & Rademaker, 1998; Glanz et al., 1999; Miller et al., 1999	
Perception of being at high risk for melanoma/ skin cancer	Pincus et al., 1991; Berwick et al., 1992; Friedman et al., 1995; Hall et al., 1997; Robinson et al., 1997a	Leary & Jones, 1993	Mermelstein & Riesenberg, 1992			
Perception by parents that children are at high risk for melanoma/skin cancer					Buller et al., 1995; Miller et al., 1999	
Family history of skin cancer	Hourani & LaFleur, 1995					
Know people who had skin cancer	Keesling & Friedman, 1987; Leary & Jones, 1993					

Table 11. Reasons given for using or not using effective sunscreens

Reason	Adults		Adolescents		Children	
	Yes	No	Yes	No	Yes	No
Know dangers of exposure to sun	Hill *et al.*,1984; Keesling & Friedman, 1987; Kawada *et al.*, 1989; Berwick *et al.*, 1992; Vail-Smith & Felts, 1993 (I); Bourke *et al.*, 1995; Buller *et al.*, 1995; Michielutte *et al.*, 1996; Newman *et al.*, 1996; Glanz *et al.*, 1999	Leary & Jones, 1993; Hillhouse *et al.*, 1996	Banks *et al.*, 1992; Hughes *et al.*, 1993; Wichstrom, 1994			
Parents know dangers of sun exposure					Grob *et al.*, 1993 (I); Bourke & Graham-Brown, 1995; Zinman *et al.*, 1995; Glanz *et al.*, 1999	Maducdoc *et al.*,1992; Buller *et al.*, 1995
Children know dangers of sun exposure					Rademaker *et al.*, 1996 (I); Donavan & Singh, 1999	Kubar *et al.*, 1995; Boldeman *et al.*, 1996
Positive attitude to sunscreen/sun protection	Hillhouse *et al.*, 1996; McGregor & Young, 1996 (I)		Grob *et al.*, 1993 (I); Hughes *et al.*, 1993		Donavan & Singh, 1999; Martin *et al.*, 1999	
Prevent sunburn	Hill *et al.* 1984; Kawada *et al.*, 1989; Vail-Smith & Felts, 1993 (I)		Grob *et al.*, 1993 (I)		Maducdoc *et al.*, 1992; Grob *et al.*, 1993 (I)	
Knowledge about sunscreen product (e.g., reapplication)	Kawada *et al.*, 1989; Pruim *et al.*, 1999	Leary & Jones, 1993				
Negative attitude to tan	Newman *et al.*, 1996					
Compliance with social norms or peer group	Kawada *et al.*, 1989; Hillhouse *et al.*, 1997		Banks *et al.*, 1992; Wichstrom, 1994		Rademaker *et al.*, 1996 (I); Martin *et al.*, 1999	
Part of deliberate sunbathing/assist tanning	Hill *et al.*, 1984 Vail-Smith & Felts, 1993 (I)		Grob *et al.*, 1993 (I); Wichstrom, 1994; Eiser *et al.*, 1995			

Table 11. (Contd)

Table 11. (Contd)

Reason	Adults		Adolescents		Children	
	Yes	No	Yes	No	Yes	No
Allows more burn-free hours in sun	Pincus et al., 1991; Autier et al., 1999 (I)		Grob et al., 1993 (I)			
Positive attitude to tanning	McGregor & Young (1996) (I)	Berwick et al., 1992	Wichstrom, 1994			
Parents insist on sunscreen use			Banks et al., 1992			
Parents remind children to use sunscreen					Donavan & Singh, 1999	
Parents practise prevention (use sunscreen)					Foltz, 1993; Buller et al., 1995; Zinman et al., 1995; McGee et al., 1997; Robinson & Rademaker, 1998; Glanz et al., 1999; Miller et al., 1999	

Reasons not to use

Reason	Adults		Adolescents		Children	
	Yes	No	Yes	No	Yes	No
Have skin that does not burn easily	Stender et al., 1996a (I)					
Already have protective tan	McGee et al., 1995 (I)					
Not outdoors enough to warrant use	Berwick et al., 1992 (I); McGee et al., 1995 (I); Stender et al., 1996a (I)					
Use other sun protection instead	Berwick et al., 1992 (I); McGee et al., 1995 (I)					
Judged that sun too mild to need sunscreen	McGee et al., 1995 (I)					
Sunscreen retards desired tan	Kawada et al., 1989; Berwick et al., 1992 (I), Robinson, 1992; Gerbert et al., 1996		Robinson et al., 1997b			
Negative attitude to sunscreen	Hill et al., 1984; Hillhouse et al., 1996					
Sunscreens a nuisance	Berwick et al., 1992; Gerbert et al., 1996; Hill et al., 1984					

Reason	Adults		Adolescents		Children	
	Yes	No	Yes	No	Yes	No
Reason not to use						
Sunscreens too expensive	Gerbert *et al.*, 1996; Vail-Smith & Felts, 1993 (I)	Stender *et al.*, 1996a (I)				
Sunscreens greasy or have an odour	Gerbert *et al.*, 1996; Vail-Smith & Felts, 1993 (I)	Stender *et al.*, 1996a (I)				
Forget	Marlenga, 1995; McGee *et al.*, 1995					
Not masculine	Hill *et al.*, 1984					
Is 'dorky' or 'uncool'	Lowe *et al.*, 1993 (I) (especially males); Nguyen *et al.*, 1994 (I)					

'Yes', studies in which significant associations were reported between reason and sunscreen use or in which an association was inferred (I) because a proportion of the sample stated the reason for use
'No', studies in which the stated reason for use was tested but not found

being outdoors long enough or the sun not being strong enough to warrant use) and using an alternative form of protection. The most clearly articulated reason for not using sunscreens was that they retard the acquisition of a sought-after tan. A generally negative attitude to sunscreens was found to predict no use. A number of studies identified the objections to sunscreens as considering them a nuisance, expensive, greasy, have an odour and easy to forget. One study reported that men who found sunscreens 'unmasculine' were less likely to use them (Hill & Boulter, 1996). In two studies, adolescents perceived sunscreens as 'uncool' or 'dorky' (Lowe *et al.*, 1993; Nguyen *et al.*, 1994)

It might be expected that subjects with a history of skin cancer (other than melanoma) would be more inclined to use sunscreens than the average population (Whiteman *et al.*, 1994; Harth *et al.*, 1995; Hall *et al.*, 1997), but two studies in Queensland, Australia, do not support that assumption (Green *et al.*, 1999a,b; Pruim *et al.*, 1999). It might also be expected that patients with conditions that require protection from the sun would use sunscreens. Yet, sunscreen use was reported by less than 50% of British renal transplant recipients, who are at higher risk for non-melanoma skin cancer (Seukeran *et al.*, 1998), and only 50% of Puerto Rican patients with systemic lupus erythematosus, a disease that may be exacerbated by sunlight, reported sunscreen use (Vila *et al.*, 1999).

Children's sunscreen use was predicted by the parents' use of sunscreens and other solar protection, the parents' perception of their child's risk of melanoma/skin cancer and parental reminders. While there is evidence of a strong parental effect on sunscreen use among children, little evidence is available concerning the children's own knowledge and attitudes.

Strategies to increase sunscreen use
A number of interventions have been conducted to promote sun protection in general and sunscreen use in particular, in which the effect on sunscreen use was measured. These programmes can be broadly classified as targeted to particular population groups (Tables 12 and 13) or to the community as a whole (Table 14). Studies were excluded if they addressed formative research only, had no data on sunscreen use or did not report the impact on sunscreen use. A study in children in which drawing was used at interview after a test was also excluded.

Interventions were conducted in a variety of settings. School programmes were the most common (11 studies), and the results of programmes at beaches and pools (five studies) and other recreational settings were also reported. Work sites and clinical settings were less often targeted for intervention. Two localized community interventions were also considered to be targeted interventions: one in which an educational brochure was available for general use and another targeted to households in one suburb. The targeted interventions were generally short-term programmes aimed at improving sun protection behaviour among specific high-risk groups, including children, adolescents, beachgoers, outdoor workers and patients with non-melanoma skin cancer. The programmes incorporated a range of strategies, from brief educational presentations or packages aimed at increasing knowledge or specific recommendations for sunscreen use, to integrated programmes with multiple components to promote sustainable behavioural change by developing supportive social and physical environments for sun protection.

Most programmes incorporated some educational elements designed to increase awareness about skin cancer and the benefits of sunscreen use (Fig. 23). Strategies designed to influence social norms for sunscreen use were commonly directed at children and included peer-led programmes, role modelling and parental involvement or home activities. A few promoted strategies for sustainable change by encouraging the development of policies on sun protection in organizations such as schools, recreational programmes and lifesaving clubs. Programmes were led by medical experts in a few settings.

Twenty-one of the 28 studies reported at least some measure of outcome with regard to sunscreen use, although proxies for behaviour were used in some studies. For example, two studies measured intention to use sunscreen rather than actual use.

Nine of the 16 targeted interventions were successful in increasing sunscreen use. The designs of the more targeted interventions were generally adequate, involving either quasi-experimental or randomized controlled trials, although a few had weaker designs, with either no control group or no or a limited pre-intervention test, and few reported the impact on sunscreen use. The interventions were successful across a range of settings, including schools, beaches or pools, recreation sites, clinics and households. Two others changed factors that are precursors to behaviour, i.e. beachgoers' intention to use sunscreen (Detweiler et al., 1999) and care-givers prompting use of sunscreens by youths (Parrott et al., 1999).

The intensity and duration of the targeted intervention appeared to affect the success of programmes. Thus, successful programmes tended to be longer, have multiple components or be supported by broader community-based programmes. Two brief, school-based programmes consisting of only one class session had no impact on behaviour (Mermelstein & Riesenberg, 1992; Buller et al., 1997) even though they included some interactive components such as discussions, worksheets and take-home bags to involve parents. The duration of the intervention did not appear to improve sunscreen use in two studies, a 4-month educational package for schoolchildren (Hughes et al., 1993) and a 41-day intervention at swimming pools with role models, incentives and free sunscreen (Lombard et al., 1991), but an Australian study (Girgis et al., 1993) provides some evidence that solar protection scores were increased after school-based interventions of longer duration with more interactive learning techniques.

Distributing educational brochures has had mixed success. Detweiler et al. (1999) found that brochures could promote the intention to use sunscreens. Moreover, brochures with specific reco-mmendations for sunscreen use appeared to be more effective than general recommendations for sun protection. A comic book brochure with specific recommendations for using sunscreens SPF ≥ 8 was successful in changing the use of sunscreens by Hawaiian householders (Putnam & Yanagisako, 1982). A brochure promoting general awareness of sun protection and, specifically, a 'SunSmart Siesta' to holiday-makers had no effect on their sunscreen use, although sun avoidance during peak UV radiance increased (Segan et al., 1999).

Other components of successful strategies involve increasing the perception of risk for developing skin cancer. An intervention in which adolescents were shown computerized photo-images of their own faces with superimposed ageing and skin lesions was successful in improving both the frequency of sunscreen use and application of sunscreen (Novick, 1997). Education about skin cancer risk and specific recommendations for sun protection in a medical

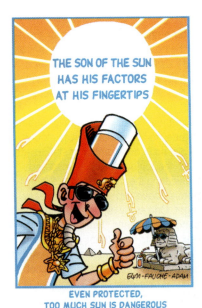

THE SON OF THE SUN HAS HIS FACTORS AT HIS FINGERTIPS

EVEN PROTECTED, TOO MUCH SUN IS DANGEROUS

Figure 23 Educational brochure aimed at improving sun-exposure behaviour

Table 12. Impact of targeted interventions on sunscreen use

Reference	Location	Study design and setting	Sample size	Population group	Duration of intervention	Strategy	Sunscreen use outcome	Other outcomes
Australia								
Dobbinson et al. (1999)	Australia, Victoria, 1997, 1989	Beaches Cross-sectional/ post-test comparison with control group	n = 129 VIC & n = 134 NSW lifesavers	Lifesavers on patrol	10 years	Incentives provided to clubs to develop sun protection policies and comply with adequate protection while on patrol. Awareness training for juniors	Sunscreen use in VIC greater than in NSW Regular use in sun 97% vs 85%, p < 0.001 When no sun, 76% vs 54%, p < 0.001	More VIC than NSW lifesavers used hats, shirts, and shelter/shade in sun. (No difference in shirt use when not in sun)
Segan et al. (1999)	Australia, Victoria, November 1993	Tourism in Queensland Randomized controlled trial	21 flights to Queensland on Saturdays & Sundays n = 373	Tourists aged ≥ 17	Pre-flight test Post-holiday test (most < 2 weeks)	Brochure provided information and sun protection recommendations, e.g., 'SunSmart Siesta Plan'	Sunscreen use not significantly different from control group	Fewer mean days spent outside between 11:00 and 14:00 (controls, 3.7, intervention 3.2, p < 0.001) Hats, clothing, shade use not signifcant
Canada								
Gooderham & Guenther (1999)	Canada, London, Ontario, 1998	Schools pre-/post-test	35 schools (pre-test n = 244)	Grade 4 students 9–11 years	1 month before intervention 1-h class, 35-min slide show, worksheets. Post-test Follow-up at 1 month	Interactive 'sun awareness' class session, slide presentations, (incidence, risks and prevention), activity book	Increase in 'always' use of sunscreen SPF > 15 (T1 69%, T2 88%, p < 0.001) Increase in winter and summer use	Significant increase in use of hats, long-sleeved shirts, trousers, sunglasses
United Kingdom								
Hughes et al. (1993)	England, 1990	7 schools, post-test only (intervention and control groups)	n = 543 (262 matched tests 1 & 2)	School students 12–16 years	Educational package May–June Post test in July Follow-up test in September	Workbook with sun protection tips; education on UVR and skin cancer Components assessed Workbook and either video, poster design, homework or discussion	No impact on sunscreen use	No impact on other sun behaviour

Table 12. (contd)

Reference	Location	Study design and setting	Sample size	Population group	Duration of intervention	Strategy	Sunscreen use outcome	Other outcomes
USA								
Putnam & Yanagisako (1982)	USA, Hawaii. October 1981	Community Pre-/post-intervention Repeated cross-sectional samples	n = 304	Residents of suburb (reporting for household) ≥ 18 years	Pre-test December 1980–February 1981 Package distributed to households. Post-test (October 1981) 4 months after distribution	Comic book emphasized increased risk for skin cancer among whites and gave recommendations for sun protection (use of SPF ≥ 8, protect skin during peak UVR), education on how to check skin and when to seek medical advice	38.5% of readers changed their use of SPF ≥ 8 sunscreen after reading book

Readers significantly more likely than non-readers to use sunscreen ($p < 0.0005$) but not other sun protection | 44% of readers changed their avoidance of sun exposure 10:00–14:00

30% of readers wore protective clothing |
Robinson (1992)	USA, Chicago 1983–89	Medical Longitudinal (no control group)	n = 1022	NMSC patients Not reported	Phase 1:2 weeks and 6 months before operation Phase 2 annual follow-up with written material	Recommended daily sunscreen use, ceasing tanning, minimizing time outside peak UVR	Daily SPF ≥ 15: Before operation, 0; 1 year, 12%; 2–6 years, 25%	Decreased tanning after 1 year Increased clothing use with increased outdoor activity after 2–6 years
Robinson et al. (1998b)	USA, Chicago, May 1990–September 1991	Medical Pre-/post-intervention	178 pairs	Patients and helpers 30–60 years	NMSC patients & helpers surveyed pre- and post-intervention (~ 1 year after surgery)	Education and recommendations provided in brochure and verbally by staff. Emphasizing ceasing tanning, avoiding outdoor activities 10:00–14:00, wearing protective clothing, using SPF ≥ 15 sunscreen	Increased sunscreen use ($p = 0.01$ for patients, $p = 0.013$) for helpers	Helpers ($p = 0.018$) and patients ($p = 0.02$) decreased hours spent outside. Helpers ($p = 0.001$) also decreased use of indoor tanning devises
Lombard et al. (1991)	USA, Virginia, 1991	Pools Pre/post	2 private swimming pools	Public 1–16 years ≥ 16 years	Pre: 15 days Intervention phase. 41 days of observation	Sun protection competition and feedback, posters, fliers Lifesaver role modelling Provision of free sunscreen	No change in mean quantity of sunscreen used at either pool	Increase in children's use of protective behaviour (6.5% to 27%) Increase in adults' sun protection (22% to 38%)

Table 12. (contd)

Reference	Location	Study design and setting	Sample size	Population group	Duration of intervention	Strategy	Sunscreen use outcome	Other outcomes
Mermelstein & Riesenberg (1992)	USA, Chicago, 1992	10 schools Randomized controlled trial	$n = 1703$	Students 14–17 years	Pre-test. Intervention, 1 session. Post-test	Education video, discussion of barriers to sun protection, work sheet to assess personal risk for skin cancer	No effect on intention (likelihood) to use sunscreen	No effect on intention (likelihood) to use other sun protection behaviour
Buller *et al.* (1997)	USA, Tucson, Arizona, 1993	3 schools Quasi-experimental	$n = 318$	Grade 4 students	Pre-test, brief 2 x 1-day intervention (1 h curriculum & fair). Post-test and 3-month follow-up test	Interactive learning activities	Neither intervention affected children's intention to use sunscreen	Neither intervention affected intention to use hats or lip balm
Glanz *et al.* (1998b)	USA, Hawaii, 1995	Recreational settings for children (three YMCAs, one summer fun site, one pool) Pre/post intervention	Parents	Children 6–8 years and staff	Base-line 4-week intervention Follow-up	Staff given manual on activities, sun protection, policy development guidelines. Programme provided sunscreen and sun protective environment. Children given activities for home and incentives for sun protection. Monitoring and feedback on children's sun protection behaviour. Parents given educational brochures	Increase in sunscreen use: parents 61% to 63%, children 68% to 75%	Compositive sun protection scores significantly improved for parents and children, not staff. Shade use increased: parents 46% to 58%, children 23% to 38%
Detweiler *et al.* (1999)	USA, New England, 1996	Public beach Pre-/post-intervention (no control group/ randomly assigned to treatment)	$n = 217$	Beachgoers (76% women) 18–79 years	Beachgoers completed pre-test questions before reading brochure and post-test questions (in sealed section) after reading brochure	Prospect theory: message framing	Beachgoers who read brochures highlighting potential 'gains' are more likely than those reading brochures highlighting potential 'losses' to use and reapply sunscreen and request free sunscreen	Not measured

Table 12. (contd)

Reference	Location	Study design and setting	Sample size	Population group	Duration of intervention	Strategy	Sunscreen use outcome	Other outcomes
Weinstock *et al.* (1988)	USA, 1996	Public beach Randomized controlled trial	n = 2324	Beachgoers	Baseline, 12- and 24-month follow-up	Intervention: pamphlet, free sunscreen, sun damage and skin sensitivity checks	Difference between intervention and control group, p = 0.02 at 12 months increasing at 24 months	Sun protection index, p = 0.001 Sun avoidance, p = 0.004 at 12 months At 24 months, hat use also significant, p=0.03
Novick (1997)	USA, Long Island, New York, 1997	2 day camps Randomized controlled trial	n = 30	Female students 13–28 years	5 weekly tests included logs of sunscreen application and measured weight of supplied sunscreen. Intervention images shown on 2 days in week 4	Subjects shown computerized photographic images of themselves. Two intervention groups shown altered images: either aged only or aged and disfigured with lesions	Increased use of sunscreen and more thorough application of sunscreen post-test	No change in mean time spent outside
Dietrich *et al.* (1998)	USA, New Hampshire, 1998	Public beaches Part of multi-component community randomized controlled trial	10 towns randomly assigned	Children aged 2–11 years at beach	Baseline and 1-year follow-up	Educational materials: avoid sun, cover up (hats, clothes), use SPF > 15, encourage family/friends to use	Increase in intervention towns from 0.56% pre-test to 0.76% post-test (mean; applied to at least one body part)	No change in clothing or shade use, children with any protection increased from 0.53% to 0.74% Change in control group was from 0.66% to 0.72%.
Parrott *et al.* (1999)	USA, Georgia, 1999	8 youth soccer participants Pre-/post intervention	n = 12 coaches, n = 50 parents, n = 61 players	Coaches 33–64 years Parents 31–56 years Youths 8–14 years	Pre-test: curriculum manual presented to coaches during focus group meeting. Post-test	Education on skin cancer, and how to protect skin (including how to choose and use sunscreen)	More parents prompting youths to wear sunscreen and role modelling More coaches preceiving they were able to encourage youths to wear sunscreen	No change in wearing of other sun protection items

VIC, Victoria State; NSW, New South Wales State; NMSC, non-melanoma skin cancer

Table 13. Targeted interventions in which effect on sunscreen use was not reported separately

Reference	Location	Study design and setting	Sample size	Population group	Duration of intervention	Strategy	Sunscreen use outcome	Other outcomes
Australia								
Girgis et al. (1993)	Australia, New South Wales, 1993	School Randomized controlled trial/ diary	11 schools n = 612	School-children 9–11 years	4-week curriculum. 1 × 30-min lecture. Control group	Curriculum: interactive Lecture: didactic 'Skin Safe' booklet distributed to both groups	Not reported	Significant (p < 0.01) difference in protection score at post-test Increased sun protection in curriculum group
Girgis et al. (1994)	Australia, New South Wales, 1994	One electrical supply company (12 depots) Randomized controlled trial	n = 142	Outdoor workers 22–63 years (mean, 40)	Pre-test. 1-week inter-vention Post-test at 1 month	30-min lecture and presentation; brochure included education on increased risk of outdoor workers for skin cancer; sun protective clothing available at workplace	Sunscreen use not reported separately	Solar protection scores increased in intervention group (p < 0.02) and remained stable in control group (p = 1.0). Group difference at post-test was significant (p = 0.04)
USA								
Lawler (1989)	USA, 1989	Community Process evaluation only		General population	Available through American Cancer Society	Education booklet on sunscreen products and prevention strategies		
Reding et al. (1995)	USA, Wisconsin, 1991–92	School Quasi-experimental	n = 401	Third-grade students	Pre-test. Two 30–40 min presentations ~ 1 week apart on how and when to protect. Post-test & 6-month follow-up test	Education only	No sunscreen use measures	Increased knowledge No sun protection behaviour measured

Table 13. (contd)

Reference	Location	Study design and setting	Sample size	Population group	Duration of intervention	Strategy	Sunscreen use outcome	Other outcomes
Friedman et al. (1995)	USA, Texas, 1992	Worksite Longitudinal	n = 324	Hospital employees average, 41 years	Pre-test before clinical screening (May 1992). 4–7 month follow-up surveys	5-min screening and 15-min educational video on prevention, early detection and treatment	Analysis of predictors of intention to use sunscreen. Change in intention after test not reported	
Grant-Petersson et al. (1999)	USA, New Hampshire, 1997–99	Multi-component community-wide intervention in small towns (population 4000–12 000). Process evaluation from randomized controlled trial	24 elementary schools, 31 child-care centres	School-children 2–9 years	Schools, 2-year intervention Child-care centres, 1–2 year intervention	Schools held ~3 h of class lessons. Child-care centres held two 'SunSafe' theme days. Materials included 'SunSafe' manual (activities, reading lists, etc), cartoon video, cover-up video. ABCs guidelines 'Avoid the sun. Block the sun using SPF 15 + sunblock. Cover-up using hats and protective clothing. Speak out to family and friends regarding sun protection. Parental activities	Individuals' sunscreen use not measured	Individuals' other sun protection behaviour not measured

Table 14. Impact of large-scale community interventions

Reference	Location	Study design and setting	Sample size	Population group	Duration of intervention	Strategy	Sunscreen use outcome	Other outcomes
Australia								
Hill *et al.* (1993)	Australia, Melbourne, 1987–89	Community Cross-sectional/ trends	1988 n = 1655 1989 n = 1397 1990 n = 1376	Melbourne residents 14–69 years	On-going community-wide intervention. Surveys of adult residents 1988, 1989, 1990	'Slip! Slop! Slap!' school education programmes and annual summer public media campaign. Programme further developed into large-scale multi-component programme 'SunSmart' (1988), with strategies including lobbying manufacturers to reduce sunscreen costs	1988–90 Increased sunscreen use if outside > 15 min 11:00–15:00: males, 10% to 14–15% ($p < 0.05$); females, 16% to 20–24% ($p < 0.001$)	1988–90 Fewer residents spending > 15 min outside 11:00–15:00: males 85% to 72–76% ($p < 0.001$); females, 69% to 54–66% ($p < 0.05$) Increased hat use among males and females ($p < 0.001$) Increased clothing coverage index: males, 0.68 to 0.65–0.72 ($p < 0.01$); females, 0.68 to 0.63–0.69 ($p < 0.01$)
Borland *et al.* (1990)	Australia, Victoria, 1988–89	Community Media Pre-post-intervention (repeated cross-sectional sample)	Pre-campaign n = 560 Post-campaign n = 605	Victoria residents ≥ 14 years	Summer campaign	'SunSmart' campaign	29% reported increased sunscreen use	22% hats 13% shirts 4% shade
Canada								
Rivers & Gallagher (1995)	Canada, 1991–93	Community Cross-sectional/ trends	n = 1681	Screening participants 2–87 years (median, 45 years)	On-going public and media campaign Surveys of screening participants 1991, 1992 and 1993	Annual media campaign and distribution of educational materials. 'Living with Sunshine' school curriculum. Community screening during 'Sun Awareness Week'	Sunscreen use increased in males and females Usual use of sunscreen by 60% of males and 77% of females in 1991 and 63% males and 79% of females in 1993	Other sun protection not measured

Table 14 (contd)

Reference	Location	Study design and setting	Sample size	Population group	Duration of intervention	Strategy	Sunscreen use outcome	Other outcomes
USA								
Miller *et al.* (1999)	USA, Massachusetts, Falmouth, 1994–97	Community Pre-/post-intervention	$n = 401$ pre-test $n = 404$ post-test	Households with children ≤ 13 years	Two random surveys of households at pre-test and and after 3 years of intervention	Multi-component community intervention (incorporated community activism, publicity campaign, distribution of sun protection educational materials and targeted interventions) Strategies include awareness raising, role modelling by parents and institutionalizing sun protection	At post-test more parents reported children used sunscreen For children aged 6–13, increase in use significant with regular use, when outside, at beach and continuous use at beach (36% to 53%, $p < 0.001$). For children aged < 6, increase significant only for continous use at beach (47% to 70%, $p < 0.001$) More parents bought and used sunscreen. Fewer parents sunbathed	Other sun protection behaviour generally consistent at both pre and post-test Increase in use of shirts at beach among children 6–13 years Decreased incidence of sunburn in children
Geller *et al.* (1997)	USA, 1995	Community Cross-sectional	58 cities $n = 700$ adults, 185 television stations, 54 newspapers	Residents ≥ 18 years	1994–95 post-test national survey of stations, newspapers and resident population	71% stations and 61% newspapers reported UVR index in 1994 and 1995	Regular sunscreen use associated with awareness of UVR index	64% aware of UVR index 38% changed sun protection 40% perceived UVR index helped choose when to tan
Robinson *et al.* (1997a)	USA, 1996	Community Cross-sectional/ trends	1986 $n = 1012$ 1996 $n = 1000$	Residents ≥ 18 years	Public education programmes initiated in 1983; annual media campaign in May since 1985 Surveys of residents 1986 and 1996	Campaign includes print, television and radio messages on risks of sun exposure and benefits of sun protection	Sunscreen use increased from 35% to 54%	Increased regular use of tanning lamps/booths from 2% to 6%

setting were effective in raising the perception of susceptibility to skin cancer of patients treated for non-melanoma skin cancer and their helpers, and this was associated with increased sunscreen use (Robinson, 1992; Robinson & Rademaker, 1995).

One intervention study among outdoor workers (Girgis et al., 1994) and one among schoolchildren (Girgis et al., 1993) affected sun protection behaviour, but sunscreen use was reported only as part of a composite solar protection score. The impact of one intervention at swimming pools in which clients were given incentives and role modelling of lifeguards is also unclear, although the authors reported that the sun protection score improved when two or more sun protection measures were taken together, with no change in the mean quantity of free sunscreen used at the pools (Lombard et al., 1991).

Few studies of large-scale community interventions were reported. These represent long-term commitments from communities to the control of skin cancer, and the interventions were generally evaluated subsequently in cross-sectional population surveys. The programmes evaluated included the 'Slip! Slop! Slap!' and 'SunSmart' campaigns in Victoria, Australia (Borland et al., 1990; Hill et al., 1993), the 'Sun Awareness' programme in Canada (Rivers & Gallagher, 1995), UVR index forecasting in the USA (Geller et al., 1997), the Melanoma Skin Cancer Detection and Prevention Program in the USA (Robinson et al., 1997a) and the Falmouth Safe Skin Project in Massachusetts, USA (Miller et al., 1999). The 'Sun Awareness' programme used strategies for improving community knowledge about skin cancer and sun protection, which included mass media, distribution of educational brochures and development of a school curriculum for sun protection. The UVR index forecasting and the Melanoma Skin Cancer Detection and Prevention Program are based on televi-

sion and print media messages on sun protection. The Sun Awareness programme also included strategies aimed mainly at improving community knowledge of skin cancer and sun protection. In contrast, the Falmouth Safe Skin Project and the 'SunSmart' programme are multi-component programmes encompassing regular mass media campaigns and local interventions, involving working with various groups to institutionalize sun protection by creating supportive social and physical environments. Five of the large-scale community interventions had a positive impact on sunscreen use at a population level. No effect on sunscreen use was seen in a study in which the UVR index was reported on television and print media nationally in the USA, although sunscreen use was associated with increased awareness of the forecasts (Geller et al., 1997).

Compensatory behaviour

As noted above, sun-protective behaviour to some extent involves choices among alternative behaviours, not all of which are completely effective in protecting the skin from UVR. Hence, to the extent that increased sunscreen use leads to reduced use of other forms of sun protection, net exposure to UVR may increase.

Sunscreens are designed primarily to prevent sunburn. Most sunburns in children and adults occur during intentional exposure to the sun (Hill et al., 1992; McGee et al., 1995; Melia & Bulman, 1995; Autier et al., 1998). Although use of sunscreens during unintentional exposure can reduce the occurrence of sunburn (Hill et al., 1993; Green et al., 1999a), the situation is different for intentional exposure, and usual use of sunscreens, or use of sunscreens with a higher SPF, during intentional exposure seems to have little impact on the occurrence of sunburn (Wulf et al., 1997; Autier et al., 1999; McCarthy et al., 1999).

A double-blind study of intentional exposure to the sun indicated that peo-

ple who use high-SPF sunscreens stay in the sun longer than those who use lower-SPF products (Autier et al., 1999). These investigators assigned French and Swiss volunteers aged 18–24 to use SPF 10 or SPF 30 sunscreen while on their summer holiday, assumed to consist of ≥ 15 days in a sunny region. The sunscreens were packaged identically, and 44 people were randomized to receive SPF 10 sunscreen and 43 to SPF 30 sunscreen. Analysis at the end of the summer revealed that the mean duration of the holidays was similar in the two groups, at 19 and 20 days, respectively. The number of skin reddening episodes was also comparable. However, those people randomized to the SPF 30 sunscreen had spent more hours per day in the sun (4.6) than those randomized to SPF 10 sunscreens (4.0). Similarly, the mean accumulated hours of exposure to the sun during the holiday was significantly greater for the subjects randomized to SPF 30 sunscreen (73 h) than those to SPF 10 (58 h). This study suggests that use of sunscreens by people who intentionally expose themselves to the sun reflects a desire to avoid sunburn rather than total exposure to UVR, and that guarding against skin cancer may be at best a secondary motive. The studies of beachgoers also lend support to the idea that sunbathers' use of sunscreens is driven by factors other than a desire to protect against skin cancer. It is possible that the increasing popularity of sunscreens will lead people who wish to be maximally protected to reduce their overall protection by over-reliance on sunscreens.

Cross-sectional surveys of comparable samples from the same population at different times indicate how people adjust various components of their sun protection behaviour. In Victoria, Australia, representative samples of 14–69-year-olds were interviewed during three successive summers covering a period when a major sun protection campaign was under way, and the point prevalence of sun protection behaviour was measured (Hill *et al.*, 1993). Over this period, the use of sunscreens increased from 10% to 15% by men and from 16% to 28% by women. The prevalence of hat wearing rose from 23% to 32% among men and from 14% to 20% among women. The mean proportion of the body that was clothed did not decrease, but the proportion of people out of doors between 11:00 and 15:00 decreased. Surveys in Queensland, Australia, using the same method, four years apart (Baade *et al.*, 1996) showed an increase in sunscreen use (odds ratio, 1.7) at the same time as increases in shade seeking (odds ratio, 1.3) and hat wearing (odds ratio, 1.5), and both the proportion of people who went outside and the average time spent outside between 11:00 and 15:00 decreased. Likewise, in a Canadian study of screening participants in an on-going public education campaign (Rivers & Gallagher, 1995), increased sunscreen use was found, but other protective behaviour did not appear to have been measured.

In an evaluation of a community intervention in the USA (Miller *et al.*, 1999), children aged 6–13 years were reported by their parents to have increased sunscreen use but engaged in less sunbathing. At the beach, however, they were less likely to wear a shirt but more likely to use a sunscreen. An intervention study at swimming pools in the USA showed changes in children's non-sunscreen protective behaviour but no change in the amount of freely available sunscreen taken from dispensers (Lombard *et al.*, 1991). An inverse correlation between sunscreen use and the wearing of clothes was found for European children engaged in intentional exposure to the sun (Autier *et al.*, 1998). One year after an educational intervention in an elementary school in the USA, increases were reported in the use not only of sunscreens but also of hats, long-sleeved shirts, long trousers and sunglasses (Gooderham & Guenther, 1999).

Australian coastal lifeguards studied 8 years apart reported increased use of SPF ≥ 15 sunscreens while on duty (Fig. 24) and increased use of shade and hats (Dobbinson *et al.*, 1999). In a study in the USA, young women who were shown motivational material on photo-ageing increased their use of sunscreens without changing the amount of time spent outside (Novick, 1997).

In a study of intentional exposure to the sun by people aged ≥ 40 who were randomized to apply an SPF ≥ 15 sunscreen or a placebo moisturizer (Cockburn *et al.*, 1997), the levels of other sun protection behaviour, including time spent outdoors, were similar among those given sunscreen and those not given sunscreen. This result contrasts with the pattern reported in the study of Autier *et al.* (1999) and suggests that the way in which different sun protection behaviours are 'balanced' by individuals depends on personal characteristics and motivations.

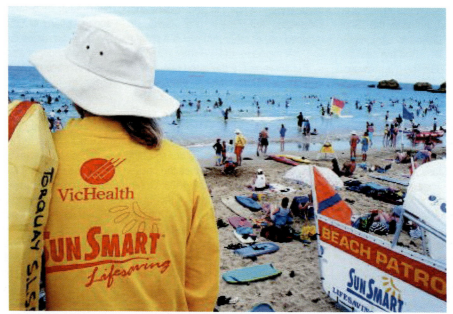

Figure 24 T-shirt and sign advertising the 'SunSmart Campaign' on a beach in Australia

Chapter 4

Metabolism of sunscreens in various species

In order to achieve the stated SPF (2 mg/cm²) of a sunscreen preparation, about 35 ml are needed for a whole-body application for adults. If it is applied at the recommended frequency, at least twice this amount could be applied during a day at the beach. During other periods, sunscreens may be applied to sun-exposed sites such as the face, hands and arms for extended periods or used daily in cosmetic preparations. Ideally, sunscreens should remain on the skin surface, so that they can be washed off, or should be bound only to the non-viable epidermis (stratum corneum). Relatively little is known about the percutaneous absorption and metabolism of sunscreens. Since they might be used daily throughout life, it is clearly important that any interactions that sunscreens may have within viable skin and systemically should be assessed. The percutaneous absorption of sunscreens has been studied in humans and animals in vivo. Ex-vivo techniques, in which viable excised skin is used as a membrane in a diffusion chamber and test material is collected in a receptor fluid, have also been used.

Humans
Organic sunscreen ingredients
para-*Aminobenzoic acid*
Arancibia *et al.* (1981) studied the percutaneous absorption and pharmacokinetics of three topical sunscreen preparations containing 5% PABA in six male volunteers. A dose of 20 g of sunscreen was applied to the face, neck, trunk and upper extremities (at approximately the recommended level of application) in the

early morning. Urine samples were taken before application and at periods 2–48 h after application and were analysed for PABA and its acetylated derivative. The cumulative urinary excretion of total PABA at 48 h ranged from 16 to 96 mg, which represented 1.6–9.6% of the applied dose. No difference was found between the three preparations. Most of the recovered PABA (70–90%) was in the acetylated form. When the volunteers received a 500-mg oral dose of PABA, acetylated PABA represented 50–82% of the recovered compound (it is not stated at which time this analysis was carried out, but elimination after oral administration was rapid, with a half-time of 56 min). The authors stated that significantly ($p < 0.05$) more acetylation, a common metabolic pathway for many drugs, occurred after topical application than after oral administration, perhaps because of slow, sustained presentation to metabolizing enzymes.

Wester *et al.* (1998) compared the percutaneous absorption of [14C]PABA in human skin *in vivo* and in an isolated, perfused porcine skin flap. In each case, 10 cm² of skin were treated with PABA delivered at a dose of 21.5 µg/cm² in 50 µL ethanol. In the five volunteers, the site was washed 24 h after application and tape-stripped on day 7; the volunteers collected their urine over 7 days. With the pig skin, venous effluent was collected every 30 min for 8 h, and then the skin surface was washed and tape-stripped, and the remainder of the tissue was digested. The urine of the volunteers contained 12% ± 6.3% (SD) of the applied dose; 30% ± 13%

was recovered from the skin surface wash and 0.56% ± 0.47% from the stratum corneum by tape-stripping. In a comparison with urinary excretion after intravenous injection in rhesus monkeys, in which the systemic availability is assumed to be 100%, it was estimated that 15% ± 8.4% PABA had been absorbed percutaneously. In the pig system, 5.9% ± 3.7% (perfusate + skin) had penetrated viable tissue. These results show that absorption of PABA through human skin is under-estimated in the perfused porcine skin flap. Determination of the percutaneous absorption of other compounds in the two systems gave more comparable results.

Ethylhexyl salicylate
The penetration of 5% (w/w) [14C]ethylhexyl salicylate in an oil-in-water emulsion and a hydroalcoholic formulation through human epidermis was evaluated *in vitro* after application of 'a finite dose', a target of 5 mg/cm², and 'an infinite dose', a target of 100 mg/cm². [3H]Sucrose was added to the formulations to allow monitoring and confirmation of the integrity of the membrane. Samples were taken from the receptor fluid between 2 and 48 h and assessed by 14C-scintillation counting. The results (Table 15) show that < 1% of the applied dose penetrated the epidermis, and the amount remaining bound to the epidermis represented 11–33%, depending on the experimental conditions. In a similar study with a finite dose of [14C]salicylic acid in an oil-in-water vehicle, the total penetration (1.6 µg/cm²) was similar to that of ethylhexyl

Table 15. Percentage (± SE) recovery of 5% (w/w) ethylhexyl salicylate and metabolites in various body compartments 48 h after dosing, depending on vehicle and dosing protocol

Medium	Finite dose		Infinite dose	
	Oil-in-water	Hydroalcoholic	Oil-in-water	Hydroalcoholic
Receptor fluid	0.65 ± 0.16	0.59 ± 0.09	0.47 ± 0.22	0.23 ± 0.05
Wash	37 ± 5.3	36 ± 6.0	34 ± 3.1	44 ± 7.4
Epidermis	17 ± 1.3	33 ± 4.7	12 ± 1.4	14 ± 2.4
Improved recovery technique				24 ± 7.8
Total	54 ± 5.5	70 ± 6.8	46 ± 2.2	83 ± 6.4

Modified from Walters *et al.* (1997)

salicylate in the same vehicle. The authors suggested that non-specific epidermal esterases may have converted ethylhexyl salicylate to salicylic acid. If that is so, the penetration of the sunscreen may have been even less than that estimated (Walters *et al.*, 1997).

Benzophenone-3

The percutaneous absorption of benzophenone-3 in a sunscreen containing 6% benzophenone-3, 7.5% ethylhexyl methoxycinnamate, 5% ethylhexyl salicylate and 7% octocrylene (all v/v) was studied in nine healthy volunteers with a mean age of 29 years. The product was applied to the forearms at six times (12 mg/cm^2) the application density for SPF assessment (2 mg/cm^2) and left for 12 h, after which it was washed off. Urine samples were taken just before application and for 48 h after application. Analysis for benzophenone-3 and its metabolites in urine (the authors do not mention analysis for the other ingredients) showed a steady increase over the 48-h period in all volunteers, and the authors estimated that 1–2% of the applied benzophenone-3 had been absorbed over 10 h (Hayden *et al.*, 1997). This study has been criticized on the grounds of the very high application density of the sunscreen (Agin *et al.*, 1998). Furthermore, the urinary concentrations may be an underestimate of skin penetration, as tissue-bound sunscreen and metabolites, unknown urinary metabolites and

excretion via other routes cannot be assessed.

Various organic ingredients

The epidermal penetration of the active 'chemical' ingredients of six sunscreen products was evaluated *in vitro* over 8 h. In the system used, heat-separated epidermis acts as a membrane in a Franz diffusion cell in which there is a donor and a receptor chamber. Of five 'chemical' absorbers assessed, only benzophenone-3 was found in the receptor fluid at concentrations representing up to 10% of the applied dose. Up to 14% of the applied dose of other sunscreen ingredients remained in the epidermis (Jiang *et al.*, 1999).

The percutaneous penetration of five sunscreens was assessed in fresh skin discarded at surgery from women aged 17–65 years. The samples were 344-μm dermatome slices which were placed on static diffusion cells containing only receptor fluid. Sunscreens containing ethylhexyl methoxycinnamate (5%), benzophenone-3 (4.9%), benzophenone-4 (6.9%), ethylhexyl triazone (4%) and octocrylene (8%) were applied at 3 mg/cm^2 and left for 16 h. They were then washed off, the stratum corneum was tape-stripped 16 times, and the viable epidermis was heat separated from the dermis. The sunscreen content of the tape (stratum corneum), epidermis, dermis, receptor fluid and washing solution was determined by high-perfor-

mance liquid chromatography (HPLC), which resulted in recovery rates of 93–97%, depending on the ingredient. With the exception of benzophenone-3, the quantity in the receptor fluid was low or below the limit of detection. The largest amounts of all ingredients were found in the stratum corneum, with very little in the viable epidermis or the dermis (Potard *et al.*, 1999).

The transdermal absorption of sunscreens was assessed in human skin *in vivo*. Saturated solutions of sunscreens in a glycol–water mixture were placed in a glass chamber attached to the skin of the arm for 1 h, and percutaneous absorption was modelled from decreases in the sunscreen concentration in the vehicle. The authors estimated the amount of sunscreen absorbed over the whole skin surface (1.8 m^2) within 1 h. Benzophenone-3 and isoamyl-*para*-methoxycinnamate were absorbed to the greatest degree, at rates of 80 and 89 mg/h, respectively. This approach does not yield information on the degree of accumulation in tissue compartments nor on systemic accumulation (Hagedorn-Leweke & Lippold, 1995).

The penetration of 5% benzophenone-3, 7.5% ethylhexyl methoxycinnamate and 3% ethylhexyl salicylate in two vehicles (an emulsion gel and petroleum jelly) was evaluated *in vitro* in 600-μm slices of skin in static Franz diffusion chambers, and the concentrations of the ingredients were determined in a skin surface wash, the whole epidermis including stratum corneum, the dermis and the receptor fluid 2 min, 30 min, 2 h and 6 h after application. Benzophenone-3 was the only ingredient detected in the receptor fluid, a maximum of about 5% of the dose being found at 2 and 6 h when it was applied in petroleum jelly. Benzophenone-3 was also found in the dermis at all times, with a maximum of about 2% in petroleum jelly at 6 h. The concentrations of the ingredients were also evaluated *in vivo* in the stratum corneum at various depths. The highest concentrations were found 30 min after application, with slightly lower values at 2 and 6 h (data not given). The initial one to five tape strips contained the highest concentrations of all ingredients, with much higher values in the emulsion gel vehicle (~ 35% of the applied dose) than in petroleum jelly (~ 10% of the applied dose). The values for the three sunscreen ingedients were about the same in a given vehicle at a given depth of stratum corneum (Treffel & Gabard, 1996).

Gas chromatography with mass spectrometry was used to assess the presence of five sunscreen ingredients —isoamyl-*para*-methoxycinnamate, benzophenone-3, 4-methylbenzylidene camphor, ethylhexyl dimethyl PABA and ethylhexyl methoxycinnamate — in the breast milk of six women who had used sunscreens or skin-care products or used public swimming pools. Benzophenone-3 was detected in four of six samples at concentrations of 16–420 ng/g of fat. A concentration of 20 ng/g was reported in the milk of one woman who had not used sunscreens during the summer of the study. Two samples contained ethylhexyl methoxycinnamate at concentrations of 28 and 47 ng/g of fat. No other sunscreen ingredient was detected (Hany & Nagel, 1995).

Inorganic sunscreens

TiO_2 and ZnO are generally considered to be harmless pigments that cannot enter the skin and are largely unaffected by optical radiation. TiO_2 is, however, a semiconductor which can absorb light and, under certain conditions, generate free radicals which can cause cell damage (Wamer *et al.*, 1997). Therefore, TiO_2 particles used in sunscreen preparations are often coated with other materials, such as aluminium and silicon, to reduce any potential photoreactivity. This coating has been shown to be efficient, remaining stable even after application to the skin and subsequent UV irradiation (Van der Molen *et al.*, 1999). The literature on the potential of inorganic sunscreens to penetrate the skin shows some confusion, as in most cases the metal, Ti or Zn, and not the metal oxide was identified, whereas the metals themselves are not photoactive.

Titanium dioxide

As Ti has been found in biopsy samples, it has been inferred that TiO_2 can penetrate the skin (Dupre *et al.*, 1985; Dundas & Laing, 1988; Moran *et al.*, 1991; Tan *et al.*, 1996). In a pilot study, Tan *et al.* (1996) assessed the percutaneous absorption of microfine TiO_2 in a sunscreen containing 8% of this agent through 16 samples of skin from 13 patients (aged 59–82 years) who were due to undergo skin surgery. The product was applied twice a day for 2–6 weeks before surgery. The recovery of TiO_2 from tissue, excluding the stratum corneum (removed by stripping), was 0.0 to about 4.5 μg/g of wet weight, with a mean value of about 1.6 μg. The values in skin from nine untreated cadavers of unspecified age were equal to ($n = 1$) or lower than ($n = 7$) this mean value in eight of nine samples, but the other showed a value close to the maximum of the treated group. When this outlier was excluded, the treated group had higher ($p = 0.0006$) values than the controls, but inclusion of the outlier removed this difference ($p = 0.14$). These data, although inconclusive, suggest that TiO_2 penetrates the stratum corneum. It should be noted that the mean age of the study population was 71 years; furthermore, the samples were taken from skin at a site destined for surgery. In a study of the percutaneous absorption of TiO_2 particles by X-ray microanalysis in combination with scanning electron microscopy, no Ti was found in deeper layers of the skin (Van der Molen *et al.*, 1997).

TiO_2 and ZnO in a sunscreen formulation applied to human skin removed during plastic surgery was found to be restricted to the surface, with no intercellular or intracellular penetration (Dussert *et al.*, 1977). The skin was prepared for examination immediately after application, however, and studies of the time-course of penetration were not performed.

Zinc oxide

No evidence for percutaneous absorption of Zn was found from a topically applied sunscreen product containing 40% ZnO in a controlled cross-over study carried out with six normal volunteers aged 21–24 years, who received ZnO in a white petrolatum base over a large surface area. The serum concentration of Zn was assessed at 1, 2 and 3 h (Derry *et al.*,1983). In contrast, evidence of percutaneous absorption of Zn was found 48 h after topical application of a sunscreen containing 25% ZnO to five healthy volunteers aged 22–54 years (Agren, 1990). Zn was assessed in epidermis and blister fluid after the raising of suction blisters, a process that takes 2–3 h and is likely to compromise the integrity of barrier function. Analysis of epidermis *per se* yields no information on the barrier function of the stratum corneum.

Non-sunscreen chemicals present in sunscreens

Citropen and bergapten

Sunscreens containing bergamot oil were applied to human volunteers at a concentration of 3.2 mg/cm^2 in an oil-in-water emulsion and at 1.4 mg/cm^2 in an oil vehicle. Suction blisters were raised 100–220 min after application, and the fluid was assessed by HPLC for 5,7-dimethoxycoumarin and 5-methoxy-psoralen. This approach, which subjects the skin to trauma, does not provide reliable information on natural percutaneous absorption; however, it can be estimated that about 0.2% of each compound was recovered in the oil–water emulsion and about 0.07% of each in the oil vehicle (Treffel et al., 1991).

Vitamin E (α-tocopherol acetate)
The percutaneous absorption of α-tocopherol acetate was assessed in 11 patients aged 36–77 years with actinic keratoses. The patients rubbed a cream containing this ingredient into the skin of their forearms twice daily (morning and night) for 3 months. Before the main study, the patients applied a placebo containing the base cream only for 1 month. Skin biopsy samples were taken for analysis at the end of the 3-month period and (presumably) at the end of the 1-month period to provide baseline data. Similarly, blood samples were taken. Analysis of plasma from all subjects showed no difference during the baseline and treatment periods in the concentrations of free α-tocopherol (13 ± 6.3 (SD) and 13 ± 6.1 μg/mL, respectively) or α-tocopherol acetate (2.1 ± 0.9 and 2.5 ± 1.3 μg/mL, respectively). The analysis of four lots of randomly pooled biopsy samples showed a substantial increase in the concentration of α-tocopherol acetate (baseline, 5.9 ± 12 (SD) μg/g; all values 0 except one outlier; treated, 260 ± 200 μg/g) but no difference in the concentration of α-tocopherol or γ-tocopherol. These data indicate that α-tocopherol acetate is not metabolized to the free form of α-tocopherol in plasma or skin (Alberts et al., 1996).

Experimental models

Animal models are widely used to study percutaneous adsorption. The pig in particular is considered to be suitable because its skin is similar to that of humans.

Micro-Yucatan pig
Gupta et al. (1999) studied the percutaneous absorption of radiolabelled ethylhexyl methoxycinnamate and benzophenone-3 through excised micro-Yucatan pig skin sliced at 250–300 μm and placed in diffusion cells. The sunscreens were dissolved in either a hydroalcoholic or an oil-based (diisopropyl adipate) vehicle. Analyses were conducted on the receptor fluid to assess penetration, washes of skin to assess remaining sunscreen, stratum corneum (from tape strippings) and the viable tissue, which was digested. Analyses of the stratum corneum showed that, in each vehicle, it retained more ethylhexyl methoxycinnamate than benzophenone-3. The maximum concentrations in the stratum corneum were reached at 1 h and remained fairly constant for the 10-h duration of the experiment. Removal of the stratum corneum before sunscreen application resulted in much greater total penetration of both sunscreens in both vehicles. When the ratios of retained: penetrated dose of sunscreens alone and in combination were compared (Table 16), the higher the ratio, the more sunscreen remained in the stratum corneum. In both vehicles, the ratio was higher for ethylhexyl methoxycinnamate than benzophenone-3, and for both sunscreens the ratio was higher when they were applied in combination than when applied alone. The ratios were significantly different for each sunscreen alone or in combination in the hydroalcoholic vehicle but not in the oil vehicle. The formulation can thus markedly affect the pharmacokinetics of sunscreens.

Rat
Fischer 344 rats were treated topically on shaved skin with up to 800 μg of benzophenone-3 in ethanol or 50 μg in a lanolin/white petrolatum base. Up to 39% of the compound was recovered from the urine 72 h after application. Benzophenone-3 was also detected in internal

organs. The results were similar with the two bases (El Dareer et al., 1986).

In a study of the distribution and metabolism of benzophenone-3, rats were given a single topical application on a limited area of shaved skin. As the animals were not restrained, however, intake may have occurred during grooming. Plasma samples from one group were analysed at various times between 5 min and 48 h. Animals in another group were killed 6 h after administration and the content of various tissues was analysed. For a third group, urine and faeces were analysed for periods up to 168 h after administration. The parent compound and its metabolites were detected in plasma within 5 min, with peak absorption at 2.5 h. The plasma time-course was biphasic, with half-times of 1.3 and 15 h (Okereke et al., 1994).

In a study of the effect of two daily applications of benzophenone-3 at 100 mg/kg bw in a petroleum jelly base for 4 weeks, blood samples were taken on day 16, and reduced glutathione concentrations were assessed. The treated rats had a significantly lower concentration than those given the vehicle only, suggesting that reduced glutathione is involved in the metabolism of benzophenone-3 in rats. However, the contribution of unintended intake during grooming in these studies is not known (Okereke et al., 1995).

A study of the metabolism of benzophenone-3 after oral administration to rats is described even though sunscreens are not taken orally. The animals were given 100 mg/kg bw, and three metabolites, 2,4-dihydroxybenzophenone (the major metabolite), 2,2'-dihydroxy-4-methoxybenzophenone and 2,3,4-trihydroxybenzophenone, were identified in free and conjugated forms by HPLC. The parent compound and its metabolites (free and bound) were detected after 6 h in most tissues, and all were detected in plasma 5 min after administration. Both benzophenone-3 and its metabolites were excreted primarily in urine, and faeces were a

Table 16. Distribution of benzophenone-3 and ethylhexyl methoxycinnamate in a hydroalcoholic vehicle when applied individually or in combination to micro-Yucatan pig skin in a diffusion chamber

Compartment	Benzophenone-3		Ethylhexyl methoxycinnamate	
	Alone	With ethylhexyl methoxycinnamate	Alone	With benzophenone-3
Receptor (% applied dose)	1.8	0.32	0.48	0.36
Viable skin (% applied dose)	12	11	13	7.1
Penetrated (receptor + viable skin) (% applied dose)	14	11	13	7.5
Retained (in stratum corneum) (% applied dose)	24	34	58	55
Retained:penetrated	1.7	3.1	4.5	7.4

Modified from Gupta *et al.* (1999)

secondary route of excretion. The authors suggested that *O*-dealkyation is the major pathway of metabolism of this compound (Okereke *et al.*, 1993).

The pharmacokinetics of benzophenone-3 was investigated in blood samples taken at various times after oral administration to male rats at a dose of 100 mg/kg bw. Some free benzophenone-3 was detected, but the majority was bound to plasma protein and could be detected only after acid hydrolysis. The compound was absorbed rapidly from the gastrointestinal tract and was detected in the blood 5 min later. The peak plasma concentration (26 μg/mL) was found at 3 h. Elimination was biphasic, with half-times of elimination of 0.88 and 16 h. This two-compartment model of elimination has been associated with distribution to the tissues. In some studies, animals were killed 6 h after administration and the tissue distribution of benzophenone-3 was assessed. The highest concentrations were found in the liver and kidneys, which accounted for 6.5% and 0.97% of the initial dose, respectively. When excretion in urine and faeces was assessed for up to 96 h, urine was found to be the major route of excretion, with a peak at 6–12 h.

Hydrolysis of urine samples with β-glucuronidase showed that the main form was a conjugate with glucuronic acid; however, acid hydrolysis revealed other forms of conjugation. Faecal excretion was largely complete within 24 h, and about 50% of the benzophenone-3 was in a conjugated form (Kadry *et al.*, 1995).

Zinc oxide administered as a suspension or mixed into the adhesive layer of tape was shown to penetrate the skin into the blood within 1 h of application to intact skin of Sprague-Dawley rats (Hallmans & Liden, 1979).

Hairless guinea-pig

In a study of the dermal absorption and metabolism of [^{14}C]PABA *in vitro*, 200-μm sections of skin were obtained by microtome and placed in a diffusion cell with HEPES-buffered Hanks balanced salt solution, which ensured their viability for 48 h. Experiments were also carried out with distilled water, which made the skin non-viable. PABA was applied in ethanol at a dose of about 2 μg/cm^2. The skin surface was washed 24 h later and left for a further 24 h to allow any remaining absorbed compound to enter the receptor fluid. Analysis 48 h after appli-

cation showed that 5% of the total dose was in the receptor fluid and 21% in skin maintained under physiological conditions. Significantly more absorption occurred with water as the receptor fluid, 19% of the total dose being found. When skin was maintained under physiological conditions, the acetyl derivative accounted for most (61% of absorbed dose) of the PABA in the receptor fluid, but the parent molecule predominated in the skin (86% of absorbed dose). In both compartments, only small amounts of the acetyl derivative were recovered when water was used as the receptor fluid. These studies show that the skin readily metabolizes PABA (Nathan *et al.*, 1990).

Rabbit

The percutaneous uptake of ^{65}ZnO was estimated by γ-radiation counting in a small study: 20–25% of the total zinc applied remained in the skin 6 or 24 h after a single or double application. Autoradiography indicated that little ^{65}Zn was present in the epidermis, but large amounts were present in the subdermal muscle layer. Only trace amounts were observed in the dermis, but there was evidence of Zn in hair follicles (Kapur *et al.*, 1974).

Chapter 5

Cancer-preventive effects of sunscreens

Human studies

Many epidemiological studies have been conducted to assess the relationship between exposure to the sun and the risks for cutaneous melanoma and non-melanocytic skin cancer. Some of these investigations have also involved obtaining information on sunscreen use. Since use of sunscreens was not the primary question addressed in most studies, the information collected about use is often not optimal, so that it is often not known exactly when the agent was used, what quantities were used, the type of sunscreen or the frequency of use. Additional important considerations that must be kept in mind when interpreting the results of observational (cohort and case–control) studies of the relationship between use of sunscreens and skin cancer are outlined below.

First, there are problems of confounding. Sunscreens are most commonly used by people whose skin is sensitive to the sun (e.g. burn easily), expose their skin to the sun and do not protect their skin in some other way. These people are also those at highest risk of developing skin cancer. Thus, the relationship between use of sunscreens and skin cancer is confounded by sensitivity to the sun, exposure to the sun and lack of use of other protection against the sun. To deal with this confounding effectively, accurate measurements of sensitivity, lifetime exposure and other sun protection behaviour are required. Accurate measurements of sun sensitivity are difficult to obtain. There may also be confounding between sunscreen use and a past history of skin cancer or of a benign

sun-related skin lesion, which indicate an increased risk for skin cancer, if use of sunscreens was recommended at the time these lesions were diagnosed or treated.

Second, the characteristics of sunscreens and sunscreen use that make them potentially efficacious are rarely adequately measured, either because of poor study design or poor recall. If sunscreens are efficacious, their efficacy almost certainly depends on a high SPF rating and proper use. Proper use includes application some time before engaging in outdoor activities, applying sufficient sunscreen to obtain the

protection implied by the SPF value and re-application periodically during outdoor activities. If these are not documented, potentially efficacious use will be diluted by non-efficacious use, and a protective effect, if present, may be missed.

In the light of these and other considerations, it will be important in evaluating observational studies of sunscreens that the information shown in the box be available, in addition to that generally needed to assess the quality of a study.

Most of the evidence about the value of sunscreens for cancer prevention has

---

Information required for evaluation of epidemiological studies on sunscreens

- the period of study (earlier studies are less likely to cover experience with potentially efficacious sunscreens);

- distinction of potentially efficacious sunscreen use from use of related products (e.g. 'suntan lotions') that are unlikely to be efficacious;

- adequate measurement of sunscreen use, including, ideally, when use began and ended, frequency of use, amount usually used, the SPF of the sunscreen usually used and exposed sites normally protected;

- measurement of cutaneous sensitivity to the sun and adequate control for this variable in the analysis;

- measurement of patterns of sun exposure throughout life and control for this variable in the analysis;

- measurement of use of other protective measures against the sun and control for this variable in the analysis;

- measurement of past history of skin cancer or benign sun-related skin lesions and control for this variable in the analysis.

come from cohort and case–control studies. Relatively few randomized trials have been conducted to assess the use of sunscreens for preventing cancer, because it is commonly believed that skin cancers develop only after long-term exposure to UVR. In addition, cutaneous melanoma, the most serious type of skin cancer, is less common than other skin cancers. Precursor lesions lend themselves better to the randomized trial design (see p. 80) because they have a short latency; however, a recent study of the use of sunscreens in the prevention of squamous-cell carcinomas (Green et al., 1999a) indicates that the problem of latency in studying cancer may not be insurmountable.

Cutaneous melanoma

No randomized trials or cohort studies have been reported on use of sunscreens and the risk for cutaneous melanoma (Fig. 25).

Case–control studies

Fifteen case–control studies have been conducted to examine the association between use of sunscreens and the risk for cutaneous melanoma (Table 17).

Klepp and Magnus (1979) assessed the use of 'sun lotion or oil' among 78 hospitalized patients with cutaneous melanoma and 131 controls who were being treated at the same institution in Norway (Norwegian Radium Hospital) for Hodgkin disease, non-Hodgkin lymphoma, testicular cancer or bone or soft-tissue sarcoma. The case and control

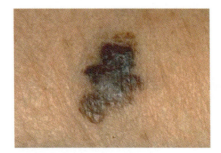

Figure 25 Melanoma of the trunk

cancers were diagnosed between 1 January 1974 and 1 May 1975, and the patients completed a written questionnaire [response rates not reported]. Patients who reported using such compounds 'sometimes, quite often or almost always' had a higher risk for melanoma (relative risk [RR], 2.3; 95% confidence interval [CI], 1.3–4.1) than those who had almost never used them. The elevated risk was seen only for males (RR, 2.8; 95% CI, 1.2–6.7) and not for females (RR, 1.0; 95% CI, 0.42–2.5). [A potential weakness of this study is that the term 'sun lotion or oil' was used rather than 'sunscreen', and this may have been interpreted as referring to compounds meant to promote tanning, such as 'tanning oils', or to moisturizing lotions used while in the sun or to sunscreens.]

Graham et al. (1985) conducted a case-control study of cutaneous melanoma in Buffalo, New York, USA, among 404 patients seen sequentially between 1974 and 1980. The controls were 521 patients with other cancers (gastrointestinal tract, respiratory, breast and reproductive neoplasms and Hodgkin disease and non-Hodgkin lymphoma) seen at the same institute. All interviews were conducted by nurses face-to-face [participation rates not reported]. The main purpose of the study was to evaluate the relationship between exposure to the sun and risk for melanoma, but the subjects were also asked about their use of 'suntan lotion' and of 'sunscreening lotion'. An elevated risk for cutaneous melanoma was seen among men who reported having used suntan lotion (RR, 1.7; 95% CI, 1.1–2.7) or sunscreen lotion (RR, 2.2; 95% CI, 1.2–4.1). No increased risk was detected with use of these products among women. [The strengths of the study include its large size and use of a specific question about sunscreen preparations; the potential weakness is the lack of data on sun sensitivity and on the duration and frequency of use of sunscreens.]

Herzfeld et al. (1993) conducted a case–control study of cutaneous melanoma of the trunk among men in upstate New York, USA, in order to determine the cause of the rapidly increasing incidence of tumours at this site. All 394 newly diagnosed cases ascertained between 1 January 1977 and 31 December 1979 were eligible for the study, and 324 participated in a telephone interview, although 38% of these interviews were with other respondents, usually the subject's wife. The overall participation rate was 82%. The major focus of the investigation was outdoor recreational activity, freckling, hair colour, sensitivity to the sun and use of 'suntan lotion'. Control subjects were selected by random-digit dialling, in which the area code and first three digits of the telephone exchange were matched with those of patients, and limited to white male respondents over the age of 18. The response rate among controls was estimated to be 65%. Before adjustment for host factors and exposure to the sun, patients who 'always' used suntan lotion were shown to have an increased risk for melanoma (RR, 2.6; 95% CI, 1.4–4.7) by comparison with men who used them less often or not at all. In a logistic regression analysis, however, sun lotion use was not a significant factor in risk for melanoma, although actual risk ratios are not given. The authors interpreted the elevated crude odds ratio as being due to the use of suntan lotions by sun-sensitive men at higher risk for melanoma. The authors also cautioned that 'sun lotion' may refer not only to sunscreens but also to tanning oils, as the two were not differentiated in the questionnaire. [The weaknesses of the study are use of the term 'suntan lotion' as the sole definition of exposure and use of respondents other than the patients, which makes assessment of sun sensitivity and sun exposure uncertain. Measurements of risk after adjustment for phenotype and exposure to sunlight were not given.]

Table 17. Case–control studies of sunscreen use and risk for cutaneous melanoma

Population Place/date	Type of cases/ controls	No. cases/ controls	Exposure	RR[a] (95% CI)	Comments	Reference
Norway 1974–75	Hospital cases Other cancer controls	78 cases 131 controls	Sometimes, often or almost always use sun lotion/oil	M 2.8[b] (1.2–6.7) F 1.0[b] (0.42–2.5) T 2.3[b] (1.3–4.1)	Elevated risks among males only. Sunscreens not dif- ferentiated from 'sun lotions'.	Klepp & Magnus (1979)
USA 1974–80	Hospital cases Other cancer controls	404 cases 521 controls	Used sunscreening Used suntan lotion	M.2.2[b] (1.2–4.1) M 1.7 (1.1–2.7) F 'No added risk'	Elevated risks among males only	Graham et al. (1985)
USA 1977–79	Population cases and controls	324 male trunk melanoma cases 415 controls	Always used 'suntan lotion'	2.6[b] (1.4–4.7) Not significant after control for 'tendency to sunburn and water sports'	'Suntan lotions' and 'sunscreens' not differ- entiated in questionnaire	Herzfeld et al. (1993)
Sweden 1978–83	Hospital cases Population controls	523 cases 505 controls	Often used sun protection agents	1.8[b] (1.2–2.7)		Beitner et al. (1990)
Canada 1979–81	Population cases and controls	369 trunk and lower limb melanomas 369 controls	Used sunscreen almost always	1.1 (0.75–1.6)	Highest risk in those using sunscreen 'only for first few hours' RR, 1.62 (1.04–2.52)	Elwood & Gallagher (1999)
Australia 1980–81	Population cases and controls	507 cases 507 controls	Used sunscreens ≤ 10 years	1.1 (0.71–1.6)		Holman et al. (1986)
USA 1981–86	Population cases and controls	452 cases 930 controls	Always used sun- screens	All cutaneous melanoma 0.62[b] (0.49–0.83) Superficial spreading melanoma (SSM) 0.43 (CI not available)	Study involved only women aged 25–59 at diagnosis. CI estimated. RR for SSM adjusted for host factors and sun exposure	Holly et al. (1995)
Denmark 1982–85	Population cases and controls	474 cases 926 controls	Always used sunscreens	1.1[b] (0.8–1.5)		Osterlind et al. (1988)
Australia 1987–94	Population cases Controls from same school	50 cases 156 controls All children < 15	Always used sunscreens	2.2 (0.4–12) on holidays 0.7 (0.1–6.0) at school		Whiteman et al. (1997)
Sweden 1988–90	Population cases and controls	400 cases 640 controls	Almost always used sunscreens	Trunk 1.4 (0.6–3.2) Other sites 2.0 (1.1–3.7)	No information on duration of use	Westerdahl et al. (1995)
Spain 1989–93	Hospital cases Hospital visitors	105 cases 138 controls	Always used sunscreens	0.2 (0.04–0.79)		Rodenas et al. (1996)

Table 17 (contd.)						
Population Place/date	Type of cases/ control	No. cases/ controls	Exposure	RR^a (95% CI)	Comments	Reference
Spain 1990–94	Hospital cases and controls	116 cases 235 controls	Used sunscreen	0.48 (0.34–0.71)	Inadequate description of measurement of sunscreen use	Espinoza Arranz *et al.* (1999)
Europe 1991–92	Hospital cases Neighbourhood controls	418 controls 438 controls	Ever use psoralen sunscreens Ever use sunscreens	2.3 (1.3–4.0) 1.5 (1.1–2.1) M 1.8 (1.1–2.7) F 1.3 (0.87–2.0)	Highest risk for sun-sensitive subjects using sunscreens to tan: RR, 3.7 (1.0–7.6)	Autier *et al.* (1995, 1997b)
Austria, 1993–94	Hospital cases and controls	193 cases 319 controls	Often used sunscreen	3.5 (1.8–6.6)		Wolf *et al.* (1998)
Sweden 1995–97	Population cases and controls	571 cases 913 controls	Always used sunscreen Used sunscreens to spend more time sunbathing	1.8 (1.1–2.9) 8.7 (1.0–76)		Westerdahl *et al.* (2000)

^{a} Relative risk estimates adjusted for phenotype and sun-related factors where possible
^{b} Crude relative risk ratio only available

Beitner *et al.* (1990) evaluated the roles of solar exposure and pigmentation in cutaneous melanoma and also examined sunscreen use among 525 patients with melanoma who had been referred to the Department of Oncology at the Karolinska Hospital in Stockholm, Sweden. This patient sample represented 64% of all newly diagnosed cases of cutaneous melanoma in the population of Stockholm County between February 1978 and December 1983. Patients with melanoma were compared with 521 controls matched for age and sex who were selected from the population registry of Stockholm County. The reported response rates were 99.6% among cases and 96.2% among controls, leaving 523 case and 505 control responses available for analysis. Data were collected from a postal questionnaire which included questions on sensitivity to the sun, eye and hair

colouring, frequency of sunbathing, erythema and use of 'sun protection agents'. After control for age, sex and hair colouring, subjects who reported using protective agents 'often or very often' had an increased risk for cutaneous melanoma (RR, 1.8; 95% CI, 1.2–2.7) when compared with those who reported never having used these agents. The authors noted that the elevated risk for melanoma among patients who used sunscreens might be due to the fact that such use allows extended exposure to the sun. [The lack of specificity of the term 'sun protection agents' and the lack of specific categories of frequency of use are a weakness in this study.]

The Western Canada Melanoma Study was a case–control investigation undertaken to determine the relationship between phenotypic factors, history of tanning and sunburn, exposure to sun-

light and risk for cutaneous melanoma in the four western provinces of Canada. All newly diagnosed cases among people aged 20–79 ascertained between 1 April 1979 and 31 March 1981 in the cancer registries of Alberta, British Columbia, Manitoba and Saskatchewan were approached for a face-to-face interview (Elwood *et al.*, 1984). For each case, one control was selected from the subscriber lists of the provincial medical services plan and frequency matched by sex, age (5-year age group) and province of residence. The rates of participation were 83% among cases and 59% among controls. Analysis of a subset of cases of melanoma on intermittently sun-exposed sites (trunk, lower limbs) and their controls (369 pairs) provided information about use of sunscreens on these sites during outdoor activity (Elwood & Gallagher, 1999). The risk of people who reported using sunscreen 'almost always' was very similar to that of people reporting using sunscreens 'sometimes' (RR, 1.1; 95% CI, 0.75–1.6). Those who reported use 'only in the first few hours' of solar exposure had an increased risk for cutaneous melanoma (RR, 1.6; 95% CI, 1.0–2.5) after adjustment for hair, eye and skin colouring, propensity to burn and exposure to the sun. [The potential weaknesses of this study are that the information on sunscreens is relevant only to sites intermittently exposed to sunlight and the categorization of frequency of use of sunscreens is nonspecific.]

Holman *et al.* (1986) conducted a large case–control study to examine the relationship between phenotype, sunlight and cutaneous melanoma in Western Australia in the early 1980s. All cases of this cancer diagnosed in people under the age of 80 in the accessible regions of Western Australia between 1 January 1980 and 5 November 1981 were eligible for inclusion in the study. A total of 507 patients were interviewed about outdoor recreational activities and occupational exposure to the sun. Information was also collected on skin reactions to sunlight, skin and hair colouring, freckling and the number of raised naevi on the arms for each subject. A total of 507 control subjects randomly selected from the Commonwealth Electoral Roll and public school system and matched to the cases by sex and 5-year age group were interviewed with the same standardized questionnaire as used for the cases. Of those approached for interview, 90% of cases and 69% of controls completed the questionnaire. Frequency and duration of sunscreen use were evaluated. People who had used sunscreens for less than 10 years did not have a reduced risk for cutaneous melanoma (RR, 1.1; 95% CI, 0.71–1.6), nor was any reduction seen for those who had used the compounds for 10–15 years (RR, 1.2; 95% CI, 0.78–1.7), after control for pigmentary traits and sensitivity to the sun. Frequency of use likewise

did not appear to be related to risk, as people who had used sunscreens during more than one-half of episodes of exposure had a relative risk of 1.1 (95% CI, 0.76–1.6) when compared with those who had 'never or hardly ever' used sunscreens. In the absence of control for fair pigmentary traits and sun sensitivity, a positive relationship was seen between use of sunscreens and the risk for cutaneous melanoma. The authors noted that this underlined the importance of good assessment of phenotype in evaluating the protective value of sunscreens against skin cancers. In addition, the authors point out that the lack of a protective effect of sunscreens in this study might be due to the fact that effective sunscreens were not available in Australia at the time when most of the subjects were in their teens and early 20s, the period of life when the protection afforded by sunscreens might be most valuable. [The strengths of the study include the control for sensitivity to the sun and the availability of information on the frequency and duration of use of sunscreens. A weakness of the study is the use of several nonspecific categories of exposure to sunscreens.]

Holly *et al.* (1995) studied factors associated with cutaneous melanoma in northern California, USA. Women in one of the five counties in the San Francisco Bay area in whom cutaneous melanoma was diagnosed between 1 January 1981 and 31 December 1986 and were aged 25–59 at diagnosis were included. Although the primary aim of the investigation was to evaluate the effect of oral contraceptive use and pregnancy-related factors on the risk for this disease, detailed information was also collected on exposure to sunlight, phenotypic factors and sunscreen use 5 years before diagnosis. The controls were residents of the same geographic areas as the patients and were identified by random-digit dialling. The response rates were 79% for patients and 77% for controls. Women who reported using

sunscreens 'almost always' had a lower risk for cutaneous melanoma than those who reported that they never used these agents [RR, 0.62; 95% CI, 0.47–0.83]. [These results were not controlled for phenotype or exposure to sunlight.] When the risk for superficial spreading melanoma (the commonest type of melanoma) was assessed after control for sun sensitivity and sunburn history before the age of 12, the risk of women who 'almost always' used sunscreens was lower [RR, 0.43; *p* < 0.001, CI not reported] than that of women who never used them. The authors concluded that use of sunscreens was strongly protective against melanoma, after adjustment for sensitivity to the sun, past history of sunburn and other host factors. [This study is unusual in showing the highest levels of risk for melanoma among women with the least solar exposure, after control for sun sensitivity. A potential weakness of the study is the lack of specific categories of frequency of use of sunscreens.]

Osterlind *et al.* (1988) evaluated the relationship between solar exposure and phenotype and the risk for melanoma, excluding lentigo maligna melanoma, in 474 patients in eastern Denmark aged 20–79 whose cancers were diagnosed between 1 October 1982 and 31 March 1985. All of the patients completed a face-to-face interview in their homes to assess occupational and recreational exposure to the sun, including holidays on the Mediterranean Sea, history of sunburn, sensitivity to the sun and use of sunscreens. The controls were selected from the population register of residents of the same area, and a total of 926 were matched to the cases by sex and 5-year age group and interviewed. The participation rates were 92% for cases and 82% for controls. In comparison with the incidence of melanoma among people who had never used sunscreens, a small, nonsignificant increase in risk (RR, 1.3; 95% CI, 0.9–1.7) was seen for people who had used them for less than

10 years or for more than 10 years (RR, 1.2; 95% CI, 0.9–1.5). Frequency of use was not associated with the risk for melanoma (RR, 1.1; 95% CI, 0.8–1.5) among people who always used them when compared with those who had never or hardly ever used them. Although the study did not find a protective effect of sunscreens, the authors cautioned that effective sunscreens were not available to the patients when they were young. [The strengths of the study include good control for sun sensitivity, high participation rates and the availability of information on duration and frequency of use of sunscreens.]

Whiteman et al. (1997) conducted a case–control study in Australia to evaluate the risk factors for melanoma in young people in whom cutaneous melanoma was diagnosed when they were less than 15 years old during the period 1987–94. The cases were ascertained through the Queensland Cancer Registry. Of 61 eligible patients, 50 completed an interview, and the parents of a further two deceased patients completed surrogate interviews. The exposures of interest were sunlight, history of sunburn, family history of melanoma and characteristics of sun sensitivity. Participants were also asked about use of sunscreens while on holidays and while at school. Data were collected on facial freckling and naevus density at the age of 5. After control for tanning ability, freckling (Fig. 26) and number of naevi, patients who had 'always' used sunscreens while on holiday had a nonsignificant elevated risk (RR, 2.2; 95% CI, 0.4–12) for cutaneous melanoma when compared with those not using sunscreen. Use of sunscreens while at school was associated with a non-significant reduced risk (RR, 0.7; 95% CI, 0.1–6.0). [Because this was a relatively small study (only 11 patients reported 'always' using sunscreens on holiday and only two reported using them at school), the relative risk esti-

mates have wide confidence intervals. A weakness of this study is the nonspecific categorization of the frequency of use of sunscreens.]

Westerdahl et al. (1995) conducted a case–control study of melanoma in southern Sweden, in which they reported the effects of sunscreen use. A total of 454 cases of melanoma diagnosed between 1 July 1988 and 30 June 1990 among residents of the Southern Sweden Health Care Region aged 15–75 were ascertained through the regional cancer registry. Of these, 400 completed and returned a postal questionnaire. The 400 cases were compared with 640 healthy controls selected at random from the National Population Registry and matched to cases by age (within 1 year), sex and parish of residence. The response rates for cases and controls were 88% and 70%, respectively. Data were collected on exposure to sunlight, constitutional factors, freckling, naevi and use of sunscreens. When compared with people who never used sunscreens, those who used them 'almost always' had a relative risk for melanoma of 1.8 (95% CI, 1.1–2.8) after adjustment for history of sunburns, history of frequent sunbathing during the summer, number of raised naevi, freckling and hair colour. Similar risk ratios were seen for men and women. Evaluation of risk by use before the age of 15, at 15–19 and > 19 years showed elevated odds ratios at each age similar to those of people 'always using' sunscreens. The risks for trunk melanomas were similar to those for melanomas of the extremities and head and neck (RR, 1.4; 95% CI, 0.6–3.2 and RR, 2.0; 95% CI, 1.1–3.7, respectively) after adjustment for sunburns, frequent sunbathing, freckling and naevi. [A weakness of the study is the nonspecific measure of frequency of sunscreen use.]

A study of melanoma was conducted by Rodenas et al. (1996) in Andalusia, Spain. All patients in this Mediterranean

population with cutaneous melanoma diagnosed during 1989–93 and who had been referred to the Dermatology Centre at the University of Granada Hospital were ascertained, and 105 of these agreed to participate in the study. Visitors to patients in wards other than dermatology were recruited as controls, and 138 agreed to take part in the study. The response rates were 80% for cases and 69% for controls. Exposure to sunlight, skin sensitivity to sunlight, medical history, use of sunscreens and personal and family history of cutaneous diseases were recorded at a personal interview, and each subject was examined by a dermatologist, at which time naevus density, freckling and skin and hair colour were assessed. Only 6% of the controls but 36% of the patients had sun-sensitive skin. People who reported 'always' using sunscreens had a decreased risk for cutaneous melanoma (RR, 0.20; 95% CI, 0.04–0.79) after adjustment for age, skin colouring, sun sensitivity, naevi, and recreational and occupational exposure to sunlight. [It is uncertain whether use of sunscreens by the control subjects was typical of that of

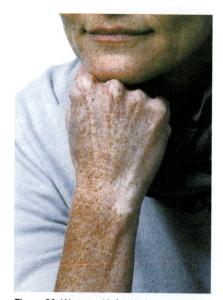

Figure 26 Woman with freckled complexion

the Spanish population, and the overall prevalence of sunscreen use in this study was low.]

A relatively small hospital-based case–control study of melanoma carried out in Madrid, Spain, included 116 patients with melanoma referred between January 1990 and January 1994 and 235 control patients admitted to the same hospital because of emergencies unrelated to cancer or skin disease (Espinosa Arranz et al., 1999). Data on exposure to the sun and use of sun-protection agents, including sunscreens, were collected by personal interview; sensitivity to the sun was recorded, and freckles, naevi and other actinic lesions were counted during a physical examination. Use of sunscreens, represented as a simple 'yes' or 'no' dichotomy, appeared to protect against melanoma. The relative risk of persons with 'no' use with reference to 'yes' use was 2.1 (95% CI, 1.4–2.9) after adjustment for sensitivity of the skin to the sun and number of naevi. The risk for melanoma was strongly related to the sensitivity of the skin to the sun, with a relative risk of 20 for those who always burned and never tanned with reference to those who always tanned and never burned (p for trend, < 0.001). Of the control subjects, 4.6% always burned and never tanned, and 48% always tanned and never burned. [The main weakness of this study is the lack of an adequate description of how sunscreen use was measured. It is uncertain what 'yes' and 'no' referred to exactly, because the question asked is not given. Use of sunscreens by the emergency department patients chosen as controls may not have been typical of that of the general population.]

Autier et al. (1995) conducted a case–control study of melanoma in five collaborating referral centres in Belgium, France and Germany. All cases diagnosed in white patients in the centres between 1991 and 1992 were eligible,

and these patients were invited to participate in the study; face-to-face interviews were conducted in the patients' homes. Of the 456 eligible patients, 418 (91.7%) participated. Neighborhood controls were selected within the municipality of residence and frequency matched to cases by broad age ranges (20–39, 40–59, ≥ 60) and by sex. The rate of participation among controls was 78%. The focus of the study was exposure to solar and artificial UVR, and data were collected on recreational and occupational exposure and on host factors and phenotype. Sunscreen use was assessed from the answers to questions about the use of agents containing tanning accelerators such as psoralens and use of non-psoralen-containing sunscreens. Subjects who had ever used psoralen-containing sunscreens had an increased risk for cutaneous melanoma after control for age, sex, hair colouring and number of weeks spent each year in sunny destinations (RR, 2.3; 95% CI, 1.3–4.0), and the risk was found particularly among people who reported no history of sunburn. Use of psoralen-containing sunscreens was relatively uncommon. People who had ever used non-psoralen-containing sunscreens also had an increased risk after adjustment for the same factors (RR, 1.5; 95% CI, 1.1–2.1) when compared with subjects who had never used these agents. Use of sunscreens appeared to be associated with an increased risk among subjects with either light or dark hair. Similarly, both sun-sensitive and sun-insensitive individuals showed an increased risk with use of sunscreens. Use of sunscreens tended to be associated with a higher risk for melanoma among people who sunbathed than in those who did not. The highest risk among sunscreen users was that of subjects with no history of sunburn after the age of 14. Use of clothing rather than sunscreen appeared to be protective. The authors suggested that the increase in risk associated with sunscreen use is due to the fact that

their use allows greater duration of exposure to UVR and particularly UVA. [A potential weakness of this study is the categorization of sunscreen use into 'ever' and 'never'.]

The study of Wolf et al. (1998) was designed to evaluate the association between phenotype, exposure to sunlight, use of sunscreens and the risk for cutaneous melanoma. The cases were those of 193 Austrians in whom cutaneous melanoma was diagnosed between June 1993 and July 1994 and who were treated at the Department of Dermatology at the University of Graz. The controls were 319 patients with no history of skin cancer who were treated at the same university clinic during the same period. Each case and control patient completed a questionnaire designed to elicit information on occupational and recreational exposure to the sun, history of sunburns and use of sunscreens [response rates not reported]. Data were also collected on eye, hair and skin colouring, sun sensitivity and freckling and other factors. [It is not clear whether the data were collected by postal or telephone questionnaire or at a face-to-face interview.] After adjustment for skin colouring, sunbathing and history of sunburn, patients who reported having 'often used' sunscreens had a significantly increased risk for melanoma (RR, 3.5; 95% CI, 1.8–6.6) when compared with those who never used such agents. The investigators concluded that use of sunscreens does not prevent melanoma. [Potential weaknesses of the study include lack of information on response rates for cases and controls and on the way in which the questionnaire was administered and the use of patients with other dermatological conditions as controls. The information on frequency and duration of sunscreen use was non-specific.]

Westerdahl et al. (2000) studied the association between sunscreen use and risk for melanoma in a population-based case–control study of 571 patients aged

16–80 in whom cutaneous melanoma was diagnosed between 1995 and 1997, and 913 healthy controls. The 674 eligible cases were identified in the Regional Tumour Registry of the South Swedish Health Care Region. For each case, two healthy controls matched by sex, age and parish were selected by random sampling from the National Population Registry of residents of the same Region. Eligible cases and controls were sent a comprehensive questionnaire, and 584 patients (86%) and 1028 controls (76%) completed it. After exclusion of 13 cases with no matched control and 115 controls with no matched case, the final sample comprised 571 patients (84% of eligible cases) and 913 controls (68% of selected controls). The questionnaire elicited information on medical history, medicaments, constitutional factors, educational level, UVR exposure, smoking habits and alcohol use. Detailed information was collected on sunscreen use (any use, use the first time in the sun each year, regular use, SPF of the sunscreen used, sunburns, age at first and last use, reason for using sunscreens), UVR exposure (sunbathing habits, holidays in sunny places, sunburns, use of sunbeds, outdoor employment, residence in a sunny climate) and constitutional factors such as skin phototype, hair and eye colour, naevi and freckles. The median SPF of the sunscreens used by patients and controls was 6 (range, 2–25). A significantly increased risk for melanoma was found for regular use ('always') of sunscreens (RR, 1.8; 95% CI, 1.1–2.9), after adjustment for hair colour, history of sunburns and frequency and duration of sunbathing. The risk for melanoma was significantly increased among subjects who reported using sunscreens with a SPF < 10 (RR, 2.9; 95% CI, 1.2–20), when compared with people who did not use sunscreens, and for subjects who had not experienced sunburn while using sunscreens (RR, 1.9; 95% CI, 1.0–3.7).

The risk was even higher for subjects who reported using sunscreens in order to be able to spend more time sunbathing (RR, 8.7; 95% CI, 1.0–76), and, in an analysis by subsite, was significantly increased only for melanoma of the trunk (RR, 2.5; 95% CI, 1.2–5.2).

Squamous-cell carcinoma
Randomized trials
Green et al. (1999a) evaluated the use of sunscreens in the prevention of squamous-cell carcinoma of the skin in the Nambour Skin Cancer Prevention Trial (Table 18; Fig. 27). A total of 1850 residents aged 20–69 in the town of Nambour, Queensland, Australia, were invited to participate in a randomized trial of the value of daily application of SPF-16 sunscreen and use of 30-mg β-carotene supplements in the prevention of skin cancer. A total of 1647 eligible subjects attended the baseline survey for assessment of cancer risk factors, and a dermatologist conducted a full skin examination of each person in 1992. All clinically diagnosed skin cancers detected on initial examination were then removed. A total of 1621 of the 1647 subjects subsequently agreed to be randomized to one of four study groups: sunscreen and β-carotene, sunscreen and placebo, no sunscreen and β-carotene and no sunscreen and placebo. Participants randomized to sunscreen were instructed to apply the agent to their head and neck, arms and hands every morning, and re-application was recommended after heavy sweating, bathing and long solar exposure. Those randomized to no sunscreen were instructed to continue their usual use of sunscreens. The code that identified the group of each subject was known only to the principal investigator and to those who packaged the β-carotene tablets for distribution. None of these individuals had any contact with the study subjects. Participants attended a clinic every 3 months to assess their compliance with the study protocol and to receive new

sunscreen, β-carotene or placebo. The weight of sunscreen returned to the study centre at 3-month intervals was noted, and a random subgroup of sunscreen users kept 7-day diaries on three occasions to record the frequency of sunscreen application and sun exposure. At follow-up clinics held in 1994 and 1996, the subjects were again examined by dermatologists, and all skin cancers diagnosed and removed were examined histopathologically by a single pathologist. The subjects reported any lesions that had been removed in the intervals between the clinics, and study personnel obtained the relevant clinical reports and pathology reviews. Reported skin cancers were counted only when verified from medical records. Skin cancers diagnosed within 1 year of the start of the trial were not counted as they were considered to represent latent disease at baseline. In 1996, after 4.5 years of follow-up, 1383 trial subjects remained in the study, and 789 new skin cancers had been diagnosed in 256 study subjects. Since lesions diagnosed in 1992 were not included for the reasons noted above, the analysis was limited to 758 new lesions diagnosed in 250 subjects after 1993. No protective effect was found against squamous-cell carcinoma in subjects randomized to β-carotene (RR, 1.2; 95% CI, 0.89–1.4). The relationship with sunscreen use was analysed for all subjects, regardless of β-carotene use, as no interaction was seen between the two interventions, but concentrated only on skin cancers that occurred on body sites where sunscreen

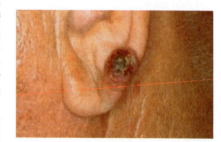

Figure 27 Squamous-cell carcinoma of the ear

Table 18. Randomized trial in Nambour, Australia, of risk for non-melanocytic skin cancer among 1383 subjects randomized to daily sunscreen use or no sunscreen

Tumour	No. of cases	Exposure	Rate ratio (95% CI)
Squamous-cell carcinoma	Sunscreen arm: 28 tumours in 22 subjects Non-sunscreen arm: 46 tumours in 25 subjects	Daily sunscreen application to head, neck, arms and hands	*SCC lesions* RR, 0.61 (0.46–0.81) *SCC participants* RR, 0.88 (0.50–1.6)
Basal-cell carcinoma	Sunscreen arm: 153 tumours in 65 subjects Non-sunscreen arm: 146 tumours in 63 subjects	Daily sunscreen application to head, neck, arms and hands	*BCC lesions* RR, 1.0 (0.82–1.3) *BCC participants* RR, 1.03 (0.73–1.5)

From Green *et al.* (1999a)

had been applied (head and neck, arms and hands). A total of 28 new squamous-cell carcinomas were detected in the group given sunscreen and 46 in those not given sunscreen (RR, 0.61; 95% CI, 0.46–0.81), a statistically significant difference. These lesions were seen in 22 participants given sunscreen and 25 not given sunscreen (RR, 0.88; 95% CI, 0.50–1.6). The authors concluded that sunscreen use could be of significant benefit in protecting against squamous-cell carcinoma. They noted that because no placebo sunscreen was used, the comparison group was less than ideal, reducing the ability of the study to detect an effect of daily sunscreen application. [The strengths of this study are that it is large and prospective and included good intermediate assessment of sunscreen use and solar exposure.]

A supplementary report by Green *et al.* (1999b) noted that the solar exposure of people given sunscreen did not differ from that of people who did not receive sunscreen. This observation was made in a randomly selected sample of 175 participants who wore UVR-sensitive polysulfone strips on 4 separate days, 2 in the summer and 2 in the winter. In addition, the prevalence of sunburn was lower among those receiving sunscreen than among those

not receiving it. These findings suggest that the reduction in the incidence of squamous-cell carcinoma seen in the group given sunscreen was probably due to attenuation of the UVR by the sunscreen rather than to alterations in sun-related behaviour. The finding also suggests that use of high-SPF sunscreens by an older population in day-to-day activities may not result in longer exposure to the sun.

Cohort studies
Grodstein *et al.* (1995) examined the factors involved in squamous-cell carcinoma in a cohort of 107 900 female nurses, 197 of whom had had a histologically confirmed diagnosis of squamous-cell carcinoma. Once those with lesions on the anus, vulva and vagina had been excluded, 191 remained for analysis. The analysis showed that use of sunscreens over a 2-year period by women who spent 8 h or more per week in the sun was not protective by comparison with no use of such agents (RR, 1.1; 95% CI, 0.83–1.7). The authors noted that long-term use might produce different results.

Case–control studies
Table 19 summarizes the results of studies of non-melanocytic skin cancer in relation to use of sunscreens.

Pogoda and Preston-Martin (1996) completed a population-based case–control study among women in Los Angeles County, USA, to evaluate whether the use of lip coverings lowered the risk for lip cancer. A total of 74 women age 25–74 in whom lip cancer was diagnosed between 1978 and 1985 were interviewed, as were 105 female controls identified by random-digit dialling who were frequency matched to cases by decade of birth. The response rates of patients and controls were 57% and 66%, respectively. The rate was low because the prolonged retrospective case-finding period meant that 13% were deceased and a further 13% could not be located by the study personnel. Major items of interest on the etiologic questionnaire were the effects of complexion, sunlight exposure, and use of lip coverings on risk. After adjustment for complexion, history of skin cancer and cigarette smoking, women with low mean sun exposure who applied lip covering more than once per day had a slightly lower risk than similarly exposed women who did not use it or applied it only once per day (estimated RR, 0.77 [95% CI, 0.24–2.5]). Women heavily exposed to the sun appeared to have had greater protection from more than one application per day than similarly exposed women who did not use lip coverings

Table 19. Case–control studies of sunscreen use and non-melanocytic skin cancer

Place/date	Type of cases/control	No. cases/controls	Exposure	RR[a] (95% CI)	Comments	Reference
California, USA 1978–85	Lip cancer cases and population controls	74 cases 105 controls	Lip covering > 1/day High UVR conditions	Estimated RR, 0.41 (95% CI not available)	Lip covering likely to be coloured lipstick in most cases	Pogoda & Preston-Martin (1996)
			Lip covering > 1/day Low UVR conditions	Estimated RR, 0.77 (0.24–2.5)		
Australia 1987–88	Basal-cell carcinoma cases and controls from population cohort	226 cases 102 controls	Use of SPF > 10 sunscreen half the time or more in the 10 years before diagnosis 1–9 years ≥ 10 years	1.8 (1.1–2.9) 1.1 (0.69–1.7)		Kricker et al. (1995)
			Use of SPF > 10 sunscreen half the time or more 11–30 years before diagnosis 1–9 years ≥ 10 years	1.2 (0.69–2.1) 0.72 (0.40–1.3)		
Australia 1987–94	Squamous-cell carcinoma cases and controls from population cohort	132 cases 1031 controls	Use of SPF > 10 sunscreen Age 8–14 Age 15–19 Age 20–24	0.61 (0.08–4.7) 1.9 (0.82–4.4) 0.99 (0.44–2.2)		English et al. (1998a)
Spain 1990–92	Hospital cases of non-melanocytic cancer and hospital controls	260 cases 552 controls	Use of solar protective creams	Males 0.6 (0.3–1.1) Females 0.7 (0.4–1.4)	Cases of basal-cell and squamous-cell carcinoma combined in analysis	Suarez-Varela et al. (1996)

Relative rate of naevi ≥ 2 mm in children in highest quartile of sunscreen use adjusted for sun exposure index, sex, study

[a] Relative risk estimates for phenotype and sun-related factors where possible

(estimated RR, 0.41; 95% CI not available). [The relevance of the results of this study are difficult to assess, as much of the lip covering worn by the women is likely to have been cosmetic coloured lipstick rather than sunscreen. Although lipstick is not a chemical sunscreen, the study does suggest that attenuation of UVR can be effective in preventing lip cancer.]

The relationship between exposure to the sun and squamous-cell carcinoma was addressed in a study in Geraldton, Western Australia, to evaluate whether the timing of exposure to sunlight was important (English et al., 1998a). The cases included both prevalent cases from 1987 and new squamous-cell carcinomas diagnosed up to 1994. Thus, 132 patients and 1031 controls, some of whom had basal-cell carcinoma, were available for analysis. Use of sunscreens with SPF-10 or more was examined in three age groups, 8–14, 15–19 and 20–24.

Subjects who reported use of sunscreens at age 8–14 appeared to have a slightly reduced risk for squamous-cell carcinoma (RR, 0.61; 95% CI, 0.08–4.7), although this was not statistically significant. Those who had used sunscreens at the age of 15–19 had a relative risk of 1.9 (95% CI, 0.82–4.4), and those who had used sunscreens at 20–24 had a risk of 0.99 (95% CI, 0.44–2.2) by comparison with subjects who had not used them. Although the small sample size limits the power of this study, overall, no strong protective effect of sunscreens was evident. [The strengths of this study include the complete examination of each subject by a dermatologist, close annual follow-up for new lesions and good assessment of exposure to the sun. The weaknesses include the relatively nonspecific description of exposure to sunscreens.]

Suarez-Varela *et al.* (1996) conducted a case–control study in Valencia, Spain, to evaluate protective measures against non-melanocytic skin cancer in a Mediterranean population. The study population comprised 260 cases of skin cancer treated at La Fe University Hospital between 1990 and 1992, and 552 controls recruited from among other patients at the same institute and from an old-age centre within the hospital's area of coverage. The controls were frequency matched to cases by sex and age (± 5 years). Use of 'solar protective creams' appeared to be associated with a protective effect among both men (RR, 0.6; 95% CI, 0.3–1.1) and women (RR, 0.7; 95% CI, 0.4–1.4). The authors noted that few of the subjects used sunscreens and consequently the power of the study is low. [The authors did not analyse the data by histological type of skin cancer, and separate risk estimates were not available for squamous-cell and basal-cell carcinoma. In addition, the sun exposure and sunscreen use of persons in an old-age centre may not be typical of those of the Spanish population.]

Basal-cell carcinoma
Randomized trials
In the study described above, Green *et al.* (1999a) also evaluated the role of sunscreen in the prevention of basal-cell carcinom (Fig. 28; Table 18). No protective effect against this tumour was found in persons randomized to β-carotene (RR, 0.89; 95% CI, 0.64–1.1), and no significant effect of daily sunscreen use was seen. Thus, 153 new tumours were

found in the group receiving sunscreen and 146 in the group not given sunscreen (RR, 1.0; 95% CI, 0.82–1.3). The tumours occurred in 65 persons randomized to daily sunscreen use and 63 randomized to no sunscreen (RR, 1.0; 95% CI, 0.73–1.5).

Cohort study
In an analysis of 771 cases of basal-cell carcinoma in a cohort of 73 366 nurses, Hunter *et al.* (1990) demonstrated that those who usually used sunscreens when outdoors during the summer had an elevated risk for this tumour when compared with those who did not use these agents (RR, 1.4; 95% CI, 1.2–1.7). Sunscreen use was analysed only among study participants who had spent 8 h per week or more outdoors. The authors noted that the relative risk declined after adjustment for hair colour, childhood sensitivity to the sun and history of sunburn and suggested that the continued presence of an elevated risk was probably due to further, unmeasured confounding.

Case–control study
Kricker *et al.* (1995) conducted a case–control study of basal-cell carcinoma in Geraldton, Western Australia (Table 19). A cohort of 4103 subjects aged 40–64 were recruited and given a physical examination, and those 226 in whom a basal-cell carcinoma had been diagnosed at the examination in 1987 or in the previous year constituted the cases for the analysis. Controls were selected from among members of the same cohort who did not have a basal-cell carcinoma (although several had had a squamous-cell carcinoma). A total of 1021 controls matched to cases in three strata were chosen: women, men aged 40–54 and men aged 55–64. Age appeared to have little effect on the incidence or prevalence of basal-cell carcinoma among women in this cohort. Subjects who had used sunscreens one-half the time or more while

in the sun during the 1–9 years prior to diagnosis had a higher relative risk for basal-cell carcinoma than those who had never used sunscreens or had used them less than half the time (RR, 1.8; 95% CI, 1.1–2.9) during the same period. The risk persisted after adjustment for sex, age, ability to tan and site of the lesion. No change in relative risk was found for those who had applied sunscreens more than half the time throughout the decade preceding diagnosis (RR, 1.1; 95% CI, 0.69–1.7) by comparison with those who had not used them or had used them less than half the time. Relatively few subjects had used sunscreens in the period 11–30 years before diagnosis. The risk of those who had used sunscreens for 1–9 years during this period was similar to that of those who had not used them or had used them less than half the time (RR, 1.2; 95% CI, 0.69–2.1). People who had used them for 10 or more years in the interval 11–30 years before diagnosis had a RR of 0.72 (95% CI, 0.40–1.3). The authors concluded that there was little evidence that use of sunscreen protects against basal-cell carcinoma. They noted that the elevated risk of those who had used sunscreens for 1–9 years in the 10 years before diagnosis was probably artefactual and was due to the fact that people identified as being at higher risk in the years before diagnosis may have been advised to use sunscreens. [The strengths of this study include the complete examination of each subject by a dermatologist, close annual follow-up for new lesions

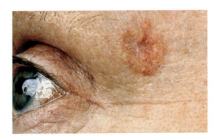

Figure 28 Basal-cell carcinoma

and good assessment of exposure to the sun. The weaknesses include the relatively nonspecific description of exposure to sunscreens.]

Precursor lesions

Melanocytic naevi

Naevus counts are the strongest individual predictors of risk for cutaneous melanoma (Fig. 29) (Holman & Armstrong, 1984; Holly et al., 1987; Grob et al., 1990) and are likely to be the precursors of many melanomas (Skender-Kalnenas et al., 1995). Therefore, a number of investigations have been conducted to explore the causes of acquired melanocytic naevi. The results have demonstrated a positive relationship between exposure to sunlight and naevus density (Pope et al., 1992; Harrison et al., 1994; Kelly et al., 1994). Several of these studies have also addressed the question of whether sunscreen use can modify the risk for acquiring melanocytic naevi (Table 20). Most such studies have been carried out in children, as most neonates are born with no naevi and develop their highest naevus density by adolescence. The maximal density may be reached at an earlier age in areas with a great deal of sunlight, such as Australia (Gallagher et al., 1990; English & Armstrong, 1994a,b; Kelly et al., 1994).

Randomized trials: One randomized trial has been conducted to evaluate whether use of sunscreens can reduce the development of naevi in children (Gallagher et al., 2000). The study was conducted in six elementary schools in Vancouver, Canada, in which 696 children in grades 1 and 4 (ages 6–7 and 9–10, respectively) were ascertained, and 458 (66%) were enrolled in the trial. The naevi on the children were counted at enrolment, and each child was randomized to receive sunscreen (SPF 30, broad spectrum) or no sunscreen but allowed to continue usual use. Both groups were followed for 3 years, during which time

their sun exposure was assessed. Of the children who were recruited, 86% completed the trial, when their naevi were counted again. Analysis of the data for white children showed a modest reduction in the median number of new naevi (the outcome measure) among those randomized to sunscreen use by comparison with those receiving no sunscreen (median counts, 24 and 28; $p < 0.05$). Further modelling of the data demonstrated an interaction between freckling and the intervention, suggesting that sunscreen use was more effective in preventing new naevi in children who freckled than in those who did not. Measures of exposure to sunlight showed little difference between the two groups, indicating that the differences in counts of new naevi in the two groups were not due to differences in exposure.

A further trial to evaluate use of sunscreens in preventing naevi in children is under way in Australia (Milne et al., 1999a,b).

Cohort studies: In an unusual cohort study, with retrospective assessment of exposure to sunshine and sunscreen use and prospective recording of changes in naevus counts, Luther et al. (1996) examined the risk factors for the development of naevi in a cohort of 866 German children. The children were examined in 1988, and 377 underwent a second physical examination in 1993. The number of naevi more than 2 mm in diameter was counted at each examination on all body sites except the scalp, and the counts in 1988 were subtracted from those in 1993 to obtain the outcome measure, the number of new naevi. Freckling, sun sensitivity, hair and skin colouring, exposure to the sun during holidays, history of sunburn and use of sunscreens were assessed from responses to the questionnaire. After elimination of the records of 20 children with the darkest skin, data on the 357 remaining subjects (41%) showed

relationships between high naevus count, sun sensitivity and days of intense exposure to the sun. In a univariate analysis, regular use of sunscreen was associated with an increased risk for having a large number of new naevi (RR, 1.8; 95% CI, 1.0–3.3) by comparison with children who had never used sunscreens. The final logistic regression model of factors accounting for the development of new naevi did not contain sunscreen use. The authors noted that children who had used sunscreens tended to have greater cumulative exposure to the sun than those who had not used them, although no data were presented to quantify this statement. [The strengths of this study are the large number of children involved and the reliability of the naevus counts. The potential weaknesses are the low subject retention over the 5-year period and the retrospective assessment of sunscreen use and sun exposure.]

Cross-sectional studies: Three cross-sectional studies have been conducted to evaluate the relationship between acquired naevi and sunscreen use among children (Table 20), and two have been conducted among adults.

Pope et al. (1992) recruited 2140 British schoolchildren aged 4–11 to study the relationship between pigmentation characteristics, sun sensitivity, freckling, sunburn history, sun exposure and the prevalence of naevi. The children either attended one of 10 primary schools in the West Midlands or were selected from the patient lists of five general practitioners in the same geographical area. The

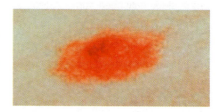

Figure 29 Dysplastic naevus of the trunk

Table 20. Studies of sunscreen use and acquired melanocytic naevi among children

Place/date	Type of study	No. of subjects	Exposure	End-point	RR[a] (95% CI)	Comments	Reference
West Midlands, Englands (dates not reported)	Cross-sectional	1130 girls and 1010 boys aged 4–11	Always or often used sunscreens	Naevi, any size; ≥ 2 mm	Not reported	Significantly higher naevus count (p < 0.001) in children using sunscreen	Pope et al. (1992)
Townsville, Australia (dates not reported)	Cross-sectional	506 children aged 1–6	Use of summer sunscreens	Naevi, any size; ≥ 2 mm	Not reported	Use of sunscreen 'not associated with naevus number or density'	Harrison et al. (1994)
Bochum, Germany 1988–93	5-year cohort study	357 children aged 1–6 at start	Regular use of sunscreens	Naevi ≥ 1 mm; ≥ 2 mm	1.8 (1.0–3.3)	Unvariate result only. Not statistically significant in multivariate model	Luther et al. (1996)
Vancouver, Canada 1993–96	Randomized trial	309 children aged 6–10 at start	Use of SPF 30 sunscreen when in the sun > 30 min	Naevi, any size	Not reported	Significantly fewer new naevi in children using sunscreen	Gallagher et al. (2000)
Belgium, France, Germany, Italy 1995–97	Cross-sectional	631 children aged 6–7		Naevi ≥ 2 mm	Trunk, 1.7 (1.1–2.6) Head and neck, 1.5 (0.86–2.5)		Autier et al. (1998)

[a] Relative to naevi ≥ 2 mm

participation rates varied among the schools from 38% to 66%. The children were examined by a nurse who was trained to identify naevi and to differentiate them from freckles. Naevi of any size, those 2 mm or more and those 5 mm or more in diameter were enumerated on all body sites except those covered by the child's underpants and the scalp. Skin, hair and eye colour were recorded, and sun exposure and use of sunscreens were assessed from answers to a questionnaire. Analysis of the data on sunscreens was not presented in detail; however, the authors noted that "children who often or always use a sunscreen in strong sunlight had more moles than those who never or sometimes use a sunscreen (p < 0.001)". [The strength of the association between use of sunscreens and number of naevi and whether this association was adjusted for sun sensitivity and sun exposure could not be determined because of incomplete reporting of the study.]

Harrison et al. (1994) studied sun exposure and the prevalence of naevi in a sample of children aged 1–6 in a cross-sectional study in Townsville, northern Australia. The mothers of the children were identified from the records of maternity wards in the two local hospitals and from lists of the mothers of children who had participated in previous studies of naevi. A total of 707 children were invited to participate in the study. After exclusion of non-respondents, those who had left the area and a few with two or more non-European grandparents, 506 children remained (72%). The naevi of the children were enumerated according to an IARC protocol (English et al., 1990), and the degree of freckling on the face and shoulders was estimated. Hair and eye colour were noted, and skin reflectance was assessed with a spectrocolorimeter. Sun exposure before examination, sun sensitivity, sunburn history and use of sunscreens were determined for each child from the answers to a questionnaire completed by the parents. No quantitative data on the relationship between sunscreen use and the prevalence of naevi is presented in the paper; however, the authors stated that 'use of summer sunscreen significantly reduced the number of sunburns ($p = 0.022$) but was not associated with annual sun exposure or with naevus number or density'. [The strength of the association between use of sunscreens and number of naevi and whether this association was adjusted for sun sensitivity and sun exposure are uncertain because of incomplete reporting of the study.]

Autier et al. (1998) conducted the most complete cross-sectional study to date on the relationship between sunscreen use and the prevalence of naevi. The investigation was conducted among elementary school children in Belgium, Germany, France and Italy. A total of 1234 parents of children aged 6–7 were approached by letter to participate in the study, and 682 agreed. Of these, 51 were eliminated from the study because the child was not of 'Caucasian' origin, the child's skin examination could not be completed or the parents could not be reached for interview, leaving 631 children (51%). Whole-body skin examinations (with the exception of the buttocks, genital area and scalp) were conducted on each child by a trained physician, who enumerated naevi 2 mm or greater in diameter. The degree of freckling on the face, arms and shoulders was also noted. Naevi were counted by the IARC protocol (English et al., 1990). Parents were interviewed in their homes by trained, non-medical, female interviewers about each child's sun exposure, sun sensitivity, sunburn history, clothing preferences and sunscreen use. Particular attention was paid to assessing holiday sun exposure by collecting data on the month of each holiday, its duration, place and latitude, whether it had been sunny

during the vacation, and the child's clothing and sunscreen use during the holiday. The frequency of sunscreen use was evaluated in categories ranging from 'never' to 'always' using such agents during each holiday. Questions were also posed about the sun exposure and sunscreen use of each child during recreational pursuits apart from holidays. Total sunscreen use on the head and neck and the trunk—sites representing constantly and intermittently exposed body sites—was evaluated. A direct relationship was seen between the prevalence of naevi and use of sunscreen on both the head and neck (RR for highest quartile of use, 1.5; 95% CI, 0.86–2.5) and the trunk (RR for highest quartile of use, 1.7; 95% CI, 1.1–2.6). The association persisted after adjustment for sun exposure, sex, study area, eye colour and sun sensitivity. A significant exposure–response gradient of naevus count with increasing sunscreen use was reported. The authors noted that since the relationship persisted after control for potential confounders, it was probably due to the fact that children who used sunscreens could remain in the sun longer than those who did not use these agents.

In a study conducted in Belgium, France and Germany in 1991 and 1992 of 438 controls selected for a case–control study of melanoma, the use of sunscreen was associated with a higher density of pigmented lesions of the skin (Autier et al., 1995). The naevus count on both arms of control subjects increased significantly from those with no sunscreen use to those who had ever used non-psoralen-containing sunscreens, with a rate ratio of 1.3 (95% CI, 1.2–1.4) after adjustment for age, sex, hair colour, number of holiday weeks spent each year in sunny resorts and sunbathing during 'the hottest hours of the day'. The increase in naevus count was greater for subjects who had ever used psoralen-containing sunscreens (RR, 2.1; 95% CI, 1.8–2.4); the adjusted

rate ratio between non-psoralen-containing sunscreen users and psoralen-containing sunscreen users was 1.6 (95% CI, 1.4–1.8).

The other study that addressed the issue of sunscreen use and the prevalence of naevi in adults is that of Dennis et al. (1996), which was conducted in Washington State, USA. The results were presented in such a way that they did not provide any information on the association between sunscreen use specifically and number of naevi, and the study was not considered further.

Actinic (solar) keratoses

Actinic keratoses are a risk factor for basal-cell carcinoma (Fig. 30) and a precursor lesion for squamous-cell carcinoma (Marks et al., 1988). They are known to be related to solar exposure and, like basal-cell and squamous-cell carcinoma, are more common in individuals with light skin and hair colouring, a propensity to freckle and sun-sensitive skin (Vitasa et al., 1990). The rate of transformation of actinic keratoses to squamous-cell carcinomas is low, however, and many of these lesions appear to regress spontaneously, particularly in the absence of exposure (Marks et al., 1986). As they are known to be potential precursors of squamous-cell carcinoma, these lesions have been used as intermediate end-points in recent studies of the use of sunscreens in preventing squamous-cell carcinoma. The relationship has been assessed in several randomized trials and one cross-sectional study (Table 21).

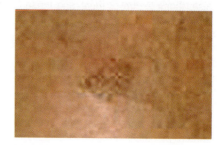

Figure 30 Actinic keratosis of the scalp

Table 21. Studies of sunscreen use and actinic keratoses

Place/date	Type of study	No. subjects	Randomization or exposure	End-point	RR[a] (95% CI)	Comments	Reference
Lubbock, Texas USA 1987–90	Randomized trial	50 persons with clinically diagnosed actinic keratoses	SPF-29 sunscreen daily vs base cream (placebo)	Average annual rate of actinic keratosis formation	Sunscreen, 21 Placebo, 28 36% reduction, $p = 0.001$	All subjects warned against solar exposure and encouraged to use hats and other mechanical protection measures	Naylor et al. (1995)
Cardiff, Wales, United Kingdom, 1988–92	Cross-sectional	560 men and women aged ≥ 60	Normally used sunscreens	Prevalent actinic keratoses or squamous-cell carcinomas	Sunscreens vs placebo, 0.56 (0.34–0.82) RR adjusted for age not given	Use of sunscreen protective in univariate analysis; in multi-variate analyses, effect largely accounted for by confounding with age	Harvey et al. (1996a,b)
Maryborough, Australia 1991–92	Randomized trial	431 persons aged ≥ 40 with 1–30 actinic keratoses	SPF-17 sunscreen daily vs base cream (placebo)	Prevalent actinic kera-toses on head, neck, hands and forearms No. of new actinic keratoses No. of remissions	Placebo vs sunscreen, 1.5 (0.81–2.2) Sunscreen vs placebo, 0.62 (0.54–0.71) Sunscreen vs placebo, 1.5 (1.3–1.8)	All participants also told to avoid midday sun and wear hats	Thompson et al. (1993)

[a] Risk ratio

Randomized trials: Naylor et al. (1995) conducted a randomized controlled trial between December 1987 and December 1990 to test the hypothesis that sunscreen use can reduce the appearance of new actinic keratoses. Fifty-three individuals with a history of prior actinic keratoses or a non-melanocytic skin cancer who had sought treatment at a university or Veterans Affairs dermatology practice in Lubbock, Texas, USA, were recruited for the trial. All of the subjects lived close enough to the clinic for follow-up visits every 3 months. The volunteers were examined, and then all actinic keratoses were removed with liquid nitrogen and non-melanocytic skin cancers were excised surgically. A detailed history of sun exposure was taken, and the subjects were randomized to receive either a broad-spectrum SPF-29 sunscreen (containing ethylhexy methoxy-cinnamate, benzophenone-3 and ethyl-hexyl salicylate) or a placebo of identical appearance containing the sunscreen base cream but without the active ingredients. The subjects were warned against overexposure to sunlight and were encouraged to use hats. Use of sunscreens other than that provided in the study was discouraged. The subjects were instructed to apply the sunscreen to all sun-exposed body sites and not to change their usual activity patterns. Participants in both groups were seen at 1 month, 3 months and every 3 months afterwards for 2 years. At each visit, new lesions identified clinically as actinic keratoses were noted and removed with liquid nitrogen, and new non-melanocytic skin cancers were removed surgically. Only lesions on sunscreen-treated areas were counted, and several actinic keratoses that appeared on bald areas of the scalp were not included. Of the 53 subjects originally enrolled in the trial, 50 visited the clinic at least once at or after 3 months, and 37 came for their final visit at 2 years. Three subjects dropped out of the study before the first 3-month visit and were excluded from the analysis. The 13 subjects who did not report for the 2-year follow-up were not included in the analysis but did not have a different outcome from those who completed the trial. The outcome of the trial was determined by comparing the annual rates of formation of actinic keratoses in the two groups. Participants given sunscreen had an average of 13.6 (SD 18.5) new actinic keratoses per year, while those given placebo had 27.9 per year (SD 31.8). The distribution of risk factors between the two groups differed, however, and when these were taken into consideration in a Poisson regression model, an expected value of 21.1 new actinic keratoses per year was estimated for the group given sunscreen on the basis of the experience of the placebo group. Thus, the annual rate of new actinic keratoses was estimated to be 36% lower for people who received sunscreen than for those who did not ($p = 0.001$). Too few non-melanocytic skin cancers were diagnosed during the 2-year trial for analysis.

Thompson et al. (1993) conducted a randomized trial to determine whether daily use of high-SPF sunscreens could attenuate the development of new actinic keratoses in subjects who already had at least one. The trial was conducted in Maryborough, southern Australia, among 588 subjects aged 40 or more, each of whom had 1–30 actinic keratoses and who were recruited in September 1991. An examination was conducted to note all actinic keratoses on a body site map,

and the subjects were randomized into one of two groups, with stratification to equalize the sex distribution and sun sensitivity. One group received an SPF-17 broad-spectrum sunscreen containing ethylhexyl methoxycinnamate and butyl methoxydibenzoylmethane, with instructions to apply 1.5 ml to the skin of the head and neck and the same amount to the forearms and hands every morning. They were told to re-apply the sunscreen during the day if necessary. Each subject kept a diary, recording the time of day they applied the sunscreen. Those in the other group received a placebo cream containing the same sunscreen base but without the active ingredients. The colour and consistency of the placebo were identical to those of the sunscreen. All subjects were instructed not to rely solely on the sunscreen but to avoid the sun in the middle of the day and to wear hats and appropriate clothing in order to moderate their solar exposure. Three follow-up examinations were made in the 7 months after recruitment, the season in southern Australia when there is the most sunlight. At each examination, total actinic keratoses, remissions and new actinic keratoses were noted, the diaries were examined, and the bottles of sunscreen were weighed. By March 1992, 431 subjects (73%) had completed the trial and were re-examined by the same physician who had seen them at the start. All actinic keratoses were recorded on a new body site map so that the physician would be unaware which lesions had been present at the start of the study. The groups were compared for the overall prevalence of actinic keratoses on the head and neck, arms and hands, the number of new actinic keratoses arising during the study and the number of actinic keratoses that regressed during the study. Subjects given the placebo had a greater increase in the mean number of actinic keratoses during the course of the study (1.0 ± 0.3 SE) than those given sunscreen (0.6 ± 0.3 SE; RR, 1.5; 95%

CI, 0.81–2.2). Fewer new actinic keratoses appeared during the course of the study among people given the sunscreen than those given placebo (mean, 1.6 versus 2.3 lesions per subject; RR, 0.62; 95% CI, 0.54–0.71). After control for sex and sun sensitivity, the likelihood of remission of actinic keratoses present at the start of the study was greater for people given sunscreen than for those given placebo (25% versus 18% of initial lesions regressing; RR, 1.5; 95% CI, 1.3–1.8). [This was a short-term investigation, and many subjects did not complete the protocol.]

Cross-sectional studies: Harvey et al. (1996a,b) completed a cross-sectional study of factors associated with actinic keratoses in an older (age 60 or more) population in Wales, United Kingdom. A random sample of 1034 men and women over the age of 60 and living in the county of South Glamorgan were sent letters of invitation to participate in a study of skin cancer. Of those invited, 560 (54%) were seen in their homes by a research registrar in dermatology (Harvey et al., 1996a), when a detailed questionnaire was completed on risk factors for non-melanocytic skin cancer and actinic keratoses, including cumulative sun exposure and sun sensitivity. The skin of the head, neck, arms (to the shoulder), legs (below the knee) and feet was examined. Polaroid photos and 35-mm slides were made of any suspected skin cancer or actinic keratosis. The physicians of any patients with a suspected non-melanocytic skin cancer were contacted directly, while those subjects with actinic keratoses were reassured that no immediate treatment was necessary and that the lesion would be reassessed at the next visit. A second visit was made 1–2 years later, and the details of treatment for any lesion removed between visits were recorded. New lesions were also noted and photographed. At the conclusion of the study, the slides of all lesions were reviewed by three consultant dermatologists, and the majority view was accepted as correct for each lesion. Of the 154 actinic keratoses diagnosed by the registrar, 135 were confirmed by the panel. The panel also appears to have added a further two lesions to this total, giving 137 actinic keratoses. Univariate analysis showed that subjects who had used sunscreen had a reduced risk for a prevalent actinic keratosis, but a multivariate analysis indicated that the inverse relationship was accounted for by the age of the subjects, as those who were older had a greater probability of having a prevalent actinic keratosis and were also less likely to have used sunscreens.

Intermediary end-points
DNA damage
The ability of sunscreens to prevent the formation of UVR-induced lesions in human skin DNA has been evaluated in a few studies. (Fig. 31)

Untanned gluteal skin sites from five healthy volunteers were treated with 2 mg/cm^2 of sunscreen (7.5% ethylhexyl methoxycinnamate and 4.5% benzophenone-3, SPF 15) or the vehicle and then exposed to solar-simulated UVR at doses up to 10 MEDs (Freeman et al., 1988). Biopsy samples were obtained within 3 min of the end of the exposure, and DNA was extracted from epidermis. After cleavage by *Micrococcus luteus* UV endonuclease, which recognizes pyrimidine dimers in DNA, an alkaline agarose gel electrophoresis method was used to quantify the number of lesions. After exposure to an equivalent dose of UVR, the number of pyrimidine dimers was 32 per 10^7 bases in untreated skin and 0.8 per 10^7 bases in sunscreen-treated skin.

van Praag et al. (1993) evaluated the effect of a sunscreen (SPF 10) in biopsy samples obtained from the UVB-exposed, sunscreen- or vehicle-treated right buttock and from the UVB-exposed,

untreated left buttock of 10 volunteers. Cyclobutyl thymine dimers were assayed in skin sections by immunofluorescence microscopy with a monoclonal antibody. A single dose of UVB resulted in significant dimer-specific nuclear fluorescence, which was abolished by pretreatment with sunscreen, indicating that the sunscreen offered good protection against UVB-induced DNA damage.

Seven male and seven female volunteers with sun-sensitive skin were irradiated with UVB (unfiltered Waldmann F 85/100 W-UV21 tubes) at a dose of 0.15, 0.15, 0.37, 0.92 or 2 kJ/m^2 over areas of the lower back measuring 2 x 3 cm. The last four areas were covered with 2 µl/cm^2 of a sunscreen of SPF 10 before irradiation (Bykov et al., 1998b). Biopsy samples from each irradiated site and from one unirradiated area were taken less than 15 min after irradiation and rapidly frozen. DNA was extracted, and UVB-induced photoproducts were measured by a post-labelling HPLC technique. Cyclobutane dimers were formed in unprotected skin at a rate of about 2.5 photoproducts per 10^6 nucleotides and

were about five times more abundant than 6–4 photoproducts. The sunscreen reduced the rate of adduct formation to about 1/20th of the value seen in unprotected skin. There was a large difference in individual response to UVB and no correlation between the photoproduct levels in unprotected and protected skin. Thus, the effective dose of solar irradiance to DNA may be highly individual, and protection against erythema by sunscreens is unrelated to protection against DNA damage.

Young et al. (2000) assessed the ability of two sunscreens with an identical SPF of 4 but with different spectral absorption profiles to inhibit photodamage in human epidermis *in situ* in eight volunteers with sun-sensitive skin (types I and II). One formulation contained ethylhexyl methoxycinnamate, a UVB absorber (λ_{max} = 308 nm), while the other contained terephthalylidene dicamphor sulfonic acid (λ_{max} = 345). The sunscreen-treated sites were exposed to 4 MEDs of solar-simulated radiation (1 MED = 20 kJ/m^2 full solar-simulated UVR spectrum), whereas control and

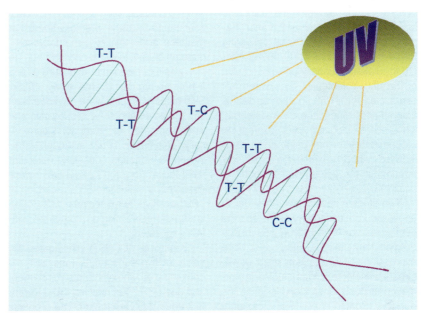

Figure 31 UV-induced cyclobutane pyrimidine dimers in DNA

vehicle-treated sites were exposed to 1 MED. Biopsies were performed immediately after UV irradiation, and the sections were analysed for thymidine dimers and 6–4 photoproducts by monoclonal antibody immunohistochemistry and image analysis. Four MEDs of solar-simulated radiation administered to skin protected by each sunscreen resulted in a comparable number of DNA lesions to that induced by 1 MED of solar-simulated radiation on unprotected skin. The authors concluded that the DNA protection factors of these sunscreens were similar to their SPFs and noted that the lack of difference between the sunscreens suggests that the action spectra for erythema and DNA photodamage are similar.

p53 *expression*
The protein TP53 plays an important role in the cellular response to DNA damage. After exposure to genotoxic agents such as ionizing radiation and UVR, wild-type TP53 accumulates and becomes immunohistochemically detectable. In human skin, UVR induces accumulation of TP53 in the epidermis. This response is rapid and transient: it is detectable as early as 2 h after irradiation, peaking at 24 h and persisting for several days (Hall *et al.,* 1993). After UV irradiation of usually unexposed skin of healthy volunteers, the pattern of expression of TP53 in the epidermis differed according to the UV wavelength: while UVA induced *p53* expression predominantly in the basal layer, UVB induced *p53* expression diffusely throughout the epidermis (Campbell *et al.,* 1993).

Two studies have shown that topical application of sunscreens decreases the overexpression of wild-type *p53* in epidermal keratinocytes (Fig. 32). The expression of *p53* and of its major downstream effector *p21* was studied in normal, previously unexposed skin of the buttocks (Pontén *et al.,* 1995) from eight volunteers of each sex aged 28–68

years, six with skin type II or III and two with type V skin. An area of 16 cm² on each buttock was irradiated with 2 MEDs of UVB of broad-band UVB–UVA (UVA SUN 3000) 15 min after application of 0.2 ml/cm² of a broad-spectrum SPF-15 sunscreen containing ethylhexy methoxycinnamate and benzophenone-3. A 3-mm punch skin biopsy sample was obtained from both treated and untreated areas before and 4, 24, 48 and 120 h after irradiation. The expression of *p53* was found to have been induced in epidermal cells 4 h after irradiation, peaked at 24–48 h and returned to nearly normal levels by 120 h. The expression of *p21* mirrored that of *p53* but disappeared at a slower rate. In addition, *p21* was induced in the papillary dermis and to a lesser extent in the reticular dermis, without concomitant expression of *p53*. In all subjects, the *p53* reaction was either absent or very weak in the sunscreen-treated areas. *p21* expression showed a pattern similar to that in unirradiated skin, indicating that it was not affected by UVR when a sunscreen had been applied.

The effect of topical application of a SPF-15 sunscreen containing benzophenone-3, butyl methoxydibenzoylmethane and ethylhexyl methoxycinnamate on chronically sun-exposed human skin was examined after exposure during a normal summer (Berne *et al.,* 1998). Skin biopsy samples were obtained from sun-protected and sun-exposed skin and were compared for immunohistochemically detectable TP53. Although large individual variation, possibly reflecting differences in sun exposure, were observed, a significant 33% reduction in TP53-positive keratinocytes was found in sun-protected skin as compared with sun-exposed skin.

Krekels *et al.* (1997) investigated the ability of two sunscreens (one SPF 10 containing ethylhexyl methoxycinnamate and one SPF 20 containing TiO₂) to protect against DNA damage. The products were applied at 2 mg/cm² to 25 volun-

teers with skin types I–III, who were then exposed for 1 or 1.5 h to natural sunshine. An increase in *p53* expression was found immunohistochemically in punch biopsy samples of unprotected skin from all subjects 24 h after exposure, although erythema was seen in only 19 of the 25 volunteers. Both sunscreens significantly reduced the fraction of cells containing TP53 in basal and suprabasal epidermal layers and the amount of TP53. The authors concluded that *p53* expression is a sensitive indicator of sun-induced dermal damage.

Krekels *et al.* (2000) investigated the DNA-protective qualities of three sunscreens with SPFs of 8, 30 and 40 applied at 2 mg/cm² to 12 volunteers with skin types I–III. An immuno-histochemical study was conducted of the induction of expression of TP53 protein in skin biopsy samples taken 24 h after exposure to 1 MED (unprotected areas) or 3 MED (protected areas) of solar-simulated radiation (exact dose not specified). The high-SPF sunscreens provided protection against both erythema and TP53 induction, whereas the SPF-8 sunscreen protected against erythema but not against TP53 expression after exposure to UVR.

Seité *et al.* (2000a) used expression of *p53* as the end-point for evaluating the protection provided by two sunscreens with the same SPF of 7 but with different UVA protection factors: one contained 7% octocrylene and 3% butyl methoxy-dibenzoylmethane and had a UVA protection factor of 7, and the other contained 3.8% ethylhexyl methoxycinnamate and 7.5% ZnO in the same oil-in-water vehicle and had a UVA protection factor of 3. Human skin biopsy samples were exposed eight times to 5 MEDs of solar-simulated radiation. Both sunscreens gave only partial protection against *p53* overexpression, but significantly fewer TP53-positive cells were found in areas covered with the sunscreen with the higher UVA

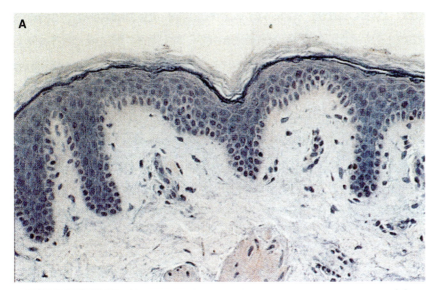

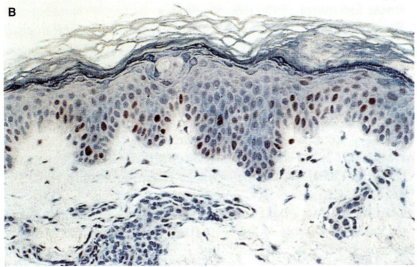

Figure 32 Accumulation of TP*3* protein in human epidermis
A, Unexposed skin shows no immunostaining against *p*53 protein; B, in sunscreen (low SPF)-protected skin, positive staining for TP53 is indicated by the dense, dark, nuclear colouration seen in both basal and suprabasal epidermal cells.

protection factor. The difference in protection by the two sunscreens was shown to be due to the difference in UVA absorption in a study in six volunteers in which *p53* overexpression was induced in their epidermis by eight exposures to 125 or 250 kJ/m^2 of UVA1 or UVA.

Sunburn cells
Sunburn cells are identified in conventionally stained epidermal biopsy samples as keratinocytes with a dense, pyknotic nucleus and a homogeneously eosinophilic cytoplasm. They represent keratinocytes that have sustained UVR-induced damage and are undergoing apoptosis (Fig. 33). As sunburn cells can be produced by sub-erythemal doses of UVR (Grove & Kaidbey, 1980), formation of sunburn cells in the epidermis is a quantifiable indicator of acute damage by UVR.

Sixteen healthy volunteers with skin types I–III were exposed to a 15-MED dose of UVR from a xenon arc solar simulator on areas of the middle of the back protected by application of 2 mg/cm^2 of a SPF-15 or SPF-30 sunscreen (Kaidbey, 1990). An unprotected area of normal skin received a dose of 1 MED and served as a control site. The SPF-30 sunscreen prevented the formation of sunburn cells in biopsy specimens more efficiently than the SPF-15 formulation, the decimal logarithm of the number of sunburn cells in 10 microscope fields being 1.1 ± 0.41 in the control area, 0.69 ± 0.41 in the area protected by the SPF-15 sunscreen and 0.16 ± 0.53 in that protected by the SPF-30 sunscreen ($p < 0.001$).

Immune suppression
UVR-induced immune suppression and its modulation by topical sunscreen application have been studied in humans, with emphasis on contact hypersensitivity, delayed-type hypersensitivity, density of Langerhans cells, release of immune modulatory molecules such as interleukin-10 or urocanic acid, natural killer cell activity and stimulation of allogeneic lymphocytes by epidermal cells.

Dinitrochlorobenzene (DNCB) is a potent contact sensitizer to which spontaneous sensitization is rarely encountered in human populations and which has been widely used for evaluating immune capacity in patients with a variety of diseases. Typically, sensitization to DNCB is induced by applying a small patch of filter paper containing 30–50 μg of the compound in acetone solution to skin in a Finn chamber and removing the patch after 48 h. The sensitization induced is tested

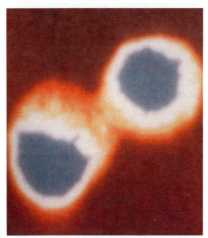

Figure 33 Apoptotic (blue) keratinocytes as a consequence of exposure to UVB

2 weeks after the first contact with DNCB by application of challenge patches containing concentrations of DNCB usually ranging from 3.125 to 12.5 µg. The challenge patches are removed after 48 h, and the contact hypersensitivity reactions are assessed 24 h later.

Whitmore and Morison (1995) used a commercially available SPF-29 sunscreen containing ethylhexyl methoxy-cinnamate, benzophenone-3 and ethylhexyl salicylate to prevent UVB-induced suppression of the induction of contact hypersensitivity to DNCB. Seventeen healthy volunteers aged 21–48 with skin type II or III were exposed to three MEDs of UVB from unfiltered fluorescent tubes on 3 consecutive days on one 16-cm^2 site on the buttock (1 MED = 1.5 kJ/m^2), with or without application of the sunscreen [amount not specified] before irradiation. One day after the last exposure, 30 µg of DNCB were applied to the irradiated site, and 2 weeks later a forearm was given a challenge dose of 3.125, 6.25, 8.8 or 12.5 µg of DNCB. A control group of nine volunteers aged 21–45 with skin type II or III underwent immunization and challenge with DNCB but were not exposed to UVB. Both the development of primary allergic

dermatitis at the sensitization site and the reaction at the elicitation sites were scored clinically. The proportion of subjects who developed a primary allergic response to DNCB at the sensitization site was reduced from 5/9 to 0/10 in the UVB-treated group (p = 0.1, Fisher's exact test), while 7/7 subjects given sunscreen plus UVB developed a primary allergic response to DNCB (p = 0.00005). The group exposed to UVB had a reduced response rate at the challenge site to all challenge doses of DNCB, except for the highest dose (12.5 µg), when compared with a control group with no exposure to UVB ($p \le 0.008$) and the group given sunscreen plus UVB ($p \le$ 0.02). The response rates to the DNCB challenge doses did not differ between the group given no UVB and that given sunscreen plus UVB.

Irritant and contact hypersensitivity responses to DNCB were studied in 160 male volunteers aged 18–60 (mean, 28 ± 9.3) with skin types II and III, who were randomly allocated to groups of 20 subjects each (Serré *et al.*, 1997). The men received an application of 2 mg/cm^2 of a broad-spectrum SPF-15 sunscreen containing 9% octocrylene, 3% butyl methoxydibenzoylmethane, 0.7% terephthalylidene dicamphor sulfonic acid and 0.3% phenylbenzimidazole sulfonic acid (UVA protection factor, 9) over a 4-cm^2 area on one buttock 20 min before a single exposure to 3 MEDs of solar-simulated radiation (1 MED = 210 ± 49 kJ/m^2). They were sensitized by application of DNCB on the irradiated skin 3 days later, and challenged 14 days later with DNCB at a dose of 3.125, 6.25, 8.8 or 12.5 µg. The reactions were read at 48 h and quantified as increases in skin thickness. Subjects in the seven control groups received either the sunscreen but no UVB, sunscreen with or without UVB but no DNCB sensitization, DNCB sensitization with or without prior UVB, UVB but no DNCB sensitization or no UVB and no DNCB sensitization. All groups were challenged with DNCB. In subjects

sensitized with DNCB, the elicitation response was linear and dose-dependent. Exposure to UVB resulted in significantly decreased responses to all doses of DNCB (p = 0.009, 0.008 and 0.004 for the doses of 6.25, 8.8 and 12.5 µg, respectively), and the percentage of positive responses to DNCB dropped from 95% to 50% (p = 0.003). Neither sunscreen nor UVB influenced the irritative response to DNCB, and prior application of the sunscreen did not modify the percentage of positive responses to DNCB (90%). Pretreatment with the sunscreen maintained a high immunization rate (85%) among volunteers exposed to UVB and restored the contact hyper-sensitivity responses to the three higher challenge doses of DNCB. Hence, an erythemal exposure to UVR significantly impairs the afferent arm of the contact hypersensitivity reaction, and the application of a high-SPF sunscreen can prevent the UV-induced suppression of induction of contact hypersensitivity.

Hayag *et al.* (1997) confirmed that sunscreens *per se* do not interfere with contact hypersensitivity and that an SPF-30 sunscreen (7.5% ethylhexyl methoxy-cinnamate, 10% octocrylene, 5% menthyl anthranilate) applied before UVB irradiation partially prevents induction of suppression of contact hypersensitivity by DNCB. This study also showed that application of a high-SPF sunscreen before UVB irradiation prevents the decrease in density of epidermal Langerhans cells at the irradiated site that usually follows exposure to UVB.

Nickel is a frequent contact allergen in the general population: up to 15% of women and 5% of men develop allergic contact dermatitis when exposed to this metal. UVR suppresses the allergic response of these individuals to patch testing with nickel, and clinical improvement of nickel allergy occurs after whole-body irradiation. This model has been developed into a technique for evaluating the immune protection afforded by sunscreens (Damian et al., 1997). A group of 29 subjects, aged 19–58 years, with skin types I–V and confirmed allergy to nickel were irradiated on the mid-back with a sub-erythemal dose of UVB (975 ± 25 J/m^2) and UVA (12.3 kJ/m^2) daily for 5 consecutive days. A sunscreen or base lotion was applied at 2 mg/cm^2 15 min before irradiation and washed off after irradiation. Three sunscreens based on cinnamate with an identical UVB protection factor of 10 but differing in their UVA protection capacity were used. After the final irradiation, nickel patches were applied to each of four segments used to test the sunscreens or the base lotion; other patches were used to test unprotected irradiated skin, and control patches were placed on adjacent unirradiated skin. A placebo patch was also included in the test array. The patches were left in place for 48 h, and the cutaneous hypersensitivity response was assessed clinically and with an erythema meter 24 h later. When the reactions of unprotected irradiated skin to nickel were compared with those of unirradiated skin, there was, on average, immune suppression of 35% ($n = 16$; $p < 0.001$). Prior application of the cinnamate sunscreen reduced but did not prevent significant UVR-induced immune suppression (mean reduction, 18%; $p = 0.004$). In contrast, immune suppression was prevented by sunscreens containing either benzophenone or ZnO (reduction, 6.7% and 10%). None of the sunscreens or their base lotion had any effect in the absence of UVR. To determine whether UVR-induced suppression of the response to nickel is specific for cell-mediated immunity or reflects suppression of nonspecific inflammation, a further 16 subjects matched for age and skin type with the group allergic to nickel were patch-tested with a skin irritant, sodium lauryl sulfate, after application of a sunscreen and an irradiation protocol identical to that of the volunteers allergic to nickel. Neither UV irradiation nor sunscreens significantly affected sodium lauryl sulfate-induced erythema. The authors concluded that nickel patch testing is a valid means of assessing UVR-induced immune suppression in humans and its modulation by sunscreens. They also concluded that, even with sub-erythemal doses, immune protection was provided only by broad-spectrum sunscreens, suggesting that UVA plays an important role in immune suppression.

Using the same approach of nickel patch-testing on irradiated and unirradiated skin of volunteers with nickel allergy, the same group of authors proposed to define the 'minimal immune suppression dose' as that dose of UVR that reduces nickel contact hypersensitivity by 20% (Damian et al., 1999). The authors concluded that the immune protection factor of a sunscreen can be evaluated by dividing the mean minimal immune suppression dose of sunscreen-treated skin by that of unprotected skin. The immune protection factor of a given sunscreen does not reflect its SPF (see p. 124).

The effects of two SPF-9 sunscreens with different absorption spectra on local and systemically induced immune suppression were evaluated with respect to the delayed-type hypersensitivity skin response after application at 2 mg/cm^2 (Moyal et al., 1997; Moyal, 1998). The first sunscreen contained two UVB (9% octocrylene, 2% phenyl benzimidazole sulfonic acid) and two UVA filters (0.7% terephthalylidene dicamphor sulfonic acid, 2% butyl methoxydibenzoylmethane), thus covering the entire range of UVR, while the second contained only the same two UVB filters and covered essentially the UVB range. Volunteers were exposed to UVA plus UVB (total dose, 58 MEDs) or UVA only (3500 kJ/m^2 over 12 exposures). The delayed hypersensitivity response was measured 48 h after application of a Multitest antigen kit on an exposed and an unexposed area. Both local and systemic immune suppression was found in all UV-irradiated groups. The second sunscreen did not prevent local or systemic immune suppression induced by UVB plus UVA, while the first reduced local immune suppression and prevented the systemic effects.

The preventive effect of two sunscreens was also measured under conditions of real solar exposure (Moyal, 1998). The sunscreens had absorption spectra covering the entire UVR range but had different SPFs and UVA protection capacity (measured by persistent pigment darkening). The first sunscreen (SPF 15, UVA protection factor 6) did not provide immune protection, while the second (SPF 30, UVA protection factor 12) significantly prevented immune suppression. These studies demonstrate that immune protection can be obtained by use of sunscreens that cover the entire UVR spectrum and with high SPF and UVA protection factors.

Neale et al. (1997) showed that use of a sunscreen (8% ethylhexyl methoxycinnamate, 2.5% benzophenone-3, 1% butyl methoxydibenzoylmethane, SPF 15) reduced the density of Langerhans cells during current but not chronic solar exposure, with a trend to greater protection at higher levels of exposure.

Partial protection against Langerhans cell depletion was also demonstrated with sunscreens containing ethylhexyl methoxycinnamate (SPF 12) or ZnO (SPF 16) (Hochberg & Enk, 1999). In the same study, both sunscreens nearly totally inhibited UVB-induced interleukin (IL)-10 mRNA expression.

The trans to cis isomerization of urocanic acid in the epidermis is considered to play an important role in the mechanism of UVR-induced immune suppression. Krien and Moyal (1994) investigated the effects of applications of 2 mg/cm^2 of sunscreens on the UVR-induced cis-urocanic acid formation in groups of volunteers aged 19–48 who were given single or multiple irradiations with either UVB (0–1.5 MEDs from a FS20 Westinghouse lamp with a peak emission at 313 nm) or UVA (100–300 kJ/m² from a Uvasun 5000 sunlamp, 335 nm, with a WG335 filter) or UVB plus UVA (1 MED on day 1, with a 25% increase each day until day 5 from a xenon arc lamp filtered with a WG305 filter). The sunscreens tested were two with SPFs of 3 and 4.5 and containing a UVB filter (3 and 5% ethylhexyl methoxy-cinnamate) and one with an SPF of 3 containing a broad-spectrum UVA filter (5% terephthalylidene dicamphor sulfonic acid). The rate of *cis*-urocanic acid formation was reduced by topical application of sunscreen; the reduction increased with increasing SPF, and broad-spectrum UVB plus UVA sunscreens were the most effective in reducing *cis*-urocanic acid formation in the stratum corneum.

Application of a broad-spectrum sunscreen lotion (8% ethylhexyl dimethyl PABA, 2% benzophenone-3, 2% butyl methoxydibenzoylmethane, SPF 15) did not protect against changes in natural killer (NK) cell activity induced by solarium lamps (Hersey *et al.*, 1987).

Another end-point for studying modulation of UVR-induced immune suppression is the mixed epidermal cell–lymphocyte reaction, in which epidermal cells are used to stimulate allogeneic lymphocytes *in vitro,* which is abrogated by UVR. van Praag *et al.* (1991) studied 32 patients with a variety of dermatoses (predominantly psoriasis) who were undergoing routine treatment with whole-body UVB irradiation (19 patients) or psoralen plus UVA therapy (13 patients). The interval between the last treatment and the start of the experiment was at least 1 year. The patients received treatment with UVR three times a week for 4 weeks, providing total doses of 72–392 kJ/m² of UVA and 5.8–34.6 kJ/m² of UVB. Immediately before each irradiation, one of two broad-spectrum sunscreens (SPF 6 and

15) or their vehicles were applied to the right forearm. The SPF-6 sunscreen contained butyl methoxybenzoylmethane, 4-methylbenzylidene camphor and phenyl-benzimidazole sulfonic acid, whereas the SPF-15 sunscreen contained these three ingredients plus ethylhexyl dimethyl PABA. Ten healthy volunteers received local UVB irradiation of the forearm. Epidermal sheets were obtained from the forearms by the suction blister method 48 h after the last irradiation, and epidermal cells inactivated by 20 Gy were used to stimulate allogeneic peripheral blood cells from two volunteers. Neither the tested sunscreens nor their vehicles prevented the UVR-induced suppression of the alloactivating capacity of epidermal cells. [The authors made no attempt to characterize the populations of epidermal cells in these studies.]

In a further study by the same group (Hurks *et al.,* 1997), 40 healthy volunteers with skin phototypes II and III were exposed to 1–2 MED of UVB for 4 days. In this study, the mixed epidermal cell–lymphocyte reaction responses were significantly increased by UVR irradiation, and this enhancement was associated with an influx of CD36⁺DR⁺ macrophages into the irradiated skin. Application of the SPF-15 sunscreen used in the previous experiment, either directly onto the irradiated skin or onto a quartz slide to prevent penetration of the sunscreen into the stratum corneum, prevented the increased responses and the influx of CD36⁺DR⁺ cells.

[These conflicting results from the same group of investigators show that the ability of sunscreens to interfere with UVR-induced modulation of cell-mediated immune responses depends critically on the irradiation protocol and on the end-points measured, which may involve different mechanisms of UVR-induced immune modulation.]

Experimental systems

Since a wide variety of artificial sources of UVR and methods were used in

the reported studies in experimental animals, criteria were drawn up to define studies that are relevant for examining protection against solar-simulated UVR (Fig. 34):

- The source of radiation should not include wavelengths outside the solar spectrum.
- The UVR dosimetry should be adequate.
- The amount of sunscreen applied should be quantified.
- Adequate control treatments should have been included.
- The experimental protocol should be consistent.

Studies in which sources of UVR were used which contain bands outside those that reach the earth's surface (e.g. UVC) are useful for proof of principle and for determining mechanisms of action, and the Working Group decided to summarize them in the text but not in the tables.

In most of the experimental studies, a single, arbitrary regimen of exposure to UVR was used to induce a biological response, such as skin cancer or immune suppression, and sunscreen was applied to investigate a possible protective effect. Although protection was observed in most studies, others showed 'no protection' (e.g. against immune suppression) and yet others showed 'total' or 'complete' protection (e.g. against carcinogenesis). Such absolute statements usually reflect limitations of study design rather than an

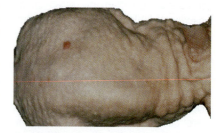

Figure 34 Solar elastosis induced in a hairless mouse after repeated exposure to solar-simulated UVR

adequate evaluation of protection against a UVR-induced biological effect. For instance, 'total protection' against photocarcinogenesis is commonly seen in a small group of animals over a limited period of observation and is often proved incorrect in an adequately expanded study. The main problem with most studies is that a dose–effect relationship is not determined, which would allow determination of any reduction in the effective exposure to UVR achieved by filtering through the sunscreen. Therefore, these studies do not allow quantification of a protection factor for photocarcinogenesis or another end-point.

Cancer and preneoplastic lesions

Studies of the potential of sunscreens to protect against photocarcinogenesis in experimental animals, mainly hairless mice, (Fig. 35) have evolved in complexity, both with the creation of more sophisticated UVR absorbers and with the evidence for a contributory role of UVA in photocarcinogenesis. A reduction in photocarcinogenesis in skin exposed to UVR through a topical sunscreen has not been difficult to demonstrate. In most studies, mice were irradiated daily with UVR at doses lower than, or approximately equal to, 1 MED through a sunscreen that provided several-fold protection from erythema. The large increases in the SPF values of commercial sunscreens has increased the difference between the effective dose of UVR received by unprotected control mice and the sunscreen-treated groups in experimental testing for protection against photocarcinogenesis. Humans are increasingly likely to expose themselves to multiples of their MED on sunscreen-protected skin, with an unknown and untested concomitant effect on photocarcinogenesis.

In addition, as new active sunscreen ingredients have been developed, with absorption spectra spanning both the UVB and UVA wavebands, it has become more

difficult to obtain comparative data on protection against carcinogenesis. It is all the more important that solar simulation, rather than unfiltered UVB radiation sources, be used, firstly to remove the environmentally irrelevant but carcinogenic UVC waveband, which may be relatively effectively absorbed by many UVB-absorbing sunscreen ingredients and thus confound measurements of the relevant protectivity, and secondly to account for variably efficient UVA absorbance by the sunscreen and the influence of the transmitted UVA wavelengths.

Of the active sunscreen ingredients that have been tested for anti-photocarcinogenic properties in animals, the simplest is the UVB absorber PABA; esterified derivatives of PABA (glyceryl and ethylhexyl dimethyl PABA) were developed later in response to the photosensitization reported by human PABA users (see p. 133 and Funk et al., 1997). Another compound, ethylhexyl methoxycinnamate, remains one of the most popular UVB absorbers, and a number of other chemicals offer a broader absorption spectrum, covering a portion of the UVA waveband. Many contemporary sunscreens contain TiO_2 and/or ZnO, which are purported both to absorb and scatter UVR broadly. Experimental photocarcinogenesis has been induced by chronic exposure to UVR applied either as a constant daily

dose or as periodically incremented daily doses, which can be done without burning the unprotected control animals because of the adaptive responses of the skin (i.e. epidermal hyperplasia and keratinization). Incremental exposures result in much larger cumulative doses of UVR, but whether the adaptive responses of sunscreen-irradiated skin are activated to the same degree as those of unprotected skin and whether they are involved in protection from photocarcinogenesis has not been examined.

Studies with radiation sources including UVC

In a landmark study, at a time when the sunburn spectrum was known to span 280–310 nm but the photocarcinogenesis action spectrum was still unknown, Knox et al. (1960) reported the first evidence for protection from UVR-induced carcinogenesis in experimental mice. The ears of Swiss albino mice were irradiated with a mercury arc lamp after application of 10% benzophenone-4 for five months. The sunscreen protected against tumour development, but the study was marred by the reported burning and necrosis of the unprotected ears and is not useful.

In later studies, more realistic UVR sources were used. Flindt-Hansen et al. (1990a) examined the effect of a 5%

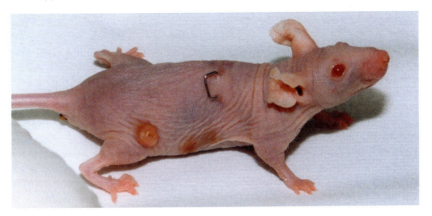

Figure 35 Hairless mouse with multiple skin tumours

PABA solution in a vehicle of 70% ethanol, 5% glycerol and water applied to the dorsal skin immediately before irradiation in groups of 30 female hr/hr hairless mice aged 8–12 weeks. The animals were exposed on 5 days per week for 30 weeks to an incremental regime of unfiltered UVB radiation from a Philips TL40 W/12 lamp. The initial sub-erythemal exposure (1.55 kJ/m^2) was increased up to 8 weeks by a maximum factor of 2.3, and the cumulative dose at 30 weeks was 490 kJ/m^2. This resulted in a mean time to tumour onset of about 22 weeks for unprotected mice, and all had acquired tumours ≥ 1 mm in diameter by 30 weeks, with an average tumour yield of 4.5. In contrast, only 12% of the PABA-protected mice had tumours by 40 weeks, with an average tumour yield of 0.16. The yield of histologically identified squamous-cell carcinomas was reduced from 2.7 to 0.04. The vehicle alone did not affect tumour induction. The dorsal skin of the mice was excised and weighed at the end of the study to verify that PABA had reduced the total tumour weight per mouse; however, no difference was seen for PABA-irradiated mice and unirradiated controls. [The significantly increased skin weight in unprotected mice may have been due partly to chronic hyperplasia induced by UVB.] The overall rate of survival was approximately 93%, so that the mice did not die of their tumours during the study.

This model was also used to examine the effect of intermittent sunscreen application in UVB-irradiated female hairless mice (Flindt-Hansen et al., 1990b). The same 5% PABA sunscreen was applied during weeks 16–26, accounting for one-third of the 30-week application of UVB. The sunscreen significantly reduced both the incidence of tumour-bearing mice at 40 weeks, from 100% of the unprotected mice to 67%, and the average tumour yield from 4.3 to 1.8. The treatment also significantly reduced the

average yield of squamous-cell carcinomas from 2.7 to 0.8 per mouse, and the proportion of the total tumour load that had progressed to squamous-cell carcinoma.

Using the same protocol on groups of 30 mice, Flindt-Hansen et al. (1989) examined the effect of PABA in which 40% photodegradation had been induced in vitro by exposure in 70% ethanol and 5% glycerol in water to 270 kJ/m^2 UVB from an unfiltered Philips TL40 W/12 light source. Although photoproducts were identified by both mass and UV spectroscopy, the photolysis induced only insignificant alterations in the absorption spectrum of the sample. The photodegraded PABA sunscreen did not induce tumours when applied alone for 30 weeks without UVB irradiation and was as effective as intact PABA in protecting against UVB-induced carcinogenesis (time to first tumour, number of tumours, number of squamous-cell carcinomas, weight of dorsal skin) when used as a daily sunscreen during 30 weeks of irradiation.

Kligman et al. (1980) performed the first comparative study of the tumour-protective activity of two sunscreens containing ethylhexyl PABA, at a concentration of 2% alone or at a concentration of 7% with 3% benzophenone-3, which provided SPFs of 2 and 15, respectively, as determined by standard methods on human skin. Groups of 20 albino (Skh-I) and 20 pigmented (Skh-II) hairless mice [sex and age not specified] were irradiated after application of either sunscreen, with a constant daily exposure of 1.85 kJ/m^2, from a bank of unfiltered UVB tubes (nine Westinghouse FS420 lamps) three times per week for 30 weeks. [The volume of sunscreen applied and the composition of the vehicle were not specified.] The unprotected mice, which received no topical treatment with the vehicle, developed large numbers of tumours, which caused the deaths of 75% of the Skh-I mice and 33% of the

Skh-II mice at 40 weeks. These mortality rates obviated detailed analysis of the tumour load. The pigmented Skh-II mice were markedly more resistant to irradiation than the albino Skh-I mice, developed a tan, and showed an extended latent period for appearance of the first tumour (21 weeks compared with 19 weeks for Skh-I); 67% survived to week 40 compared with only 25% of Skh-I mice. Markedly fewer Skh-II mice produced tumours with a diameter > 4 mm (3/23 mice compared with 6/10 Skh-I mice), although the average tumour yield at 40 weeks was approximately 13 tumours per mouse for both strains. At 30 weeks, when the survival rate was still high (83% overall), all of the unprotected irradiated mice had tumours, whereas the SPF-2 sunscreen reduced the tumour incidence to 22% (50% at 40 weeks) and the tumour yield to less than 2.0 per Skh-I mouse and prevented the appearance of tumours in Skh-II mice. The Skh-II mice developed only slight hyperpigmentation. The SPF-15 sunscreen was more effective, and prevented both tumour appearance and hyperpigmentation within the time of the study.

As part of a larger study in which 5% of an iron chelator (2-furildioxime) was incorporated into the sunscreen, Bissett and McBride (1996) irradiated groups of five Skh:HR-1 hairless mice [sex and age not specified] 2 h after application of 0.1 mL of 5% ethylhexyl PABA in ethanol and propylene glycol. [This interval is somewhat lengthy.] The protection factor of the sunscreen was determined to be 7.2 in shaved guinea-pig skin exposed to a solar simulator, according to a standard method, 15–20 min after topical application. The mice received a daily dose of 0.3 kJ/m^2 (stated to be approximately 0.5 MED in mice) of unfiltered UVB three times per week for over 40 weeks from four Westinghouse FS40 lamps. The sunscreen increased the average time to tumour onset from 19 in mice given the vehicle plus UVR to 31 weeks, and reduced the average tumour yield [from approximately 13 to approximately 5.0 tumours per mouse]. The tumours were described as papillomas and squamous-cell carcinomas, but the numbers of each were not given. This larger study demonstrated synergistic protection from UVB-induced photocarcinogenesis by 2-furildioxime in combination with ethylhexyl PABA sunscreen, extending the average time to tumour onset to 77 weeks.

Recognition that UVA would probably have to be included in the radiation spectrum tested resulted in use of sources consisting of combinations of UVB and UVA fluorescent lamps. Wulf *et al.* (1982) exposed groups of 25 female *Hr/Hr* pigmented hairless mice, 10 weeks of age, to one UVB (Westinghouse FS40) and two black light lamps (Philips TL40 W/09) immediately after application of 0.1 mL per animal of one of two commercial sunscreen lotions labelled as SPF 5 and SPF 6. The animals were exposed to an incremental regime of UVR, with UVB and UVA intensities of 0.3 and 0.8 mW/cm^2, respectively, starting from 1 MED [1.8 kJ/m^2 UVB adjusted stepwise to 7.2 kJ/m^2] after 3.5 months and then remaining constant. The treatments were repeated on 4 days per week for 12 months [for a cumulative dose of 1250 kJ/m2 for UVB and 3200 kJ/m^2 for UVA]. The SPF-5 sunscreen contained glyceryl PABA and the SPF-6 contained ethylhexyl methoxycinnamate plus benzophenone-3, and therefore had greater UVA absorbance. No vehicle was used for control treatments. Observation continued until 18 months, by which time all of the unprotected UVR-exposed mice had died of skin tumours. Both sunscreens significantly delayed the average time to onset of tumours, from 205 days to 254 days for the SPF-5 product and to 284 days for the SPF-6 product, and the time of death from 86 days to 94 days for the SPF-5 product and to 128 days for the SPF-6 product. The latter therefore provided significantly

greater protection against tumour growth than the SPF-5 product, although no difference was seen between the two sunscreens in the time to death after the appearance of progressive tumours. Some toxic effects on the skin were found in mice treated with the SPF-6 product (see p. 135).

Using similar UVR sources, Gallagher *et al.* (1984) irradiated groups of 10 female HRA/Skh-1 mice after application of two samples of ethylhexyl methoxycinnamate, one of which had previously been found to induce reverse mutation in bacteria [The carcinogenicity of ethylhexyl methoxycinnamate is discussed on p. 130]. The two unfiltered UVR sources were one comprising one UVB and one UVA lamp and another comprising one UVB and three UVA lamps. Irradiation was delivered in a stepwise incremental exposure regime starting with either a 0.33 MED ('sub-erythemal') or 1 MED ('erythemal') dose daily [reaching exposures equivalent to 0.9 and 2.8 MED, respectively, in the last week]. The cumulative dose of UVB at the sub-erythemal exposure was about 18 kJ/m^2 from both sources, and that of UVA was 56 kJ/m^2 with the first source and 127 kJ/m^2 with the second. The erythemal exposure was three times greater. Groups of 20–22 mice (8–12 weeks old for the first source and 20–28 weeks old for the second) were irradiated on 5 days per week for 10 weeks 30 min after topical application to the dorsum of 0.1 mL of 50% ethylhexyl methoxycinnamate in ethanol, and then observed until day 200. The control mice received no topical application. The normal mid-dorsal skinfold thickness was not affected by the age of the mice. The sub-erythemal dose from the first source unexpectedly produced tumours slightly faster than the erythemal doses [with average times to tumour onset of 107 days and 116 days, respectively], but the first sub-erythemal regime did not induce visible or histologically evident erythema at any time. The absence of epidermal hyperplasia was

suggested to permit a greater effective dose of UVB to penetrate the skin. The erythemal dose from the second source resulted in faster tumour production than the sub-erythemal dose, which induced distinct epidermal hyperplasia histologically [with average times to tumour onset of 116 days and > 200 days, respectively]; only 40% of mice exposed to the sub-erythemal dose had tumours by day 200. More severe epidermal hyperplasia was seen histologically after the erythemal than after the sub-erythemal doses with both sources. The 50% preparation of ethylhexyl methoxycinnamate strongly protected against tumours induced by either source, and only 4/146 surviving mice acquired a persistent skin tumour after erythemal exposure. The rate of survival after UV irradiation alone was not given, but 91% of the mice exposed to ethylhexyl methoxycinnamate and UVR survived to day 200. At this time, in order to determine whether ethylhexyl methoxycinnamate had initiated any latent tumours, both irradiated and unirradiated ethylhexyl methoxycinnamate-treated mice were subjected to eight dorsal applications of 0.1 mL of 0.05% croton oil in acetone twice a week and were observed until day 300. Croton oil had no effect in 40 previously untreated control mice, significantly induced tumours on 3/16 mice that had previously received ethylhexyl methoxycinnamate alone and revealed latent tumours in 15–46% of the mice previously exposed to UVR after application of ethylhexyl methoxycinnamate.

Snyder and May (1975) gave groups of 5 or 10 hairless mice (Jackson), nine weeks of age [sex not stated], a single topical application of 0.5% 7,12-dimethylbenz[a]anthracene (DMBA) in acetone or acetone only [volume not stated] with a paintbrush as a thin coat, followed 4 weeks later by irradiation for 15 min on 3 days per week for 29 weeks with FS40 lamps [unknown number] emitting 3.0 × 10^3 W/cm^2. The cumulative dose was 240 kJ/cm^2. [If the daily exposures were consistent, the mice received 2.8 kJ/m² per day.] This protocol was developed because DMBA treatment is known to accelerate the development of squamous-cell carcinomas after exposure to UVR. Some groups of mice were treated with a sunscreen containing 5% PABA [SPF and volume not stated] or with the sunscreen base only, which contained 55% ethanol and emollients, 60 min before irradiation. The mice were observed for a further 10 weeks. The mean time to tumour onset was 35 weeks after application of DMBA plus base and 37 weeks after UVR plus base, but the tumours appeared earlier (19 weeks) after DMBA plus base plus UVR. This study demonstrated a clear co-carcinogenic synergism between DMBA and subsequent UVR, and protection against the apparent promotion of DMBA-initiated tumours by irradiation through the PABA sunscreen; however, the poor survival rate precludes reasonable quantification of the protective effect of the sunscreen.

Studies with solar-simulated UVR
The studies described below are summarized in Table 22.

An extensive study (Forbes *et al.*, 1989) of the protective effect of ethylhexyl methoxycinnamate was conducted with groups of 12 male and 12 female Skh:Hr-1 mice, 8–10 weeks of age. A mutagenic sample of ethylhexyl methoxycinnamate (see p. 137) was also included. Ethylhexyl methoxy-cinnamate was applied in 0.1 mL acetone and ethanol (1:1) at a concentration of 7.5, 50, 75 or 500 mg/mL [0.75%, 5%, 7.5% and 50%] to the rump and saddle region, and a constant dose of 600 Robertson Berger units (equivalent to an exposure of approximately 1200 sub-erythemal doses per week) of solar-simulated UVR from a filtered xenon arc source was administered 30 min after the topical applications on 3 days per week for 8 weeks. The UVR was produced horizontally, and the target area of the mice was the skin of the hind flank rather than the

mid-dorsum. The control group received the vehicle only. A regime of tumour promotion was begun 2 weeks after exposure to UVR, comprising application of 12-*O*-tetradecanoylphorbol 13-acetate (TPA) in acetone at a dose of 2 μg/mL to the dorsum three times weekly for 20 weeks. Control mice exposed to solar-simulated UVR and the sunscreen vehicle received acetone only, and one irradiated group that received ethylhexyl methoxycinnamate at a dose of 75 mg/ml was also treated with acetone only. The animals were observed for tumours until 57 weeks, at which time the survival rate was > 75% in all groups. In unprotected mice, tumours 1 mm or more in diameter began to appear from 12 weeks, and the prevalence reached 100% at 42 weeks. Treatment with TPA slightly but significantly reduced the mean time to tumour onset, from 27 to 24 weeks. Ethylhexyl methoxycinnamate delayed the appearance of tumours in a dose-dependent manner, so that the four doses resulted in progressive reductions in the maximum prevalence of 86%, 45%, 14% and 8.3%, respectively. The protective effect of the mutagenic sample of ethylhexyl methoxycinnamate was also dose-dependent, but to a lesser extent, as 50% of this sample was as effective as 7.5% of the first ethylhexyl methoxycinnamate sample. The reason for this difference was not apparent. [The SPF values of the two samples were not measured; a difference in the SPF might have accounted for the difference in the effective dose.]

In another study (Reeve *et al.*, 1985), fluorescent tubes (one UVB tube, six UVA tubes, cellulose acetate-filtered) were used as the source of solar-simulated UVR. In groups of 24–28 female hairless HRA/Skh-1 mice that received 0.1 mL of 50% ethylhexyl methoxycinnamate and 35% ethylhexyl PABA in ethanol on the dorsum 30 min before irradiation, both products protected against the effects of radiation up to 200

days after a 10-week regime of irradiation with stepwise increments of 20% per week on 5 days per week, beginning with 1 MED. The final daily dose after adaptation was 2.8 times the initial MED. The cumulative doses were stated to be 15.4 J of UVB and 294 J of UVA [which can be calculated to be 30.8 kJ/m² of UVB and 592.8 kJ/m² of UVA]. When the mice were given promotion treatment with croton oil (8 × 0.1 mL of 0.1% croton oil in acetone over 4 weeks) from day 200, latent tumours were revealed, with a 16.5% incidence in irradiated mice given ethylhexyl PABA and 39% in those given ethylhexyl methoxycinnamate by day 300. Control groups did not receive topical applications of the vehicle. Thus, even in the absence of overt tumour growth on sunscreen-protected skin, tumours were initiated and were sensitive to exogenous promotion. The difference in induction of these tumours was accounted for by the unequal photoprotection afforded by the two UVB absorbers at the tested concentrations.

In the two studies described below, sunscreens supplemented with 5-methoxypsoralen were investigated, but only the effects of the sunscreens alone are discussed. The effects of 5-methoxypsoralen are discussed on p. 131. Groups of 20 male and 20 female hairless albino mice (outbred St John's strain [age not specified]) maintained under ambient lighting free from UVR were used to test the capacity of a sunscreen containing two UVB-absorbers, 12.5 μL/mL [1.25%] ethylhexyl methoxycinnamate and 10 mg/mL [1%] 3-benzylidene camphor, in a vehicle of peanut oil, isopropylmyristate and the antioxidants butylated hydroxytoluene and butylated hydroxyanisole, to protect against photocarcinogenesis. [The SPF of the sunscreen was not given.] (Young *et al.*, 1987). Approximately 150 μL of the product or the vehicle were applied to the dorsum of mice 30–60 min before exposure to 17 kJ/m² of solar-simulated

Table 22. Effects of sunscreens on carcinogenesis induced by solar-simulated UVR in experimental animals

Strain of mouse	UV absorber	Radiation source	Cumulative dose	Average tumour incidence or multiplicity	Reference
Skh-I hairless	0.75–50% ethylhexyl methoxy-cinnamate, non- and mutagenic	Solar-simulated UVR, 3 times per week for 8 weeks, TPA x 60 at 10 weeks	14 400 Robertson Berger units	Tumour incidence: 8.3% with 50% sunscreen; 86.4% with 0.75% sunscreen; 100% in controls	Forbes *et al.* (1989)
Skh-I hairless	50% ethylhexyl methoxy-cinnamate; 35% ethylhexyl PABA	Solar-simulated UVR, 5 times per week for 10 weeks, croton oil 8 times at 200 days	30.8 kJ/m^2 UVB	Tumour incidence: 39% with ethylhexyl methoxycinnamate; 16.5% with ethylhexyl PABA; 100% in controls	Reeve *et al.* (1985)
Hairless St John's strain	1.25% ethylhexyl methoxy-cinnamate + 1% 3-benzylidene camphor	Solar-simulated UVR, 5 times per week for 45 weeks	90 kJ/m^2 UVB	Tumour multiplicity: 1.09 with sunscreen; 6.0 in controls	Young *et al.* (1987)
Skh-I hairless	0.5% ethylhexyl methoxy-cinnamate + 0.5% butyl methoxy-dibenzoylmethane	Solar-simulated UVR, 5 times per week for 73 weeks	146 kJ/m^2 UVB	Tumour incidence: 37% with sunscreen; 67% in controls	Young *et al.* (1990)
Skh-I hairless	5% terephthalylidene dicamphor sulfonic acid, sunburn protection factor, 4; 10% terephthalylidene dicamphor sulfonic acid, sunburn protection factor, 6; 5% ethylhexyl methoxycinnamate, sunburn protection factor, 4	Solar-simulated UVR, 5 times per week for 40 weeks	384 kJ/m^2 UVB	Average tumour latency: 22 weeks with ethylhexyl methoxy-cinnamate; 26 weeks with 5 or 10% terephthalylidene dicamphor sulfonic acid; 20 weeks in controls	Fourtanier (1996)
Skh-I hairless	9.5% ethylhexyl methoxycinna-mate, sunburn protection factor, 6; 7.0% ethylhexyl PABA, sunburn protection factor, 6	Solar-simulated UVR, 5 times per week for 12 weeks	360 MED solar-simulated UVR (sun-screen) or 60 MED solar-simulated UVR (vehicle)	Tumour multiplicity; 1.7 with ethyl-hexyl PABA; 8.0 with ethylhexyl methoxycinnamate; 17.5 in controls	Domanski *et al.* (1999)
C3H	10% octocrylene + 2% phenyl-benzimidazole sulfonic acid, SPF 16; 8% ethylhexyl methoxycinna-mate + 2% phenylbenzimidazole sulfonic acid, SPF 15; 9% octo-crylene + 0.3% phenylbenzimida-zole sulfonic acid + 0.7% tere-phthalylidene dicamphor sulfonic acid + 3% 3-benzylidene camphor, SPF 15; 10% octocrylene + 0.2% phenylbenzimidazole sulfonic acid + 3.25% terephthalylidene dicamphor sulfonic acid + 1.5% 3-benzylidene camphor, SPF 22	Solar-simulated UVR, 5 times per week for 70 weeks	1589 kJ/m^2 UVB	Tumour incidence: 15% with sunscreens; 100% in controls	Anantha-swamy *et al.* (1999)

Table 22 (contd)					
Cumulative	Average tumour incidence or	Reference	Cumulative dose	Average tumour incidence multiplicity	Reference
Skh-I hairless	5% ethylhexyl PABA; 10.8% ethyl-hexyl methoxycinnamate	DMBA + solar-simulated UVR 5 times per week for 6 weeks	72.9 kJ/m² UVB	Tumour incidence: 81.3% with ethylhexyl PABA; 30.8% with ethylhexyl methoxycinnamate; 85.7% in controls	Reeve et al. (1990)
C3H haired (shaved)	8% ethylhexyl methoxycinnamate, sunburn protection factor, 4; 7.2% TiO₂, sunburn protection factor, 7	DMBA + solar-simulated UVR 5 times per week for 32 weeks	571 kJ/m² UVB	Tumour incidence: 0% with ethylhexyl methoxy-cinnamate or TiO₂; 87% in controls	Bestak & Halliday (1996)

SPF, sun protection factor (in humans); DMBA, dimethylbenz[a]anthracene

UVR (290–400 nm), supplying a daily UVB dose of about 0.4 kJ/m². The treatments were continued on 5 days per week for 44–46 weeks, when the rate of survival was approximately 70%, and tumour growth was monitored. Half of the mice were retained for further observation until week 60. All the final tumours were classified histologically, and the data were analysed statistically. Some ventral tumours occurred, a common characteristic in this mouse strain, and were considered to be unrelated to the treatments. Male mice had slightly more tumours by week 25 than female mice, but no difference was evident after this time, and there was no difference in the tumour incidence between the sexes. The sunscreen alone significantly decreased the tumour incidence and reduced the tumour multiplicity progressively, from 6.0 to 1.09 tumours/mouse at 60 weeks. The progressive incidences of malignant tumours (but not benign tumours) were also reduced by the sunscreen, from 12 (no sunscreen) to 3.

In a second study, groups of 30 female Skh-1 hairless albino mice, 8–10 weeks of age, were treated with 100 μL of sunscreen consisting of the UVB absorber ethylhexyl methoxycinnamate at 0.5% and the UVA absorber butyl methoxydibenzoylmethane at 0.5% [SPF not determined] in a vehicle of 20% ethanol in water. The mice were exposed for 20–40 min after the topical applications to 17 kJ/m² of solar-simulated UVR from a vertically mounted xenon arc source on 5 days per week for up to 73 weeks, the duration of treatment being determined by the severity of the tumour response. Tumours were monitored up to the end of the study and were then classified histologically. The rate of survival was greater than 80%. The sunscreen alone was significantly protective against photocarcinogenesis, reducing the diameter of tumours, the number of tumours per mouse and the proportion of mice with histologically identified malignancies from 67% to 37% (Young et al., 1990).

In a comparison of the ability of a newly developed broad-spectrum UVA absorber, terephthalylidene dicamphor sulfonic acid, and the predominantly UVB-absorbing ethylhexyl methoxycinnamate (not mutagenic in Ames' test) to protect from photocarcinogenesis, groups of 28 female Skh-1 hairless albino mice were treated with 5% (approximate sunburn protection factor, 4) or 10% terephthalylidene dicamphor sulfonic acid (approximate sunburn protection factor, 6) or 5% ethylhexyl methoxycinnamate (approximate sunburn protection factor, 4) in 0.1 mL of a mineral oil–glycerine–water emulsified vehicle applied to the dorsal skin (approximately 40 cm²) either 30 min before irradiation with solar-simulated UVR from a filtered xenon arc source on 3 days per week or 30 min after irradiation on 2 alternate days per week. This complex experimental design was used to identify both anti-photocarcinogenic activity and enhancement of photocarcinogenesis by the test compound according to an established protocol. However, because the mice received two or five weekly exposures to UVR without the sunscreen on the skin, the possibility of demonstrating the efficacy of the product was reduced. The weekly dose of UVB was 9.6 kJ/m²; three of the exposures were through topical sunscreen to 1.6 kJ/m² and two were through unprotected skin to 2.4 kJ/m². As the MED was determined to be 3.6 kJ/m², the daily doses were sub-erythemal. Treatment was continued for 40 weeks, and the animals were observed for a further 10 weeks. The rate of survival was > 90% at 28 weeks, at which time mice with an unacceptably large tumour load were removed. Data shown only graphically in the publication indicate that tumours began to appear in unprotected mice at 16 weeks, and 100% prevalence was seen at 25 weeks. In mice treated with 5% ethylhexyl methoxycinnamate, 50% prevalence was delayed from 20 weeks in the unprotected mice to 22 weeks, but in those treated with 5% or 10% terephthalylidene dicamphor sulfonic acid, 50% prevalence was delayed until 26 weeks. The difference between the groups was reported to be significant by a log-rank test. Analysis of the average cumulative tumour yields showed no significant protection by 5% ethylhexyl methoxycinnamate but significant protection by 5% and 10% terephthalylidene dicamphor sulfonic acid, with no difference between these two concentrations. The equal sunburn protection factor values (of 4) of 5% ethylhexyl methoxycinnamate and 5% terephthalylidene dicamphor sulfonic acid do not support the observed difference in photocarcinogenic protection (Fourtanier, 1996).

Protection from photocarcinogenesis was studied in groups [size not specified] of inbred female Skh:HR-1 hairless mice, 8–12 weeks old, irradiated with a fluorescent solar-simulated UVR source on 5 days per week for 10 or 12 weeks through 0.2 mL of sunscreen lotions (sunburn protection factor, 6, determined in mice) containing either 9.5% ethylhexyl methoxycinnamate or 7.0% ethylhexyl PABA, spread over the entire dorsal skin 15 min before exposure. The daily dose of solar-simulated UVR was 6 MED [units not given], and control mice received 1 MED of solar-simulated UVR through 0.2 mL of the base lotion after determination of the MED by the increase in mid-dorsal skinfold after 24 h under the experimental conditions. Tumours were monitored for 35 weeks; at 200 days [approximately 30 weeks], the average tumour multiplicity was 17.5 in irradiated mice given base lotion, 8.0 in those given ethylhexyl methoxycinnamate and 1.7 in those given ethylhexyl PABA. The data were not analysed statistically, but it was clear that both sun-

screens provided strong protection from photocarcinogenesis when compared with the base lotion and that ethylhexyl PABA offered greater protection than ethylhexyl methoxycinnamate (Domanski et al., 1999).

In a study to assess the relationship between protection against solar-simulated UVR-induced *p53* mutations and protection against skin cancer development, shaved female C3H/HeNCr (MTV⁻) mice were treated with complete sunscreen formulations of SPF 15 or 22. Two of these sunscreens contained UVB absorbers only (octocrylene or ethylhexyl methoxycinnamate plus phenylbenzimidazole sulfonic acid), and the other two contained UVA and UVB absorbers (octocrylene plus phenylbenzimidazole sulfonic acid plus terephthalylidene dicamphor sulfonic acid plus 3-benzylidene camphor). All were applied in the same vehicle. Groups of 16 mice, 8–12 weeks of age, were irradiated five times per week with a solar simulator (xenon arc) providing 4.54 kJ/m² UVB and 30.2 kJ/m² UVA, for 70 weeks. The sunscreens were applied 30 min before exposure at 100 μL/mouse, or approximately 2 mg/cm². All mice exposed to UVR only or vehicle plus UVR developed one or more skin tumours after 48 weeks of exposure, whereas only one mouse treated with sunscreen developed a skin tumour at this time. Although additional skin tumours developed in sunscreen-treated mice upon continued irradiation, the frequency was low, only nine of the surviving 60 mice treated with sunscreen having developed skin tumours at week 70, after a total exposure of approximately 1500 kJ/m² UVB (Ananthaswamy et al., 1999). Intermediary biomarkers found in this study are described on p. 102.

Co-carcinogenicity with DMBA: The co-carcinogenicity of DMBA and solar-simulated UVR was studied in groups of 15–16 female Skh:HR-1 mice, 20–26 weeks of age. The effect of

initiation with a single application of 50 μg of DMBA in 50 μL of acetone followed 1 week later by stepwise increments of solar-simulated UVR administered on 5 days per week from a cellulose acetate-filtered fluorescent tube source, starting from 1 MED daily, for 6 weeks, was compared in mice with unprotected skin or skin to which one of two sunscreens had been applied. The skin of the dorsum received 5% ethylhexyl PABA or 10.8% ethylhexyl methoxycinnamate in ethanolic solutions matched for absorbance at 310 nm in 0.1 mL before irradiation. The cumulative UVB dose was 72.9 kJ/m². After the treatments, the mice were observed until week 37. The rate of survival was 93%. The solar-simulated UVR regime resulted in 13.3% tumour incidence and an average multiplicity of 0.2 at 260 days [37 weeks], while DMBA resulted in 26.7% tumour incidence and 0.47 multiplicity. The combination of DMBA plus solar-simulated UVR greatly enhanced the response, so that 85.7% of mice had acquired tumours with an average multiplicity of 2.0. Irradiation through ethylhexyl PABA was not significantly protective and resulted in 81.3% tumour incidence and a multiplicity of 1.44. Irradiation through ethylhexyl methoxycinnamate, however, significantly decreased the tumour incidence to 30.8% and the multiplicity to 0.38, a response that was not significantly different from that to DMBA alone. Neither sunscreen altered the response to DMBA alone. The incidence of squamous-cell carcinoma was 7% after DMBA plus solar-simulated UVR and 13% after DMBA plus solar-simulated UVR plus ethylhexyl PABA, whereas all other treatments resulted only in papillomas during the study period. The papillomas induced by DMBA and all co-carcinogenic treatments regressed, while the papillomas induced by solar-simulated UVR alone did not (Reeve et al., 1990) (Fig. 36).

The co-carcinogenicity of DMBA and solar-simulated UVR was tested in

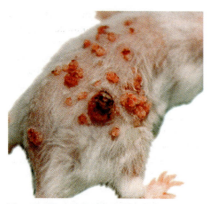

Figure 36 Experimentally induced skin papillomas on a CD1 mouse

groups of 15 shaved female C3H/HeJ mice, 10–12 weeks of age, to test sunscreens containing 8% ethylhexyl methoxycinnamate (sunburn protection factor 4 in the mouse) and 7.2% microfine TiO_2 (sunburn protection factor 7 in the mouse). Mice were initiated with 10 nmol [2.56 μg] of DMBA in 50 μL of acetone 5 days before the beginning of a stepwise incremental regime of solar-simulated UVR from a cellulose acetate-filtered fluorescent tube source (UVB irradiance, 1.7 W/m²) on 5 days per week for 32 weeks. The initial dose of solar-simulated UVR was 0.4 MED, which was increased by four weekly increments of 30%, but the exposure remained sub-oedemal throughout, giving a cumulative dose of 571 kJ/m² UVB and 11.4 MJ/m² UVA. Some groups were treated at least 10 min before irradiation with either ethylhexyl methoxycinnamate, microfine TiO_2 or the vehicle, which was an oil-in-water emulsion containing 0.1% butylated hydroxytoluene and 0.5% α-tocopherol, or the vehicle without these antioxidant additives. Tumours ≥ 3 mm in diameter were monitored until week 48. Solar-simulated UVR alone resulted in a 46% tumour incidence at 48 weeks. Whereas DMBA alone did not induce tumours, treatment with DMBA plus solar-simulated UVR resulted in a 87% tumour incidence, with an average onset of 37 weeks. The sunscreen vehicle did not alter this frequency significantly, but both ethylhexyl methoxycinnamate and TiO_2 protected against tumour development at 48 weeks. In the unprotected irradiated groups, the final average tumour multiplicity varied from 1.1 to 1.4, but the differences were not statistically analysed. All the tumours that were examined histologically were squamous-cell carcinomas, and no regressions were recorded. Thus, at low daily doses of solar-simulated UVR, both sunscreens protected from co-carcinogenesis by DMBA plus solar-simulated UVR (Bestak & Halliday, 1996).

Inorganic sunscreens: ZnO and TiO_2 of small particle size are new developments in inorganic sunscreens, and there are few adequate studies of the efficacy of these products in protecting animals against photocarcinogenesis. Groups of 30 female Skh:HR-1 mice were maintained under ambient lighting free from UVR and received an incremental regime of solar-simulated UVR from a cellulose acetate-filtered fluorescent tube source, starting with a daily dose of 1 MED and increasing in a stepwise manner to 2 MED per day, on 5 days per week for 12 weeks after topical application of 0.3 mL (2 mg/cm²) of an SPF 15 sunscreen containing aluminium stearate-coated, microfine TiO_2 as the only active ingredient. After the 12 weeks of irradiation, the mice were given topical applications of croton oil on the dorsal skin. Tumours appeared in 100% of the mice treated with solar-simulated UVR plus croton oil [although the figure in the publication indicates a 95% incidence] by 52 weeks, whereas addition of the sunscreen reduced the final incidence to 25%. The study indicates protection against photocarcinogenesis by the TiO_2 sunscreen (Greenoak et al., 1993). [The Working Group noted that the doses of UVR were not stated, and no controls receiving only the vehicle or only croton oil after solar-simulated UVR or after sunscreen alone were included.]

In a second study, a sunscreen containing 3.5% microfine ZnO plus 3.5% ethylhexyl methoxycinnamate, which had a sunburn protection factor of 7 in mice under the study conditions, was tested in the same strain of mice. The protocol was intended to simulate sunscreen use by humans previously exposed without protection to a latent carcinogenic dose of solar-simulated UVR. Thus, the mice were irradiated at selected multiples of the MED through the sunscreen (Greenoak et al., 1998). [The protocol was, however, inconsistent, the UVR was undefined and the control treatments were inadequate.]

Intermediary biomarkers

Evaluation of the preventive effects of sunscreens against UVR-induced skin cancers in animal models is labour-intensive, time-consuming and expensive. In addition, when sunscreens with high SPFs are evaluated, the animals may die before sufficient numbers of tumours are seen to distinguish differences between treatment regimens. One solution is to use priming doses of UVR without protection, but this allows only evaluation of protection against the promotion phase of the tumour process. As experiments for photocarcinogenesis necessarily last more than 1 year, a large number of animals must be included to compensate for accidental deaths. When a large number of animals is exposed, the UVR source must be powerful, and xenon arc lamps, the only source that delivers a spectrum which resembles that of the sun, are particularly expensive. This source emits a considerable amount of infrared radiation, which is difficult to filter out, and the animals must be placed far from the source. As a consequence, the amount of irradiance reaching the skin is reduced and the exposure time must be increased which may result in elimination of the sunscreen by grooming.

For these reasons, earlier, surrogate biomarkers have been used to evaluate the efficacy of sunscreens against UVR-induced skin cancer. Some biomarkers are transient (e.g. DNA damage and sunburn cells), while others are persistent (e.g. *p53* mutations). The markers may be steps in the pathway of photocarcinogenesis and therefore possibly 'causal'; they may only be related to the pathway (e.g. apoptotic cells); or they may simply be associated with exposure to UVR. Only the biomarkers that are in the pathway of photocarcinogenesis are evaluated on p. 144.

Molecular and cellular biomarkers
Studies of molecular and cellular biomarkers are summarized in Table 23.

DNA damage: The inhibition of DNA synthesis and the characteristic lesions, cyclobutane pyrimidine dimers and pyrimidine (6–4) pyrimidone, induced by direct absorption of UVR by DNA have been used to evaluate the protective efficacy of sunscreens in six studies.

In the first study, the ability of seven commercial sunscreens to protect against UVR-induced inhibition of epidermal DNA synthesis was evaluated in the hairless mouse model (HRS/J). Two hours after one exposure to UVB (0.03–1.8 kJ/m^2) delivered by Westinghouse FS20 fluorescent tubes, a significant decrease in tritiated thymidine incorporation was measured in DNA, reflecting a decrease in DNA synthesis. The maximum inhibition (70–80% below that of unexposed ventral skin) occurred at 0.15 kJ/m^2. The SPFs of the sunscreens were between 4 and 15 (claimed on the label of sunscreen product tested) or 4 and 24 (claimed by the manufacturer). A ZnO ointment was also evaluated, but the concentration of the active ingredient and the SPF of this preparation were not given. The sunscreen preparations were applied at 4 μL/cm^2 (about 4 mg/cm^2) and the ZnO ointment at 12 μL/cm^2. Statistically

significant differences in the efficacy of the sunscreens were found. The DNA protective factors, defined as the ratio of the UVR dose required to inhibit DNA synthesis by 50% with and without sunscreen, were 4.4 for the SPF 4 sunscreen, 8.4 for the SPF 6 product and 21–27.6 for the SPF 15 products. The ZnO ointment was protective at all UVR doses used. A relatively good correlation was found between the DNA protective factor and the SPF (Walter, 1981).

The ability of 1, 5 or 10% of fine-particle-size TiO$_2$, 1% PABA or 1% urocanic acid in white petroleum to prevent changes in epidermal DNA synthesis was evaluated in female hairless mice. The animals were exposed to single doses of UVB (4.4, 8.8 or 17.6 kJ/m^2) from unfiltered Toshiba FL20SE-30 fluorescent tubes, and they received approximately 2 mg/cm^2 of the sunscreens. Suppression of DNA synthesis was seen 1 h after exposure of unprotected animals. None of the sunscreens protect against the suppression induced by 8.8 kJ/m^2 UVB, except 5% TiO$_2$. DNA synthesis was strongly increased (fivefold by 4.4 kJ/m^2 and eightfold by 8.8 kJ/m^2) 48 h after exposure in comparison with the level in unexposed controls. [No data were reported for 17.6 kJ/m^2.] PABA and urocanic acid gave very little protection against this increase, whereas 1% and 5% TiO$_2$ gave complete protection. The protective effect of TiO$_2$ increased proportionately with the concentration used, and a dose of 10% TiO$_2$ was protective against the high dose of UVR (Suzuki, 1987).

The photoprotective effects against the formation of cyclobutane pyrimidine dimers of sunscreen preparations containing 8% ethylhexyl PABA, 7.5% ethylhexyl methoxycinnamate or 6% benzophenone-3 were studied in female C3H/HeNCr (MTV⁻) mice exposed to a single dose of 5 kJ/m^2 UVB from unfiltered FS40 sunlamps (fluorescent tubes). The SPFs and the absorption

spectra of the sunscreen preparations were unknown. The quantities applied were 200–250 μL/mouse. The frequency of cyclobutane pyrimidine dimers in epidermal DNA was determined by an assay sensitive for endonucleases with alkaline agarose gels. The number of cyclobutane pyrimidine dimers was reduced by 91% by ethylhexyl PABA, 86% by ethylhexyl methoxycinnamate and 67% by benzophenone-3. The vehicle had no protective effect (Wolf et al., 1993a).

Pyrimidine dimers were measured by the endonuclease-sensitive assay with alkaline sucrose gradients in epidermal DNA of female Skh:Hr1 mice. Groups of mice were exposed to single dose of solar-simulated UVR (290–400 nm) or UVA (320–400 nm) without topical treatment, or after topical application of 2 mg/cm^2 of the vehicle, a UVB absorber (ethylhexyl methoxycinnamate at 5%) or a broad-spectrum UVA absorber (terephthalylidene dicamphor sulfonic acid at 5%). The sunburn protection factor of the sunscreen preparations determined in the mouse model were similar (4). DNA protection factors were determined for both preparations and were 6.6 for ethylhexyl methoxycinnamate and 11.5 for terephthalylidene dicamphor sulfonic acid with solar-simulated UVR, and 2 and 8, respectively, with UVA. Both UVR filters were effective, but terephthalylidene dicamphor sulfonic acid was significantly more effective than ethylhexyl methoxycinnamate in protecting against the induction of pyrimidine dimers. The vehicle provided a slight but nonsignificant protective effect (Ley & Fourtanier, 1997).

Accumulation of cyclobutane pyrimidine dimers in DNA of female C3H/HeNTac mice exposed to a single irradiance of 2.5 J/m^2 per s of UVB (unfiltered Westinghouse FS20 lamp) for 1 h (about 9 kJ/m^2) was measured after application at approximately 4 mg/cm^2 of various commercial sunscreens (SPF 8, 15 or 30) or preparations containing various concentrations of PABA (5, 10,

Table 23. Molecular and cellular biomarkers of UVR-induced carcinogenesis

Animal species, strain (no. per group)	UVR source	UVR regimen	Sunscreen	Results	Reference
DNA damage					
Mouse, Skh:hr1 (9–15)	Solar-simulated UVR, 2–30 x 10^4 J/m^2, and UVA (xenon), 2–13 x 10^5 J/m^2	Single	5% terephthalylidene dicamphor sulfonic acid (sunburn protective factor, 4); 5% ethylhexylmethoxy-cinnamate (sunburn protective factor, 4)	Significant protection, with DNA protection factor > sunburn protection factor	Ley & Fourtanier (1997)
Sunburn cells (apoptotic cells)					
Mouse, Skh:hr1 (3–4)	Solar-simulated UVR (xenon), 0.11–1.8 kJ/m^2	Single	Commercial sunscreen (SPF 12); ethyl-hexyl methoxycinnamate; benzophenone-3; ZnO; talc. Pure or diluted (12.5, 25 or 50%)	No protection with 12.5% sunscreen, significant protection with 25 and 50%	Sambuco et al. (1984)
***p53* mutations**					
Mouse, C3H (20)	Filtered UVB from tubes, 4.5 kJ/m^2 per day	Repeated, 5 days per week, 12 weeks	Phenylbenzimidazole sulfonic acid, 2%; octocrylene, 10% (SPF 15)	Significant protection	Ananthaswamy et al. (1997)
			Phenylbenzimidazole sulfonic acid, 0.3%; octocrylene, 9%; terephthalylidene dicamphor sulfonic acid, 0.7%; butyl methoxydibenzoylmethane, 3% (SPF 15)	Significant protection	
Mouse, C3H (16)	Solar-simulated UVB (xenon), 4.5 kJ/m^2 per day	Repeated, 5 days per week, 16 weeks	Phenylbenzimidazole sulfonic acid; 2%; octocrylene, 10% (SPF 15)	Significant protection	Ananthaswamy et al. (1999)
			Phenylbenzimidazole sulfonic acid, 0.3%; octocrylene, 9%; terephthalylidene dicamphor sulfonic acid, 0.7%; butyl methoxydibenzoylmethane, 3% (SPF 15)	Significant protection	
			Ethylhexyl methoxycinnamate, 8%; phenylbenzimidazole sulfonic acid, 2% (SPF 15)	Significant protection	
			Octocrylene, 10%; phenylbenzimidole sulfonic acid, 0.2%; butyl methoxy-dibenzoyl methane, 1.5%; terephthalylidene dicamphor sulfonic acid, 3.25% (SPF 22)	Significant protection	

SPF, sun protection factor

15 or 20%) in a neutral cream vehicle. The UVR absorber in the commercial products consisted of combinations of benzophenone-3, ethylhexylmethoxycin-namate and ethylhexyl salicylate or ethylhexyl PABA and glyceryl PABA esters. Their protection factors in the mouse model were not determined. The SPF-8 sunscreen reduced dimer formation to 48% of the control level, but statistically significant protection was seen only with the SPF-15 (approximately 67% of control) and -30 (approximately 88% of control) products. Application of the PABA preparations resulted in a dose-dependent effect. A 10% dispersion was necessary to give significant protection (approximately 45% of controls receiving the vehicle); the 15% dispersion gave about 80% protection, and the 20% dispersion about 90% that in controls (McVean & Liebler, 1997).

The same protocol (female C3H/HeNTac mice, unfiltered FS20 sunlamps, a single dose of 9 kJ/m², cyclobutane pyrimidine dimer determination, 4 mg/cm² application of sunscreen) was used to evaluate preparations containing a single UVB absorber, 5% ethylhexyl methoxycinnamate or 5% ethylhexyl salicylate, or a single UVA plus UVB absorber, 5% benzophenone-3. The SPFs of the preparations were not measured or specified. Only the ethylhexyl methoxycinnamate preparation significantly inhibited thymine dimer formation, by about 60% compared with controls exposed without sunscreen (McVean & Liebler, 1999).

DNA damage is considered to be a transient, causal early biomarker in the pathway of photocarcinogenesis. All six studies showed protection against DNA damage by sunscreens, but only one study used solar-simulated UVR and provided information on the dose–response relationship.

p53 accumulation and sunburn cells or apoptotic cells: TP53 is expressed after DNA damage, as this protein induces transient cell cycle arrest allowing DNA repair or apoptosis to take place. The apoptotic keratinocytes produced after exposure to UVR have been called 'sunburn cells' (Fig. 37). No animal model has been used to measure accumulation of TP53 and protection by sunscreens, but the number of apoptotic cells formed after exposure to UVR has been determined in order to evaluate the efficacy of sunscreens. The cells were counted in histological sections stained with haematoxylin and eosin, except in one study (Okamoto et al., 1999) in which the terminal deoxynucleotidyl transferase-mediated UTP nick and labelling (TUNEL) technique was used.

In the first study, male hairless Skh-1 mice were exposed to increasing doses of solar-simulated UVR (290–400 nm) through a commercial SPF-12 product containing ethylhexyl methoxycinnamate, ZnO, talc and benzophenone-3. This product was applied, diluted in its vehicle to 50, 25 or 12.5% of the original concentration, at a dose of 2 µL/cm². The output of the simulator was measured with a Robertson Berger meter.

Each animal was exposed for 0, 1, 2, 4, 8 and 16 min (1.7 min corresponds to 0.96 Robertson Berger sunburn unit and is equal to 1 MED or 0.2 kJ/m²). A progressive increase in the protective effect was seen with increasing relative concentration of the sunscreen, and all treatments were significantly effective, except that with the 12.5% preparation (Sambuco et al., 1984).

In two studies, female C3H/HeN mice were exposed twice a week for 3 weeks to 4.8 kJ/m² UVB or to a single dose of UVB at 5 kJ/m² delivered by unfiltered FS40 sunlamps. Application at 200–250 µL/mouse of preparations of unknown SPF containing a single UVB absorber (8% ethylhexyl PABA or 7.5% ethylhexyl methoxycinnamate) or a single UVA plus UVB absorber (6% benzophenone-3) almost completely prevented the formation of sunburn cells, whereas the vehicle was ineffective. The three sunscreen preparations did not differ in efficacy (Wolf et al., 1994, 1995).

A further study on the effect of sunscreens on sunburn cell formation was

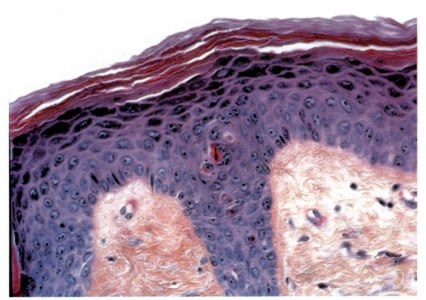

Figure 37 UVR induces keratinocyte apoptosis. The dead cells are called 'sunburn cells' and can be counted on skin sections and used to evaluate the efficacy of sunscreens.

conducted with domestic male Yorkshire pigs. The backs of the animals were treated at 0.1 mL/10 cm^2 twice a day for 3 days and 30 min before irradiation with 3–4 MED of UVB (unfiltered Westing-house FS40 fluorescent bulbs; 3 kJ/m^2). Biopsy samples were taken after 24 h, and sunburn cells were counted. PABA dissolved at 0.1% in an aqueous solution containing propylene glycol and hydroxy-propylcellulose and benzophenone-3 dissolved at 0.25% in ethanol, propylene glycol and water were protective (Darr et al., 1996).

The protection afforded by a SPF-60 commercial sunscreen [composition not given] on the induction of apoptotic cells was measured in female C3H/He mice exposed to a single dose of 0.25 or 0.5 kJ/m^2 of UVB delivered by an unfiltered Toshiba fluorescent sunlamp (FL20SE) with or without application of the sun-screen at 50 µl/mouse 30 min before exposure. Skin biopsy samples were obtained 24 h after exposure, and epi-dermal sheets were prepared by incuba-tion in EDTA and stained by the TUNEL technique. The cells were enumerated under a fluorescence microscope. The sunscreen was effective in reducing the induction of apoptic cells at both irradi-ances, with about 90% reduction when compared with unprotected animals (Okamoto et al., 1999).

Sunburn or apoptotic cells are consid-ered to be transient biomarkers of expo-sure to UVR but are not in the direct pathway of photocarcinogenesis. In five studies, sunscreens protected against the occurrence of this biomarker, but only one study used solar-simulated UVR and provided information on the dose–response relationship in hairless mice.

p53 *mutations:* Cells that acquire muta-tions at dipyrimidine sites, in particular in the *p53* gene, can expand clonally and may become a precancerous lesion. Two papers from the same authors (Ananthaswamy et al., 1997, 1999) report the results of studies of this marker.

Female C3H/HeNCr mice were exposed to repeated doses of UVB delivered by Kodacel filtered FS40 sunlamps (4.5 kJ/m^2 [2.3 MED]) on 5 days per week for 12 weeks. The efficacy of two prototype sunscreen preparations applied at 2 mg/cm^2 was measured by counting the number of *p53* mutations in exposed mouse skin. One sunscreen contained only UVB absorbers, 10% octocrylene and 2% phenylbenzimidazole sulfonic acid, while the other contained two UVA (3% butyl methoxydibenzoylmethane and 0.7% terephthalylidene dicamphor sulfonic acid) and two UVB absorbers (9% ocrocrylene and 0.3% phenylbenz-imidazole sulfonic acid). The vehicle and the SPF (15) were similar for the two preparations. After 12 weeks, 9/20 mice exposed to the vehicle plus UVR had CC→TT mutations at codon 148, 154–155 or 175–176. In contrast, only 1 of 20 mice treated with the UVB sun-screen plus UVR and 2 of 20 mice exposed and treated with the UVB plus UVA sunscreen had mutations at these codons.

In the second paper (Ananthaswamy et al., 1999), the same strain of mice and the same techniques were used to analyse *p53* mutations in epidermal DNA, but the animals were exposed for 16 weeks to solar-simulated UVR (4.5 kJ/m^2 UVB and 30.3 kJ/m^2 UVA) on 5 days per week. The dose of UVA plus UVB was 34.8 kJ/m^2 per exposure. Four sunscreens were studied: the same two sunscreens as in the previous study, a SPF-15 product containing 8% ethyl-hexyl methoxycinnamate and 2% phenylbenzimidazole sulfonic acid (UVB absorbers) and a SPF-22 product con-taining 10% octocrylene, 0.2% phenyl-benzimidazole sulfonic acid, 3.25% terephthalylidene dicamphor sulfonic acid and 1.5% butyl methoxydibenzoyl methane (UVB plus UVA absorbers). All the UVR absorbers were introduced in the same vehicle, and the products were applied at a dose of 2 mg/cm^2. Pooled data for all three codons showed the

presence of nine mutations in 16 mice treated with the vehicle (oil-in-water emulsion) plus UVR and in none of 16 mice treated with the SPF-16 (octocrylene plus phenylbenzimidazole sulfonic acid) sunscreen or the SPF-22 (octocrylene plus phenylbenzimidazole sulfonic acid plus terephthalylidene dicamphor sulfonic acid plus butyl methoxydibenzoyl methane) sunscreen. Only 1/16 mice treated with the SPF-15 sunscreen containing ethylhexymethoxy-cinnamate plus phenylbenzimidazole sulfonic acid and 2/16 of those treated with the SPF-15 sunscreen containing octocrylene plus phenylbenzimidazole sulfonic acid plus terephthalylidene dicamphor sulfonic acid plus butyl methoxydibenzoyl methane had detectable *p53* mutations. Overall, the sunscreens used in this study inhibited the number of UV-induced p53 mutations by 80–100%.

p53 mutations are considered to be a persistent biomarker in the pathway of the development of squamous-cell carci-noma. One study showed that sunscreen products protect against *p53* mutations induced by solar-simulated UVR, but the dose–response relationship was not evaluated.

Immunological end-points
It is now clearly established that UVR induces immune suppression, thus permitting the growth of tumour cells. The immunological impairment caused by UVR can be divided into local and systemic effects. Local immune suppres-sion is defined as a diminished contact hypersensitivity response to haptens, when they are applied at a UVR-irradiated site. Exposure to UVR can also result in a diminished contact hypersensitivity response when haptens are applied at a distant, unirradiated site, and this is referred to as 'systemic immune suppression'. In contrast, delayed-type hypersensitivity reactions occur when antigens are injected. The rejection of melanoma and non-

melanoma skin cancers is also altered by exposure to UVR. UVR-induced immune suppression has also been demonstrated in assays that do not involve tumour cells. In these assays, the immune system is primed to react with a certain simple chemical (the hapten) in a first contact known as sensitization or immunization (the afferent stage), which evokes a (hapten-) specific immune response. Exposure to UVR is then found to suppress the ultimate reaction. In most studies, exposure to UVR occurs before the immunization, although in a few studies it has been done after immunization, before the challenge (efferent stage).

Immunological reactions have been used to evaluate the efficacy of sunscreens. In experimental animals, UVR-induced lack of responsiveness to haptens is associated with the presence of hapten-specific T suppressor cells. The mechanism by which UVR activates the suppressor rather than the effector arm of the immune response is not completely understood; however, alterations in the number and activity of constituents of the dermal immune system (Langerhans cells and dendritic epidermal T cells) and the production of soluble factors (cytokines, neuropeptides, prostaglandins and growth factors) have been implicated. In addition, urocanic acid in the stratum corneum, when isomerized from the *trans* to the *cis* form by UVR, has immune suppressive properties. DNA damage also appears to be involved in immune suppression by UVR. The studies that have been conducted on immunological end-points are summarized in Table 24.

Langerhans cells and dendritic epidermal T cells: The role of sunscreens in preventing alterations in Langerhans cells (Fig. 38) was determined by counting ATPase-positive cells on epidermal sheets. C3Hf/HeN mice were exposed repeatedly to UVR from unfiltered fluorescent FS40 sunlamps, for 30 min/day with 3.22 kJ/m² through a commercial sunscreen containing 5% PABA as the UVR absorber. Daily treatment with the sunscreen, 'applied liberally and rubbed in', decreased the number of ATPase-positive cells from the second day of exposure for up to 11 days. In PABA-pretreated animals, a decrease was measured on days 3 and 4, but the number had returned to normal by day 7 or 8 (depending on the experiment). The morphology of the remaining cells in both unprotected and protected animals was altered (Lynch *et al.*, 1981).

HRA:Skh-1 hairless albino and HRA:Skh-2 hairless pigmented mice were exposed for 5 days/week for 4 weeks under six F40BL UVA tubes flanking a single Oliphant FL40SE UVB tube filtered with Kodacel, providing fluorescent solar-simulated UVR. The mice were unrestricted and received increasing doses of UVR, for average cumulated doses of 42 kJ/m² UVB and 811 kJ/m² UVA. Two SPF-15 sunscreen preparations were evaluated. One contained 6.5% ethylhexyl PABA plus 3% benzophenone-3, and the other 7.5% ethylhexyl methoxycinnamate plus 4.5% benzophenone-3. The vehicles (unspecified base lotions) were different. Simple solutions of 6.5% ethylhexyl PABA or 7.5% ethylhexyl methoxycinnamate in ethanol, dimethyl sulfoxide and acetone were also studied. All the products were applied at 2 mg/cm². At the end of the exposure, the mice were killed and epidermal sheets were prepared from excised skin and immunostained to detect Langerhans cells or dendritic epidermal T cells. Langerhans cells were significantly depleted in epidermis exposed for 4 weeks when compared with that from unirradiated mice. The densities of Langerhans cells in animals treated with the ethylhexyl PABA sunscreen, ethylhexyl PABA in solution, the ethylhexyl methoxycinnamate sunscreen or ethylhexyl methoxycinnamate in solution and in unexposed mice did not differ significantly, and the densities in exposed and vehicle-treated mice did not differ from those of the group receiving UVR only. Similar results were found in the two mouse strains. In contrast, ethylhexyl PABA but not ethylhexyl methoxycinnamate protected dendritic

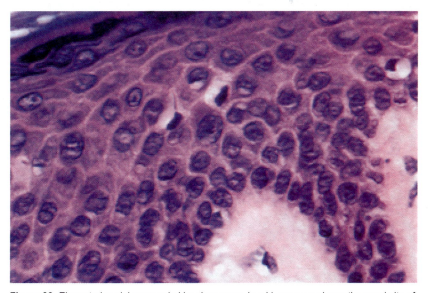

Figure 38 Elongated nuclei surrounded by clear space in mid-squamous layer, the usual site of Langerhans cells

Table 24. Immunological biomarkers of exposure to and effects of UVR

Animal species, strain (no. per group)	UVR source	UVR regimen	Sunscreen	Effect	Results investigated	Reference
Langerhans cells						
Mouse, Skh-1/Skh-2 (6)	Solar-simulated UVR (fluorescent tubes)	Repeated: 5 days per week for 4 weeks (dose increasing by 20% every week)	Commercial sunscreen: ethylhexyl PABA, 6.5%; benzophenone-3, 3% (SPF 15)	Numbers of Langerhans cells (Ia$^+$) and dendritic epidermal T cells	Significant protection	Ho et al. (1992)
		Total dose, 42 kJ/m² UVB, 811 kJ/m² UVA	Commercial sunscreen: ethylhexyl methoxycinnamate 7.5%; benzophenone 3, 4.5% (SPF 15)		Significant protection for Langerhans but not dendritic cells	
			Ethylhexyl PABA, 6.5% solution / Ethylhexyl methoxycinnamate, 7.5% solution		Significant protection / Significant protection for Langerhans but not dendritic cells	
Mouse, Skh-1 (5–14)	Solar-simulated UVR (fluorescent tubes)	Single dose, 2 MED 1 MED = 5.5 kJ/m² UVB, 530 kJ/m² UVA	1 or 2 applications	Number of Langerhans cells (Ia$^+$)	1st application / 2nd application	Walker et al. (1994)
			Ethylhexyl methoxycinnamate, 9% in lotion		No protection / Significant protection	
			Ethylhexyl methoxycinnamate, 9% in ethanol		Significant protection / Significant protection	
			Ethylhexyl methoxycinnamate, 9% in lotion	Langerhans cell function (mixed epidermal cell–lymphocyte reaction)	No protection / Significant protection	
			Ethylhexyl methoxycinnamate, 9% in ethanol		No protection / Significant protection	
Mouse, Skh-1 (10)	Solar-simulated UVR (xenon)	Single dose-effect, 2–4 MED 1 MED = 3.7 kJ/m² UVB	Terephthalylidene dicamphor sulfonic acid, 5% (sunburn protection factor 4) / Ethylhexyl methoxycinnamate, 5% (sunburn protection factor, 4)	Number of Langerhans cells (Ia$^+$)	Significant protection, less than predicted from sunburn protection factor / Significant protection, less than predicted from sunburn protection factor	Guéniche & Fourtanier (1997)
Mouse, Skh-1 and C3H (5)	Filtered UVB tubes	2 consecutive single doses of 1.8 kJ/m² each	5 commercial sunscreens: Ethylhexyl methoxycinnamate 3.5%; benzophenone-3, 1% (SPF 4) / Ethylhexyl methoxycinnamate 7%, benzophenone-3, 2% (SPF 8)	Number of Langerhans cells (Ia$^+$) in C3H mice	Significant protection, proportional to SPF / Significant protection, proportional to SPF	Beasley et al. (1998)

Table 24 (contd)

Animal species, strain (no. per group)	UVR source	UVR regimen	Sunscreen	Effect	Results	Reference
Mouse, Skh-1 and C3H (contd)			Ethylhexyl methoxycinnamate 7.5%; benzophenone-3, 4% (SPF 15)		Significant protection, proportional to SPF	Reeve (1997)
			Ethylhexyl methoxycinnamate 7.5%; benzophenone-3, 4% octyl salicylate, 5%; homosalate, 5% (SPF 30)		Significant protection (also in Skh-1 mice), proportional to SPF	
			Ethylhexyl methoxycinnamate, 7.5%; benzophenone-3, 6%; octyl salicylate 5%; octocrylene, 8% (SPF 45)		Significant protection, proportional to SPF	
Urocanic acid						
Mouse, Skh (2)	Solar-simulated UVR (fluorescent tubes)	Repeated: 5 x 6 MED or 20 x 6 MED 1 MED = 2 kJ/m² UVB plus 24.5 kJ/m2 UVA	Ethylhexyl PABA (sunburn protection factor 6) Ethylhexyl methoxycinnamate (sunburn protection factor, 6)	*trans* to *cis* isomerization	No protection No protection	Guéniche & Fourtanier (1997)
Cytokines						
Mouse, Skh-1 (10)	Solar-simulated UVR (xenon)	Single dose–effect, 2–4 MED 1 MED = 3.7 kJ/m² UVB	Terephthalylidene dicamphor sulfonic acid, 5% (sunburn protection factor, 4) Ethylhexyl methoxycinnamate 5% (sunburn protection factor, 4)	Interleukin-10 in sera	Significant protection, less than predicted from sunburn protection factor Significant protection, less than predicted from sunburn protection factor	Morison et al. (1985)
Contact hypersensitivity, delayed-type hypersensitivity, tumour susceptibility						
Guinea-pig, strain-2 (3)	Sun	Repeated: 5 h/day, 3 days	PABA, 5%	Local contact hypersensitivity to oxazolone	No protection	Fisher et al. (1989)
Mouse, HRA/Skh (10)	Solar-simulated UVR (xenon)	Repeated: 72 kJ/m² per day, 5 days	2 commercial sunscreens: Ethylhexyl PABA, benzophenone-3 (SPF 6) Ethylhexyl PABA, benzophenone-3 (SPF 15)	Systemic contact hypersensitivity to trinitrochloro-benzene	No protection No protection	Ho et al. (1992)
Mouse, HRA/Skh (6)	Solar-simulated UVR (fluorescent tubes)	Repeated: 5 days/week, 4 weeks (increasing dose) Total dose, 42 kJ/m² UVB, 811 KJm² UVA	2 commercial sunscreens (2 mg/cm²): Ethylhexyl PABA, 6.5% benzophenone-3, 3% (SPF 15) Ethlhexyl methoxy-cinnamate, 7.5%, benzophenone-3, 4.5% (SPF 15)	Local contact hypersensitivity to trinitrochloro-benzene	No protection No protection	

Table 24 (contd)

Animal species, strain (no. per group)	UVR source	UVR regimen	Sunscreen	Effect investigated	Results	Reference
Mouse, BALB/c and C3H (6)	Solar-simulated UVR (fluorescent tubes)	Repeated: 5 days/week, 4 weeks, increased by 20% (i) or 30% (ii) Total dose: (i) 70 kJ/m² UVB, 1410 kJ/m² UVA (ii) 80 kJ/m² UVB, 1580 kJ/m² UVA for BALB/c; 35 kJ/m² UVB, 682 kJ/m² UVB for C3H	(i) Ethylhexyl PABA, 8% (sunburn protection factor, 4) Ethylhexyl methoxycinnamate, 8% (sunburn protection factor 4) TiO₂, 7.2% (sunburn protection factor, 7)	Local contact hypersensitivity to trinitrochloro-benzene	BALB/c mice No protection Significant protection Significant protection	Bestak et al. (1995)
			(ii) Ethylhexyl PABA, 8% (sunburn protection factor, 4) Ethylhexyl methoxycinnamate, 8% (sunburn protection factor, 4) TiO₂, 7.2% (sun protection factor, 7)		No protection No protection No protection	
			(ii) Ethylhexyl PABA, 8% (sunburn protection factor, 4) Ethylhexyl methoxycinnamate 8% (sunburn protection factor, 4) TiO₂, 7.2% (sunburn protection factor, 7)	Tolerance	No protection No protection Significant protection	
			(ii) Ethylhexyl PABA, 8% (sunburn protection factor 4)[a] Ethylhexyl methoxycinnamate (sunburn protection factor, 4)[a] TiO₂, 7.2% (sunburn protection factor, 7)[a] ZnO (sunburn protection factor, 9)	Local contact hypersensitivity to trinitrochloro-benzene	C3H mice No protection No protection Significant protection Significant protection	
			(ii) Ethylhexyl PABA, 8% (sunburn protection factor, 4)[a] Ethylhexyl methoxycinnamate (sunburn protection factor, 4)[a] TiO₂, 7.2% (sunburn protection, factor 7)[a] ZnO (sunburn protection factor, 9)	Tolerance	No protection No protection Significant protection Significant protection	

Table 24 (contd)

Animal species, strain (no. per group)	UVR source	UVR regimen	Sunscreen	Effect investigated	Results	Reference
Mouse, C3H (5)	Filtered UVB tubes	Two single doses: 1.8 kJ/m² per day	10 commercial sunscreens: Ethylhexyl methoxycinnamate, 3.5%; benzophenone-3, 1% (SPF, 4) Ethylhexyl methoxycinnamate, 7%; benzophenone-3, 2% (SPF, 8) Ethylhexyl methoxycinnamate, 7.5%; benzophenone-3, 4% (SPF, 15) Ethylhexyl PABA, 8%; benzophenone-3, 4% (SPF, 15) Ethylhexyl methoxycinnamate, benzophenone-3 (SPF, 15) Ethylhexyl PABA, ethylhexyl methoxycinnamate, benzophenone-3 (SPF, 15) Ethylhexyl methoxycinnamate, 7.5% benzophenone-3, 4% (SPF, 15) Ethylhexyl methoxycinnamate, benzophenone-3 (SPF, 15) Ethylhexyl methoxycinnamate, 7.5%; benzophenone-3, 4.5% (SPF, 15) Ethylhexyl methoxycinnamate, 7.5%; octyl salicylate, 5%; homosalate, 5%; benzophenone-3, 4% (SPF, 30)	Local contact hypersensitivity to 2,4-dinitro-1-fluorobenzene	No protection with SPF < 15; significant protection with SPF > 15. Protection increased with quantity applied	Roberts & Beasley (1995)
	Solar-simulated UVR (xenon)	Two single doses, 2–15 MISD, dose-effect 1 MISD = 0.9 kJ/m²	Ethylhexyl methoxycinnamate, 7.5%; benzophenone-3, 4% (SPF, 15)		Significant protection with 2–7.5 MISD; no protection with 15 MISD	
		Two single doses, 2–60 MISD, dose-effect 1 MISD = 1.35 kJ/m²	Ethylhexyl methoxycinnamate, 7.5%; benzophenone-3, 4% (SPF, 15)		Significant protection with 2–30 MISD; no protection with 40 MISD	
Mouse, C3H (10–15)	Filtered UVB tubes or solar-simulated UVR (xenon)	Two single doses, dose-effect UVB: 2–15 MISD 1 MISD = 0.9 kJ/m² Solar-simulated UVR: 2–60 MISD 1 MISD = 1.35 kJ/m²	4 commercial sunscreens: Ethylhexyl methoxycinnamate, 3.5%; benzophenone-3, 1% (SPF, 4) Ethylhexyl methoxycinnamate, 7%; benzophenone-3, 2% (SPF, 8)	Local contact hypersensitivity to 2,4-dinitro-1-fluorobenzene	Significant protection against UVB, protection equal to or less than SPF Significant protection against solar-simulated UVR, protection equal to or greater than SPF	Roberts et al. (1996)

Table 24 (contd)

Animal species, strain (no. per group)	UVR source	UVR regimen	Sunscreen	Effect	Results investigated	Reference
Mouse, C3H (10–15) (contd)			Ethylhexyl methoxycinnamate, 7.5%; benzophenone-3, 4% (SPF, 15) Ethylhexyl methoxycinnamate, 7.5%; octyl salicylate, 5%; benzophenone-3, 4% (SPF, 30)			
Mouse, C3H (5–10)	Solar-simulated UVR (UVA-340 sunlamps)	Two single doses, 1–60 MISD, dose-effect 1 MISD = 1 kJ/m²	4 commercial sunscreens: Ethylhexyl methoxycinnamate, 3.5%; benzophenone-3, 1% (SPF, 4) Ethylhexyl methoxycinnamate, 7%; benzophenone-3, 2% (SPF, 8) Ethylhexyl methoxycinnamate, 7.5%; benzophenone-3, 4% (SPF, 15) Ethylhexyl methoxycinnamate, 7.5%; octylsalicylate, 5%; benzophenone-3, 4% (SPF, 30)	Local contact hypersensitivity to 2,4-dinitro-1-fluorobenzene	Significant protection, equal to or greater than SPF	Beasley et al. (1996)
Mouse, CH3 (5)	Filtered UVB tubes and solar-simulated UVR (xenon)	Repeated: 1 TISD/day, 5 days/week, 6 weeks 1 TISD = 7.5 kJ/m² UVB, 25.3 kJ/m2 solar-simulated UVR	4 commercial sunscreens: Ethylhexyl methoxycinnamate, 7%; benzophenone-3, 2% (SPF, 8) Ethylhexylmethoxycinnamate, 7.5%; benzophenone-3, 4% (SPF, 15) Ethylhexyl methoxycinnamate, 7.5% octylsalicylate, 5%; homosalate, 5%; benzophenone-3, 4% (SPF, 30) Ethylhexyl methoxycinnamate, 7.5%; octyl salicylate, 5%; octocrylene, 5%; benzophenone-3, 6% (SPF, 45)	Transplanted tumour incidence and growth	UVB: no protection with SPF 8 or 15; significant protection with SPF 30 and 45 Solar-simulated UVR: significant protection with all sunscreen	Roberts & Beasley (1997a)

Table 24 (contd)

Animal species, strain (no. per group)	UVR source	UVR regimen	Sunscreen	Effect investigated	Results	Reference
Mouse, C3H (5) (contd)			Ethylhexyl methoxycinnamate, 7.5%; octyl salicylate, 5%; homosalate, 5%; benzophenone-3, 4% (SPF, 30) Ethylhexyl methoxycinnamate, 7.5%; octyl salicylate, 5%; octocrylene, 5%; benzophenone-3, 6% (SPF, 45)	Activation of tumour antigen-specific suppressor T cells	Significant protection with both sunscreens	
Mouse, CH3 (5)	Solar-simulated UVR (xenon)	Two single doses, dose effect, 2–15 MISD Local MISD = 1.35 kJ/m^2 Systemic MISD = 6.76 kJ/m^2	2 commercial sunscreens: Ethylhexyl methoxycinnamate, 3.5%; benzophenone-3, 1% (SPF, 4) Ethylhexyl methoxycinnamate, 7%; benzophenone-3, 2% (SPF, 8)	Local and systemic contact hypersensitivity to 2,4-dinitro-1-fluorobenzene	Significant protection, greater than SPF	Roberts & Beasley (1997b)
Mouse, Skh-1 (4–24)	Monochromatic light (TL01, 311 nm)	Single dose–effect, directly on mice or on Transpore tape UVB: 21.8 kJ/m^2 = 2.8 MISD	Ethylhexyl PABA, 4.7% Ethylhexyl methoxycinnamate, 6.3% (SPF, 4)	Systemic contact hypersensitivity to 2,4-dinitro-1-fluorobenzene	Significant protection, equal to sunburn protection factor	Walker & Young (1997)
Mouse, Skh-1 (10)	Solar-simulated UVR (xenon)	Single dose effect, 2–4 MED 1 MED = 3.7 kJ/m^2 UVB	Terephthalylidene dicamsulfonic acid, 5% (SPf, 4) Ethylhexyl methoxycinnamate, 5% (SPF, 4)	Systemic contact hypersensitivity to 2,4-dinitro-1-fluorobenzene	Significant protection, less than sunburn protection factor	Guéniche & Fourtanier (1997)
Mouse, Skh-1 (20)	Solar-simulated UVR (xenon)	Single dose-effect, 0.5–16 MED, 1 MED = 30 kJ/m^2 UVB + 26.2 kJ/m^2 UVA UVA	Octocrylene, 7%; butyl methoxydibenzoylmethane, 3% (SPF, 7; UVA protection factor, 8) Octocrylene, 10%; butyl methoxydibenzoylmethane, 0.3% (SPF, 8; UVA protection factor, 3)	Systemic contact hypersensitivity to 2,4-dinitro-1-fluorobenzene	Significant protection, lower than SPF. The higher the UVA factor, the higher the immunosuppressive protection factor	Fourtanier et al. (2000)

Table 24 (contd)

Animal species, strain (no. per group)	UVR source	UVR regimen	Sunscreen	Effect investigated	Results	Reference
Mouse, C3H (5)	Solar-simulated UVR (xenon)	Single dose-effect	Octocrylene, 9%; phenylbenzimidazole sulfonic acid, 0.3% terephthalylidene dicamphor sulfonic acid; 0.7%; butyl methoxydibenzoylmethane, 3% (SPF, 15) Octocrylene, 10%; phenylbenzimidazole sulfonic acid, 0.2%; terephthalylidene dicamphor sulfonic acid, 3.25%; butyl methoxydibenzoylmethane, 1.5% (SPF, 22)	Systemic contact hypersensitivity to 2,4-dinitro-1-fluorobenzene	Significant protection, lower than sun protection factor	Ulrich et al. (1999)

SPF, sun protection factor (determined in human skin); MED, maximum erythemal dose; MISD, minimum immunosuppressive dose; TISD, effective tumour immune suppression dose
aContaining oxygen radical scavengers

epidermal T cells from the effects of UVR in both mouse strains (Ho *et al.*, 1992).

Male dd-y strain mice received a single irradiance of 0.1 or 1 kJ/m^2 UVB delivered by two unfiltered fluorescent lamp bulbs (Toshiba FL20SE-30). Before exposure, the mice were shaved and 2 mg/cm^2 of two commercial sunscreens were applied. The first contained TiO$_2$ and had a SPF of 15, and the second contained 7.5% ethylhexyl methoxycinnamate, 5% ethylhexyl salicylate and 8% ethylhexyl PABA. Skin samples were taken at intervals of 2–16 days after exposure to UVB. Adenosine 5'-diphosphate (ADP)-positive cells were counted in epidermal sheets, and the size of Langerhans cells was measured. The population of Langerhans cells was decreased and their size reduced after irradiation with 1 kJ/m^2 UVB, but the population recovered progressively to within normal limits after 16 days and the size within 8 days. Both sunscreens provided protection against the decreased number of Langerhans cells but did not prevent the shrinkage seen after the second day. Exposure to 0.1 kJ/m^2 of UVB induced little change in the Langerhans cells population (Miyagi *et al.,* 1994).

A single UVB absorber, ethylhexyl methoxycinnamate, was evaluated in female Skh-1 hairless albino mouse for its ability to inhibit UVR-induced epidermal Langerhans cells (Ia$^+$) depletion and suppression of the allo-activating capacity of epidermal cells (mixed epidermal cell–lymphocyte reaction). Ethylhexyl methoxycinnamate prepared at 9% in ethanol or a cosmetic lotion was applied before exposure to fluorescent solar-simulated UVR from a combination of two Wolf Helarium UVB/UVA tubes and six Philips TL10 UVA tubes. In experiments with a long exposure, a second application was made halfway through the irradiation. The UVR doses were multiples of 0.3–3 mouse MEDs. A single application of the UVB absorber in both vehicles at 2 mg/cm^2 gave varying degrees of protection from Langerhans

cell depletion but afforded no protection against suppression of the mixed epidermal cell–lymphocyte reaction. When the sunscreens were applied twice, there was better protection from Langerhans cell depletion and complete protection from suppression of the mixed epidermal cell–lymphocyte reaction (Walker *et al.*, 1994).

In a study described on page 99, Wolf *et al.* (1995) showed that single UVB absorbers (ethylhexyl PABA or ethylhexyl methoxycinnamate) or a single UVA plus UVB absorber (benzophenone-3) prevented the decrease in the numbers of Langerhans cells and dendritic epidermal T cells induced by a single dose of 5 kJ/m^2 UVB from unfiltered fluorescent tubes in the C3H mouse model.

Two single UVR absorbers, 5% terephthalylidene dicamphor sulfonic acid (a broad-spectrum UVA absorber) and 5% ethylhexyl methoxycinnamate (a UVB absorber), in the same vehicle were evaluated in female hairless Skh-1 mice exposed to a xenon solar simulator. The two preparations both have a sunburn protection factor determined in the mouse model of about 4 and were applied at 2 mg/cm^2 30 min before exposure to UVR. Dose–response relationships were obtained at 0, 2, 3 and 4 mouse MEDs. The end-points evaluated were inflammation, inhibition of systemic contact hypersensitivity, reaction to dinitrofluorobenzene, release of IL-10 (an immunomodulatory cytokine) in the sera and the number of Langerhans cells. The last two end-points were examined at the end of the contact hypersensitivity protocol, 13 days after exposure to UVR. Exposure to 2 MED induced a 70% decrease in the number of Langerhans cells. The vehicle had no effect. The ethylhexyl methoxycinnamate preparation protected against the effect of 2 MED but not against higher doses, whereas terephthalylidene dicamphor sulfonic acid protected against doses up to 3 MED (Guéniche & Fourtanier, 1997).

Five commercial sunscreen lotions (SPF 4, 8, 15, 30, 45) were compared for

their ability to prevent depletion of epidermal Langerhans cells after application at 2 mg/cm^2. Female C3H or hairless Skh-1 mice were exposed on two conse-cutive days to 1.8 kJ/m^2 delivered by Kodacel filtered Westinghouse FS20 sunlamps. Biopsy samples were taken 24 h after the last exposure, and epidermal sheets were stained for Langerhans cells (Ia$^+$). The number of these cells was depleted by ~ 75% in unprotected Skh1 exposed mice or those receiving placebo lotion, and the SPF 30 sunscreen completely prevented this depletion. In the C3H mice, all the sunscreens provided protection against Langerhans cell depletion, which was proportional to the labelled SPF (Beasley *et al.*, 1998).

Urocanic acid: The effect of single UVB absorbers (5% ethylhexyl PABA, sunburn protection factor, 5; and 5% ethylhexyl methoxycinnamate, sunburn protection factor, 7) in the same vehicle (a cosmetic emulsion) on the photoisomerization of urocanic acid was studied in female Skh: HR-2 pigmented mice irradiated with a single unfiltered FL40SE UVB fluorescent tube three times daily at 1 or 5 MED. Urocanic acid was extracted from dorsal epidermal scrapings obtained from skin excised immediately after irradiation. The sunscreens were applied at 3–5 mg/cm^2. Irradiation of skin that was unprotected or treated only with base lotion resulted in photoisomerization of 25% and 23% of the epidermal urocanic acid to *cis*-urocanic acid, respectively, whereas the percentage after application of ethylhexyl methoxycinnamate was 7% after three times 1 MED and 3% after three times 5 MED; that after application of ethylhexyl PABA was 2% after three times 1 MED and 0% after three times 5 MED. Thus, topical sunscreen application, independently of the nature of the UVB absorber, effectively prevented *cis*-urocanic acid formation in the epidermis in response to exposure to UVB (Reeve *et al.*, 1994).

The efficacy of some UVB absorbers against photoisomerization of urocanic acid was also evaluated in Skh:HR hairless mice exposed to fluorescent solar-simulated UVR. Neither ethylhexyl PABA nor ethylhexyl methoxycinnamate (both sunburn protection factor 6) prevented the *trans* to *cis* isomerization induced by repeated exposure (five times 6 MED or 20 times 6 MED). Between 22 and 29% photoisomerization occurred in all exposed groups (Reeve, 1997).

Cytokines: In the study of Guéniche and Fourtanier (1997) described above, the effects of sunscreens on the release of an immunomodulatory cytokine (IL-10) by UVR was studied in animals. The IL-10 in sera significantly increased in the irradiated untreated and vehicle-treated groups (from 82.7 pg/mL to 147.5 pg/mL). The groups treated with ethylhexyl methoxycinnamate were protected after exposure to 2 MED but not after 3 MED. Those receiving terephthalylidene dicamphor sulfonic acid were protected at doses up to 3 MED.

Local and systemic immune suppression and susceptibility to implanted tumours: The role of sunscreens in preventing UVR-induced immune suppression was studied in C3Hf/HeN mice sensitized with dinitrofluorobenzene 24 and 48 h after the last exposure to UVR on the unexposed or exposed back. The light sources were unfiltered Westinghouse FS40 sunlamps, and the exposure (3.22 kJ/m^2) was repeated on days 0, 1, 2, 3, 4, 6 and 7 for 30 min/day. The challenge was given 4 days after the last exposure on the footpad, and the swelling was measured 24 h later. A commercial sunscreen containing 5% PABA, applied liberally and rubbed in, failed to protect against the inhibition of local contact hypersensitivity induced by repeated doses of UVB at 3.22 kJ/m^2 (Lynch *et al.*, 1981).

PABA, ethylhexyl PABA, glyceryl PABA and benzophenone-3 in single or combined formulations, with labelled SPFs of 5–15, were applied at 0.3–0.5 mL/mouse to female C3Hf/HeN mice exposed under FS40 sunlamps for 3 or 4 weeks, and tumour growth was determined after subcutaneous transplantation of syngeneic UVR-induced tumour fragments (fibrosarcoma cells). PABA had no effect on the induction of the tumour-susceptible state after 3 weeks of exposure and treatment, and the tumour growth in the sunscreen-treated mice was equivalent to that in the unprotected animals. An almost complete lack of protection against the acquisition of tumour susceptibility after 4 weeks of UVB irradiation was also found in animals treated with the mixture of ethylhexyl PABA and glyceryl PABA, benzophenone-3 or all three products together (Gurish *et al.*, 1981).

Application of 5% PABA partially but significantly protected female C3H/HeNCR (MTV$^-$) mice against UVB-induced inhibition of systemic contact hypersensitivity to oxazolone but gave no statistically significant protection to BALB/cAnNCR mice against the induction of susceptibility to transplanted tumours. Histological evaluation of the skin showed that the sunscreen had not offered complete protection. The animals were exposed with or without sunscreen or vehicle to repeated doses of UVB from unfiltered Westinghouse sunlamps at 18 kJ/m^2 per day, for 3 days for the contact hypersensitivity or three times per week for 8 or 12 weeks for tumour susceptibility testing (Morison, 1984).

In a further study, 5% PABA applied liberally before and 2 h after exposure to UVR slightly protected female guinea-pigs exposed to sunlight (5 h per day for 3 days) against inhibition of the systemic contact hypersensitivity reaction to oxazolone and inflammation (Morison *et al.*, 1985).

The efficacy of SPF 6 and 15 commercial sunscreens containing ethyl-

hexyl PABA and benzophenone-3 in preventing systemic suppression of contact hypersensitivity to trinitrochlorobenzene was tested in inbred albino HRA/Skh hairless mice exposed to either UVB from unfiltered fluorescent tubes or solar-simulated UVR. The sunburn protection factor of the product was verified in mice and found to agree well with that on the labels of the products, which were applied at 2 μL/cm^2. Under these conditions, the two sunscreens did not prevent the suppression of contact hypersensitivity induced by either source of UVR (Fisher *et al.*, 1989).

Two commercial SPF-15 sunscreens, one containing 7.5% ethylhexylmethoxycinnamate and 4.5% benzophenone-3 and the other 6.5% ethylhexyl PABA and 3% benzophenone-3, applied at 2–3 mg/cm^2 in different vehicles were tested in inbred male Skh:HR-1 hairless albino mice exposed at 1.2 kJ/m^2 per day to a single unfiltered Oliphant FL40SE UVB fluorescent tube on 3 consecutive days. The ethylhexyl methoxycinnamate but not the ethylhexyl PABA product inhibited UVR-induced systemic suppression of contact hypersensitivity to dinitrofluorobenzene and susceptibility to transplanted tumours, but the two preparations were equally effective in preventing erythema and oedema. The tumour cells were injected 21 days after the first exposure to UVB, and tumour growth was monitored for up to 30 days (Reeve *et al.*, 1991).

The efficacy of similar commercial preparations was tested in hairless inbred albino HRA:Skh-1 mice in a study described in the subsection on Langerhans cells. The mice were sensitized by local application of trinitrochlorobenzene on irradiated skin. Neither preparation prevented inhibition of local contact hypersensitivity (Ho *et al.*, 1992).

The efficacy of 7.5% ethylhexyl methoxycinnamate was compared with that of 8% ethylhexyl PABA and 6% benzophenone-3 in four studies. The UVR source was unfiltered FS40 sunlamps. The sunburn protection factors of the products were not determined in the mouse model, and the SPFs given were rated by the manufacturer. The sunscreens were applied at doses of 200–250 μL/mouse. In two studies, UVR-induced local and systemic inhibition of contact hypersensitivity to dinitrofluorobenzene and oedema in female C3H/HeNCr mice were used as endpoints. All the sunscreens prevented oedema and suppression of local contact hypersensitivity after exposure to two or five MEDs (Wolf et al., 1993b, 1995). In another study, the sunscreens prevented oedema but only partially protected against systemic suppression of delayed-type hypersensitivity to *Candida albicans* (Wolf et al., 1993a). In the fourth study, UVR was found to enhance the growth of melanoma cells injected into the irradiated ears of mice. Mice were exposed to UVR twice a week at 4.8 kJ/m^2 for 3 weeks before injection of the tumour cells. Application of the sunscreens prevented oedema and histological damage but offered no protection against the UVR-enhanced growth of melanoma cells (Wolf et al., 1994).

In the study of the capacity of sunscreens to prevent isomerization of urocanic acid by exposure to UVR, protection against suppression of the systemic contact hypersensitivity reaction to oxazolone was also measured. Only 15% ethylhexyl PABA protected against suppression induced by three times 1 MED. When 15 MED were given, none of the concentrations of ethylhexyl PABA was protective (Reeve et al., 1994).

The ability of two organic UVB absorbers (8% ethylhexyl methoxycinnamate and 8% ethylhexyl PABA) and two inorganic sunscreens (7.2% microfine TiO$_2$ and a commercial ZnO cream) to protect the dermal immune system from 4 weeks' exposure to fluorescent solar-simulated UVR was studied in inbred female BALB/c or inbred female C3H/HeJ mice exposed to sub-erythe-

mal doses of UVR, 5 days/week for 4 weeks. Each week, the exposure time was increased by 20% (protocol (i)) or 30% (protocol (ii)). The sunburn protection factors of the formulations were measured with a solar simulator in both strains of mouse and found to vary between 4 and 9. The quantity of sunscreen applied was 2 mg/cm^2. In the experiment with C3H mice and UVR protocol (ii), oxygen radical scavengers were added to the ethylhexyl methoxycinnamate, ethylhexyl PABA and TiO$_2$ sunscreens. The end-points were local and systemic suppression of contact hypersensitivity to trinitrochlorobenzene. Tolerance, which is the failure to develop a secondary contact hypersensitivity response, was also evaluated. With protocol (i), which induced local but not systemic immune suppression or tolerance in BALB/c mice, ethylhexyl PABA exacerbated the immune suppression, whereas ethylhexy methoxy- cinnamate and TiO$_2$ protected the immune system. When the cumulative dose was increased by 12.7% (protocol (ii)), causing systemic immune suppression and tolerance, none of the sunscreens protected from immune suppression, but ethylhexyl methoxycinnamate provided partial and TiO$_2$ complete protection from tolerance. In the C3H/He mice, ethylhexyl methoxycinnamate provided some protection, whereas TiO$_2$ and ZnO provided complete protection from systemic immune suppression; ethylhexyl PABA did not protect. In this mouse strain, only TiO$_2$ and ZnO were completely effective against tolerance. Ethylhexyl methoxycinnamate was partially protective. The authors concluded that sunscreens can protect from local and systemic immune suppression, although this protection is limited and is not related to the sunburn protection factor of the sunscreens or the MED of the mouse strain. Instead, protection seemed to be provided by sunscreens with a broad absorption spectrum (Bestak et al., 1995).

Commercial sunscreens containing combinations of UVR absorbers and labelled SPFs of 4–45 were examined in five studies in female C3H/HeNHsd mice. In the first study, three UVR sources were used: unfiltered FS20 sunlamps, Kodacel filtered FS20 sunlamps and a solar simulator. Mice were exposed on 2 consecutive days. The ability of the sunscreens to prevent local suppression of contact hypersensitivity to dinitrofluorobenzene was studied. Mice protected by SPF-4 and -8 sunscreens and exposed to filtered sunlamps (1.8 kJ/m^2 per exposure) showed contact hypersensitivity responses that were significantly greater than those of the unprotected (placebo treated) control groups, whereas animals protected with SPF-15 and -30 sunscreens mounted responses similar to those of the unirradiated controls. The effects of the amount of a SPF-15 sunscreen containing 7.5% ethylhexyl methoxycinnamate and 4% benzophenone-3 on different UVR spectra were tested by comparing application of 4, 2 or 1 mg/cm^2 on one side and the three UVR sources on the other side. The two higher concentrations of sunscreen provided protection, whereas 1 mg/cm^2 did not, and the level of immune protection was related to the UVR source used, with solar simulator > filtered FS20 sunlamps > unfiltered FS20 sunlamps. The immune protection factor of the SPF-15 sunscreen was 30 for the solar simulator, 7.5 for the filtered sunlamps and 2 for the unfiltered sunlamps (Roberts & Beasley, 1995).

In the second study, the effects of four commercial sunscreen lotions of SPF 4, 8, 15 and 30 applied at 2 mg/cm^2 on the immune protection factor as measured by local suppression of contact hypersensitivity to dinitrofluorobenzene was evaluated with the same three UVR sources. The immune protection factors of the four sunscreens exceeded the labelled SPF in tests conducted with the solar simulator, but the values were significantly lower than the labelled SPF in tests with unfiltered and filtered FS20 sunlamps. The immune protection factors for the SPF-4, -8, -15 and -30 sunscreens were 15, 15, 30 and 60, respectively, in tests conducted with the solar simulator, 1, 2, 4, and 4 with the unfiltered FS20 sunlamps and 4, 8, 8 and 8 withthe filtered sunlamps (Roberts et al., 1996).

The third study evaluated the UVA-340 sunlamp, which emits a near solar UVR spectrum. The same sunscreens as used in the previous study (SPF 4–30) were evaluated in the same test for local contact hypersensitivity at the same applied dose (2 mg/cm^2). The immune protection factors obtained were 8, 15, 15 and 30, equal to or greater the level of protection predicted by the labelled SPF (Beasley et al., 1996).

In the fourth study, the influence of UVR spectrum on the tumour immune protective capacity of four commercial sunscreens (SPF 8–45; 2 mg/cm^2 applied) was evaluated. Tumour immune suppression was evaluated by the incidence and growth rate of transplanted tumours. The UVR sources were unfiltered FS20 sunlamps, Kodacel filtered FS20 sunlamps and a solar simulator. Tumours were transplanted after 6 weeks of exposure on 5 days per week to doses of 5, 7.5 or 25.3 kJ/m^2, depending on the UVR source. The tumour immune protection levels matched those predicted by the labelled SPF when sunscreen-protected mice were exposed to the solar simulator, and the SPF-30 and -45 sunscreens also blocked activation of tumour antigen-specific suppressor T lymphocytes. In comparison, when Kodacel filtered FS20 sunlamps were used, sunscreens with SPFs > 15 provided partial to complete protection with regard to tumour incidence, and all the sunscreens reduced the tumour growth rates. None of the sunscreens provided measurable tumour immune protection for mice exposed to unfiltered FS20 sunlamps (Roberts & Beasley, 1997a).

In the final study in this series, two commercial sunscreens (SPF-4 and SPF-8) were evaluated with respect to local and systemic contact hypersensitivity to dinitrofluorobenzene after exposure to a solar simulator. Dose–effect relationships were established for these two end-points, and immune protection factors were determined. These factors exceeded the SPFs, with values of 15 for local protection and 8 for systemic protection with the SPF-4 sunscreen and 15 for local protection and 15 for systemic protection with the SPF-8 product (Roberts & Beasley, 1997b).

The relationship between photoprotection against inflammation and immune suppression offered by two UVB filters (4.7% ethylhexyl PABA and 6.3% ethylhexyl methoxycinnamate) was studied in female HRA.HRII-c/+/Skh mice exposed to single doses of monochromatic UVB (Philips TL01 tubes, λ_{max} = 311 nm). A UVR dose–response curve without sunscreen was established for the two end-points. The dose of UVB for 50% immune suppression was lower than that for 50% maximal inflammation (oedema). Ethylhexyl PABA and ethylhexyl methoxycinnamate in the same vehicle totally prevented the oedema and partially prevented the systemic suppression of contact hypersensitivity to dinitrofluorobenzene induced by a single dose of UVB (21.8 kJ/m^2 or 2.8 minimum immune suppression doses). Similar responses were obtained when the sunscreens were applied topically or on a tape placed above the cages. In studies of UVB dose–response relationships for inflammation and immune suppression in mice treated topically with ethylhexyl methoxycinnamate, this sunscreen had a protection factor of 4 for both inflammation and immune suppression (Walker & Young, 1997).

In a study reported in the subsection on Langerhans cells and cytokines, Guéniche and Fourtanier (1997) studied the protection afforded by two UVR absorbers (terephthalylidene dicamphor sulfonic acid and ethylhexyl methoxycinnamate) against inhibition of systemic contact hypersensitivity to dinitrofluorobenzene induced in Skh-1 mice by various doses of solar-simulated UVR. With a UVR dose equivalent to 2 MED, the contact hypersensitivity response was inhibited by 60–70% in untreated or vehicle-treated exposed mice compared with control mice. Application of either sunscreen protected against doses up to 2 MED; at higher doses, ethylhexyl methoxycinnamate did not protect whereas terephthalylidene dicamphor sulfonic acid significantly protected the animals against doses up to 4 MED. The immune protection factors, calculated as the ratio of the minimum immune suppressive dose with and without sunscreen, were 1.6 for 5% ethylhexyl methoxycinnamate and 2.5 for 5% terephthalylidene dicamphor sulfonic acid. Thus, under these experimental conditions, the immune protection capacity of these two sunscreens is lower than their capacity to protect against UVR-induced inflammation.

The level of immune protection afforded by two broad-spectrum sunscreens with SPF 7–8 (determined for both humans and mice) but with different UVA protection levels (determined in humans by the persistent pigment darkening method as 8 or 3) was tested in female Skh-1 hairless albino mice. The two products contained the same filters against UVB (octocrylene) and UVA (butyl methoxydibenzoylmethane) in the same vehicle but at different concentrations; they were applied at 2 mg/cm^2. Solar-simulated UVR dose–response curves for inflammation and systemic suppression of contact hypersensitivity to dinitrofluorobenzene were generated and used to derive protection factors. Both sunscreens protected against suppression of contact hypersensitivity, but the product with the higher UVA protection factor gave significantly greater protection. The techniques used to determine immune protection factors gave similar results for a given sunscreen, but the immune protection factors were always lower than the SPFs (Fourtanier et al., 2000).

In a study of UVR-induced suppression of the systemic contact hypersensitivity response to dinitrofluorobenzene and protection by sunscreens, dose–response curves for UVR-induced immune suppression were generated with a xenon solar simulator in C3H/HeN mice with and without application of sunscreens. Two broad-spectrum products (SPF-15 and SPF-22) containing UVA and UBV absorbers in the same vehicle were applied 30 min before a single exposure. Both products protected, but the immune protection factors, obtained as the ratios of UVR doses inducing 50% suppression, were lower than the SPFs. The immune protection factor for the SPF-15 sunscreen was 2.3 and that for the SPF-22 product was 4.2 (Ullrich et al., 1999).

Immune suppression is considered to be in the causal pathway of photocarcinogenesis; however, an appropriate biomarker of carcinogenic risk has not been established. Most of the studies showed that sunscreens provide some protection against various end-points in UVR-induced immune suppression.

Photoageing

Chronic exposure to UVR profoundly damages the dermis and the epidermis of human and animal skin. These alterations are called 'photoageing' (Fig. 39). As they occur, like carcinogenesis, in response to cumulative exposure, evaluation of the prevention of photoageing can be used as a biomarker of protection by sunscreens against UVR-induced damage. These studies are summarized in Table 25. This biomarker is also described on p. 85.

Numerous studies have been conducted by Kligman and colleagues in Skh hairless mice of the ability of sunscreens to protect against connective tissue damage induced by repeated exposure to UVR. In the first study, two sunscreens containing 2% ethylhexyl PABA (SPF 2) or 7% ethylhexyl PABA plus 3% benzophenone-3 (SPF 15) were applied to Skh-1 and Skh-2 mice exposed to repeated doses of UVB (unfiltered Westinghouse FS20) at six human MEDs per exposure, three times a week for 30 weeks, followed by 15 weeks of observation. Skin samples were taken at 10-week intervals and were stained to reveal changes in the dermis. The unprotected, irradiated animals showed considerable dermal damage. The SPF-15 sunscreen completely prevented these changes, but the SPF-2 sunscreen was less effective. A surprising histological finding was the extent of the repair of the dermis after irradiation ceased (Kligman et al., 1982).

The second study focused on whether repair would occur if animals were protected by sunscreens after dermal damage was induced and irradiation was continued. Female albino hairless Skh-1 mice were exposed to a daily dose of UVR of 1.7 kJ/m^2 from unfiltered Westinghouse FS20 sunlamps three times weekly for 30 weeks. Commercial sunscreens of SPF 6 (5% ethylhexyl PABA) and SPF 15 (7% ethylhexyl PABA and 3% benzophenone-3) were applied after 10 and 20 weeks of irradiation. Both sunscreens, but especially the SPF 15, allowed repair of previously damaged dermis during continued irradiation (Kligman et al., 1983).

In the third study, the contributions of UVA and UVB to connective tissue damage in female albino Skh-1 hairless mice and the protection afforded by a commercial SPF-15 broad-spectrum sunscreen (7% ethylhexyl PABA and 3% benzophenone-3) was evaluated. Substantial protection against these effects was found (Kligman et al., 1985).

In the fourth study, three groups of female albino Skh-1 hairless mice received a cumulative dose of solar-simulated UVR from a xenon arc that was 10 and 16 times a previously determined minimal photoageing dose over periods of 18 and 30 weeks. Each twice-weekly exposure was designed to equal the SPF value of the first sunscreen, an SPF-7 product containing the UVB absorber ethylhexyl methoxycinnamate. The second sunscreen contained ethylhexyl methoxycinnamate and a UVA absorber (benzophenone-3) and had an SPF of 16. The third, with an SPF of 18, contained ethylhexyl methoxycinnamate, benzophenone-3 and butyl methoxydibenzoyl methane. Considerable damage to the dermal matrix was seen in the group given the SPF 7 product, with greater damage at 30 weeks than at 18. The SPF-16 sunscreen was highly protective at 18 weeks, but the damage at 30 weeks was still significant. The SPF-18 sunscreen, with the broadest spectral absorption, provided the greatest protection at both times. Thus, prevention of sunburn does not guarantee that photoageing will not occur during chronic exposure (Kligman et al., 1996).

A study was conducted in female albino Skh-1 hairless mice to determine the substantivity of sunscreen products with various SPFs and their ability to protect against chronic photodamage. Waterproof commercial sunscreens containing only ethylhexyl PABA (SPF 2) as the UVR absorber or containing ethylhexyl PABA plus benzophenone-3 (SPF 4 and 8) were evaluated. The mice

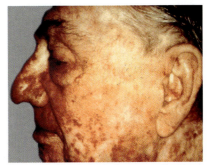

Figure 39 Elderly Australian man with extensive sun damage

Table 25. Photoageing as a biomarker of UVR-induced carcinogenesis

Animal species, strain (no. per group)	UVR source	UVR regimen	Sunscreen	Effect investigated	Results	Reference
Mouse, Skh-1 (12)	Solar-simulated UVR (xenon) and UVA (xenon or tubes)	Repeated: 3 days/week, 34 weeks with UVA at 300–1350 kJ/m² per day or solar-simulated UVR at 70 kJ/m² per day	Ethylhexyl PABA, 7%; benzophen-one-3, 3% (SPF 15)	Connective tissue damage	Significant protection	Kligman et al. (1985)
Mouse, Skh-1 (18)	Solar-simulated UVR (xenon)	Repeated: 7 MED/day (increasing doses during weeks 1 and 2), 2 days/week, 18 or 30 weeks 2.8 kJ/m² per day	Ethylhexyl methoxy-cinnamate (SPF 7) Ethylhexyl methoxy-cinnamate, benzo-phenone-3 (SPF 16) Ethylhexyl methoxy-cinnamate, benzo-phenone-3, butyl methoxydibenzoyl-methane (SPF 18)	Epidermal and dermal damage	No protection with SPF 7 Significant protection with SPF 16 and 18, but lower than predicted by SPF	Kligman et al. (1996)
Mouse, Skh-1 (12)	Solar-simulated UVR and UVA (fluorescent tubes)	Repeated: 5 days/week, 16 or 32 weeks Solar-simulated UVR: 213.5 kJ/m² per day UVA: 199–222 kJ/m² per day	Ethylhexyl methoxy-cinnamate, 2% Ethylhexyl methoxy-cinnamate, 2%; butyl methoxydibenzoyl-methane, 0.75% Ethylhexyl methoxy-cinnamate, 2%; butyl methoxydibenzoyl-methane, 2% Butyl methoxydibenzoyl-methane, 0.75%	Clinical, histological and biochemical alterations	Significant protection against clinical and histological alterations; no protection against biochemical alterations, except for third product (significant protection)	Harrison et al. (1991)
Mouse, MF1/hr (20)	UVA (xenon)	Repeated: 350 kJ/m² per day, 3 days/week, 52 weeks	Terephthalylidene dicamphor sulfonic acid 5% (SPF 5)	Clinical, histological and biochemical alterations	Significant protection	Fourtanier et al. (1992)

SPF, sun protection factor; MED, maximum erythemal dose

were exposed under unfiltered FS40 sunlamps at 0.3 kJ/m² (about 0.5 MED) three times weekly for 28, 17 and 22 weeks for the SPF-2, SPF-4 and SPF-8 products, respectively. When the sunscreens were applied 15 min or less before each UVB exposure, they protected against skin wrinkling, and an increased delay in the onset of wrinkles was seen with increasing SPF. As the time between treatment and irradiation increased (from 0 to 8 h), however, the protection afforded by all the sunscreens diminished rapidly (Bissett et al., 1991).

The protection against chronic photo-damage afforded by two single UVR absorbers, one UVB (2% ethylhexyl methoxycinnamate) and one UVA (0.75 or 2% butyl methoxydibenzoylmethane), or a combination of the two was examined in female albino Skh-1 hairless mice irradiated on the back for 8 h/day, 5 days/week for 16 weeks with fluorescent solar-simulated UVR or UVA or for 32 weeks with UVA alone. All of the UVR-exposed mice showed histological and biochemical damage, recorded as an increased proportion of type III collagen. Application of the UVB sunscreen resulted in marked protection against all non-biochemical end-points. Addition of 0.75% of the UVA absorber gave no clear advantage, but addition of 2% of the UVA absorber reduced the biochemical changes and connective tissue damage. UVA irradiation for 16 weeks caused no histological or biochemical changes, but the mice irradiated with UVA for 32 weeks showed slight dermal damage. These changes were not modified by the 0.75% UVA sunscreen (Harrison et al., 1991).

In a study in female albino MF1/hr hairless mice, sub-erythemal doses of pure UVA enhanced the numerous changes observed during chronological ageing. The photoprotective properties of a broad-spectrum UVA absorber, terephthalylidene dicamphor sulfonic acid, against UVA-induced damage were

assessed in 3-month-old albino hairless mice exposed for 1 year to 350 kJ/m² (about 0.5 MED) of UVA from a xenon source filtered through a WG 345/2 mm (Schott) filter. One group of animals received a formulation containing 5% of the sunscreen before irradiation, while another was untreated. All the changes induced by chronic exposure to UVA were reduced or abolished by the sunscreen (Fourtanier et al., 1992).

Photoageing is a persistent bio-marker of chronic exposure to UVR and is not in the pathway of photocarcino-genesis. Seven studies showed that sunscreens can reduce photoageing caused by either solar-simulated UVR or UVA. There was no clear dose–effect relationship.

In-vitro models
Measurement of optical transmission
Testing of sunscreen products to deter-mine the SPF in vivo is time-consuming and expensive in terms of volunteer time. Several attempts have therefore been made to develop a reliable in-vitro method for assessing new sunscreen formulations. A reliable in-vitro method would also permit systematic studies of the performance of sunscreens under various conditions, such as in water (e.g. water temperature, salinity and turbu-lence) or normal use (e.g. sand abrasion). Assays exist to measure the transmission of UVR through a substrate before and after application of a sunscreen. The ratio of the transmission without and with the sunscreen gives a measure of photopro-tection.

A wide range of substrates has been used to measure transmission through sunscreens. These include wool (Wurst et al., 1978; Greiter et al., 1979), pig skin (Greiter et al., 1979), lyophilized pig epi-dermis (Stamper, 1990), hairless mouse epidermis (Sayre et al., 1979, 1980; Cole & van Fossen, 1988, 1990), human stratum corneum (Kammeyer et al., 1987; Pearse & Edwards, 1993), syn-

thetic skin casts (Stockdale, 1987; Ferguson et al., 1988), surgical tape (Diffey & Robson, 1989; Sellers & Carpenter, 1992; Keeley et al., 1993), a combination of a biomembrane barrier with a biomacromolecular matrix (Gordon, 1992), roughened quartz plates (Diffey et al., 1997; DeFlandre & Lang, 1988), glass plates (Berset et al., 1996), recon-structed human epidermis (Marginean Lazar et al., 1997) and excised human epidermis (Brown & Diffey, 1986; Marginean Lazar et al., 1997; Stokes & Diffey, 1997a,b, 1999a,b, 2000).

Systems used for detection of the transmitted UVR include either a broad-band radiometer or a scanning spectroradiometer. The most reliable results are obtained when protection factors are measurement spectrored-metrically, the method being as follows. The spectral transmission of UVR through the substrate is measured on a wavelength-by-wavelength basis both with and without the sunscreen. The source of UVR must have a continuous spectrum over the wavelength range of interest (normally 290–400 nm), but the shape of the spectrum is unimportant, and there is no need to simulate the solar spectrum. Indeed, this is undesirable, since the intensity of radia-tion in the UVB region (290–315 nm) will be so low that the signal-to-noise ratio can become compromised. The trans-mittance of the sunscreen at wavelength λ nm ($T(\lambda)$) is equal to the ratio of the photocurrent measured through the substrate with the sunscreen applied to that before the sunscreen is applied. $T(\lambda)$ is usually measured in 5-nm steps from 290 to 400 nm. The SPF is then calcu-lated as:

$$\sum_{290}^{400} E(\lambda)\varepsilon(\lambda)\Delta\lambda \left/ \sum_{290}^{400} E(\lambda)\varepsilon(\lambda)T(\lambda)\Delta\lambda \right.$$

where $E(\lambda)$ is the spectral irradiance of terrestrial UVR under defined conditions, $\varepsilon(\lambda)$ is the erythema action spectrum (McKinlay & Diffey, 1987) and $\Delta\lambda$ is the wavelength step (e.g. 5 nm). The exact numerical values of the derived SPF depend on the choice of $E(\lambda)$. For example, if $E(\lambda)$ is chosen to represent midday winter sunlight at latitude 60° N, a different SPF will be obtained from that when $E(\lambda)$ is selected to represent midday summer sunlight at latitude 20° N.

The most reliable substrate is without doubt excised human epidermis, because, unlike with other substrates, interactions between sunscreen and skin are taken into account. Comprehensive studies with this *ex-vivo* substrate, yielding excellent agreement with SPFs obtained by phototesting in human volunteers *in vivo* (Stokes *et al.*, 1998), have been reported (Stokes & Diffey, 1997a,b, 1999a,b, 2000). In this method, skin is taken from the underside of the female breast during an operation for breast reduction. It is obtained by a process known as de-epidermalization, the principle of which is to remove the epidermis and epidermal appendages while leaving the deepest layers of the dermis *in situ*. The samples of skin are placed in a water bath at 60 °C for 45 s. When the epidermis is removed from the water bath, it is gently separated from the dermis by peeling. Sheets of epidermis can be stored at 4 °C for several weeks without loss of barrier function (Schaefer & Redelmeier, 1996).

DNA damage
In an *in-vitro* test system, PABA strongly protected against damage induced by UVA and UVB irradiation in calf thymus DNA in the presence of Fenton reagents. This result was attributed to the free-radical scavenging properties of PABA (Shih & Hu, 1996).

Ethylhexyl dimethyl PABA protected against broad-spectrum UVR-induced endonuclease-sensitive sites (pyrimidine dimers) in cultured human keratinocytes

if the product was not applied directly to the cells. When the sunscreen was in contact with the cells, however, a large increase in photo-induced strand breakage was seen (see also p. 137) (Gulston & Knowland, 1999).

Inhibition of semi-conservative DNA synthesis or repair synthesis
PABA and amyl dimethyl PABA spread on glass protect against semi-conservative DNA synthesis or UVB-induced repair synthesis in cultured human fibroblasts (Arase & Jung, 1986). This system is not widely used, and the results are difficult to reproduce among laboratories.

Biomarkers in cells and skin equivalents
Living cells in culture have been used to test sunscreen products and active ingredients (e.g. Marrot *et al.*, 1999). In order to mimic the three-dimensional structure of the skin, keratinocytes and fibroblasts are grown in collagen-containing matrices (Nelson & Gay, 1993; Augustin *et al.*, 1997a). The responses measured after exposure to UVR include morphological changes, cytotoxicity and the release of pro-inflammatory mediators, such as IL-1-α, tumour necrosis factor-α and prostaglandin E2. The most commonly observed result in a number of studies with various sunscreens was a relative increase in survival in the presence of sunscreen as compared with controls with no sunscreen (Nelson & Gay, 1993; Augustin *et al.*, 1997b; Sun *et al.*, 1999).

In an exploratory study with terephthalylidene dicamphor sulfonic acid, a wide range of markers, including nuclear *p53* induction in keratinocytes, melanogenesis in melanocytes, plasmid DNA damage, mutation in *Saccharomyces cerevisiae* and DNA damage as measured in the Comet assay in keratinocytes, was used to demonstrate protection against UVR emitted by a solar simulator (Marrot *et al.*, 1999).

Antimutagenicity in short-term assays
In a comprehensive study of protection against mutagenesis, Mondon and Shahin (1992) used three *in-vitro* systems — haploid and diploid cells of the yeast *Saccharomyces pombe* and Chinese hamster V79 cells — to investigate a range of mutational end-points, including specific base changes and frameshift mutations in the yeast and the broad range of mutations detected with the thioguanine-resistance marker in the rodent cell line. PABA and 4-(2-oxo-3-bornylidene)methylphenyl trimethylammonium methyl sulfate (a benzylidene camphor derivative synthesized in the laboratory) were tested for their capacity to protect against mutation induced by UVB from a Westinghouse FS20 sunlamp. Both sunscreens protected against mutation in a concentration-dependent fashion, the second being consistently more effective than PABA at equal concentrations, although absorption at equal concentrations was not determined. The authors concluded that PABA was less protective because it counteracted photosensitization. The assays were clearly effective for determining photomutagenicity and the photoprotective effects of sunscreens and indicated that the greater the sensitivity of the mutant allele to alteration, the greater the protection factor observed (Hodges *et al.*, 1977; Sutherland & Griffin, 1984).

Mechanisms of cancer prevention by sunscreens
Sunscreens absorb solar UVR and may reduce the exposure of the skin to this carcinogen. This phenomenon and its relationship to skin cancer have been investigated intensively by reference to a range of cellular and molecular changes induced by UVR and other relevant events.

Solar radiation is a complete carcinogen (IARC, 1992), and UVR is the part of the spectrum that has been implicated in skin carcinogenesis. An early step in skin carcinogenesis involves the induction of DNA damage, which then leads to a cascade of events, including cell cycle arrest, DNA repair, apoptosis, mutation and neoplastic transformation. Efficient removal of DNA lesions by cellular repair processes appears to be a critical step in the prevention of tumour formation. Errors during the repair of these lesions lead to the incorporation of wrong bases into the genetic material. The unrepaired lesions may also disrupt cellular processes by obstructing the DNA and RNA synthesizing machinery. These mistakes often result in mutation, leading to loss or inappropriate expression of the affected genes. Genetic alterations in *p53, patched (ptc), smoothened (smo)* or *sonic hedgehog (shh)* genes appear to play an important role in the development of squamous- and basal-cell carcinomas (Brash *et al.*, 1991; Ziegler *et al.,* 1993; Gailani *et al.,* 1996; Fan *et al.*, 1997; Oro *et al.*, 1997; Xie *et al.*, 1998).

The role of solar radiation in the pathogenesis of human cutaneous melanoma is more complex than that in squamous-cell carcinomas. Genetic alterations in *p16* and N-*ras* genes have been implicated in melanoma development (Kamb *et al.*, 1994; Hussussian *et al.*, 1994), and the C→T and CC→TT mutations in the *p16* gene have been detected in human melanoma cell lines (Liu *et al.*, 1995; Pollock *et al.,* 1995). The presence of these UVR-induced 'signature' mutations suggests that UVR present in sunlight plays a role in the induction of cutaneous melanomas in humans. In primary melanomas, however, only one CC→TT mutation has been described among some 25 *p16* mutations analysed (Kumar *et al.*, 1998, 1999). Mutations in the N-*ras* oncogene are also reported to play a role in melanoma development (Padua *et al.*, 1985; Keijzer *et al.*, 1989; van't Veer *et al.*, 1989).

Although commercial sunscreens were originally developed to protect against sunburn, laboratory studies have shown that some sunscreens are also efficient in protecting against UVR-induced DNA damage, skin ageing, sunburn cell formation, immune suppression and development of skin cancer in animal models (see p. 98). Sunscreens can also prevent the emergence of actinic keratoses in humans (Naylor *et al.*, 1995) and help reduce the incidence of skin cancer in patients with xeroderma pigmentosum (Kondoh *et al.*, 1994).

Because UVR-induced DNA damage, *p53* mutation, proliferation and immune suppression are key events in skin cancer development, inhibition of one or more of these events may protect against it. Sunscreens would be expected to afford protection against all these events because they should interfere with the primary event, induction of DNA damage. Of the various biological end-points used in studies of sunscreens, some represent acute effects of UVR (e.g. erythema, DNA damage and expression of *p53* and *p21*), while others represent chronic effects (e.g. *p53* mutation and skin cancer). The protective efficacy of sunscreens may vary depending upon the end-point under study.

Inhibition of UVR-induced DNA damage

UVR, particularly wavelengths in the UVC and UVB spectra, induces predominantly two types of DNA photoproducts, cyclobutane-type pyrimidine dimers (Setlow & Carrier, 1966) and pyrimidine (6–4) pyrimidone or (6–4) photoproducts (Mitchell & Nairn, 1989). Both lesions are formed exclusively in runs of tandemly located pyrimidine residues which are often 'hot spots' for UVR-induced DNA damage and mutation. Tornaletti and Pfeifer (1994) demonstrated that mutation 'hot spots' for *p53* in skin cancers are also 'slow spots' for DNA repair. In addition to pyrimidine dimers and (6–4) photoproducts, UVR induces other types of DNA lesions, such as cytosine photohydrates, purine photoproducts and single-strand breaks (Weiss & Duker, 1987; Doetsch *et al.,* 1988; Gallagher & Duker, 1989). UVA radiation and visible light (> 400–500 nm) are known to cause DNA damage indirectly by producing reactive oxygen species such as superoxide anion, singlet oxygen and hydrogen peroxide via unknown endogenous photosensitizers (Peak *et al.*, 1987). These highly-reactive, short-lived molecules produce single-strand breaks, DNA–protein cross-links and altered bases in DNA. There is some evidence that altered bases, particularly 7,8-dihydro-8-oxo-guanine (8-hydroxyguanine) are produced more frequently than single-strand breaks or DNA–protein cross-links by UVA and visible light (Tchou *et al.*, 1991, 1992; Boiteux, 1993; Pflaum *et al.*, 1994).

Because UVR-induced DNA damage is a prerequisite for initiating the process of photocarcinogenesis, inhibition of this event can protect against a wide array of events associated with skin cancer development. Several sunscreen ingredients have been tested for their efficacy to protect against UVR-induced pyrimidine dimers in human and mouse skin.

An SPF-15 sunscreen formulation containing 7.5% ethylhexyl methoxycinnamate and 4.5% benzophenone-3 reduced the number of pyrimidine dimers in human skin induced by solar-simulated UVR (Freeman *et al.*, 1988). Similarly, an SPF-10 sunscreen gave protection against UVB-induced pyrimidine dimers in human skin (van Praag *et al.*, 1993). In two later studies, the degree of photoprotection was correlated with the erythemal response (Bykov *et al.*, 1998b; Young *et al.,* 2000). One of them found an association between DNA damage and the erythemal response, whereas no association was found in the other.

Experiments in mice analogous to those in human skin have also shown that several organic sunscreen products, including ethylhexyl methoxycinnamate, benzophenone-3 and PABA and its derivatives, reduce UVR-induced DNA damage (Walter, 1981; Walter & DeQuoy, 1980; Wolf *et al.*, 1993a). Topical administration of a broad-spectrum UVA absorber containing 5% tetraphthalylidene dicamphor sulfonic acid was significantly more effective than a UVB absorber (5% ethylhexyl methoxycinnamate) in preventing the induction of pyrimidine dimers in hairless mouse skin irradiated with solar-simulated UVR (Ley & Fourtanier, 1997). In contrast, Suzuki (1987) found that 1% PABA and 1% urocanic acid afforded little or no protection against DNA damage induced by irradiation of hairless mice with a broad-spectrum UVR source (peak emission, 305 nm). [The Working Group noted that this study is hard to interpret because no attempt was made to relate the SPF to a DNA protection factor.]

Topical administration of ZnO or TiO_2 provided protection against DNA damage induced by unfiltered UVB in hairless mice (Walter, 1981; Suzuki, 1987).

Inhibition of UVR-induced p53 and p21 [Waf1/Cip1] expression

UVR induces high levels of *p53* expression (Maltzman & Czyzyk, 1984; Campbell *et al.*, 1993; Hall *et al.*, 1993; Lu & Lane, 1993; Zhan *et al.*, 1993), which in turn activates the transcription of downstream genes responsible for cell-cycle arrest at the G_1–S transition (Kastan *et al.*, 1991, 1995). The G_1–S arrest results, at least partly, from *p53* transactivation of *p21* [Waf1/Cip1], which binds to and inactivates the cyclin-dependent kinases required for cell-cycle progression (El-Deiry *et al.*, 1993; Harper *et al.*, 1993; Xiong *et al.*, 1993). Growth arrest may allow the cells to repair the DNA damage. However, *p53* can also cause apoptosis of cells with excessive unrepaired DNA damage (Reed, 1994; Ziegler *et al.*, 1994) by activation of *bax*

and/or down-regulation of *bcl-2* expression (Gillardon *et al.*, 1994; Miyashita *et al.*, 1994; Miyashita & Reed, 1995). Recent studies showed that Fas–Fas–ligand interaction is essential for the elimination of cells containing UVR-induced DNA damage (Hill *et al.*, 1999).

Because UV irradiation results in over-expression of TP53 and TP21 [Waf1/Cip1] proteins in human and mouse cells *in vitro* and *in vivo*, these two proteins have been used as indicators of DNA damage in studies of photoprotection by sunscreens. Application of 0.2 ml/cm² of a sunscreen containing ethylhexyl methoxycinnamate and benzophenone-3 to human skin 15 min before irradiation with Supavasun 3000, a broad-band UVR source, nearly eliminated UVR-induced expression of TP53 and TP21 [Waf1/Cip1] proteins (Pontén *et al.*, 1995; see also section 4.1.5 (b)). Similarly, application of an SPF-25 sunscreen containing 18% TiO_2 to human skin before irradiation with UVB (300 nm) from a monochromatic light source prevented induction of TP21 [Waf1/Cip1] protein (El-Deiry *et al.*, 1995). Repeated application of a sunscreen containing benzophenone-3, butyl methoxydibenzoylmethane and ethylhexyl methoxycinnamate to human skin before each exposure to natural sunlight for 5–9 weeks caused a 33% reduction in the number of TP53-positive cells. Surprisingly, however, a near total barrier, blue denim fabric with an SPF of 1700, resulted in only a 66% reduction in the number of TP53-positive cells in chronically sun-exposed human skin (Berne *et al.*, 1998). The protection afforded by two sunscreens with identical SPF but different UVA protection factors was compared by measuring nuclear accumulation of TP53 protein in human skin biopsy samples after chronic UV irradiation with a solar simulator. The two sunscreens only partially decreased the number of TP53-positive cells. The two sunscreens with different UVA protection factors, as determined by the persistent

pigment darkening method, provided different levels of photoprotection against nuclear TP53 accumulation. Because TP53 and TP21 [Waf1/Cip1] proteins are induced after DNA damage, it is reasonable to conclude that sunscreens prevent DNA damage and thereby prevent induction of TP53 and TP21 [Waf1/Cip1] (Seité *et al.*, 2000a).

A study was conducted to investigate whether sunscreens with different SPFs can protect against UVR-induced *p53* expression. Application of sunscreens with SPFs of 8, 30 or 40 to the buttock skin of 12 volunteers 15 min before irradiation with 3 MED of UVR from a solar simulator caused a decrease in the number of TP53-positive cells and a decrease in the intensity of immunostaining for TP53 when compared with that seen in the buttock skin of volunteers irradiated with 1 MED of UVR (Krekels, *et al.*, 2000).

Reduction of UVR-induced p53 mutations

Analyses of human skin cancers and UVR-induced mouse skin cancers for *p53* mutations have provided new insights into the molecular mechanisms by which UVR induces skin cancer. Both human and mouse UVR-induced skin cancers harbour unique mutations (C→T and CC→TT transitions) in *p53* at a high frequency (50–100%) (Brash *et al.*, 1991; Kress *et al.*, 1992; Kanjilal *et al.*, 1993; Ziegler *et al.*, 1993; Dumaz *et al.*, 1997; Ananthaswamy *et al.*, 1998). Mutations in the *p53* gene have been shown to precede the appearance of skin cancer. For example, *p53* mutations have been detected in sun-exposed skin from healthy volunteers and from skin cancer patients, and can serve as an indicator of prior solar exposure (Nakazawa *et al.*, 1994; Kanjilal *et al.*, 1995; Urano *et al.*, 1995; Ouhtit *et al.*, 1997). Furthermore, UVR-specific *p53* mutations were found in actinic keratoses (Nelson *et al.*, 1994; Ziegler *et al.*, 1994; Ren *et al.* (1996). Jonason *et al.* (1996) demonstrated that whole, mounted preparations of human skin contained clonal patches of keratinocytes with mutated TP53.

Experiments to determine the timing of *p53* mutation in relation to skin cancer development have been performed in the mouse model of photocarcinogenesis. The presence of mutant *p53*-positive clusters was reported in UVB-irradiated mouse skin well before the appearance of skin tumours (Berg *et al.*, 1996). Similarly, *p53* mutations in UVB-irradiated C3H mouse skin were detected as early as week 4 of chronic UVR irradiation, and the frequency of *p53* mutations increased progressively, reaching 50% at week 12 (Ananthaswamy *et al.*, 1997).

The finding that *p53* mutations arise early during UVR-induced skin carcinogenesis suggests that they might be used as an early biological marker of the efficacy of sunscreens in photoprotection. Several organic SPF-15 sunscreens containing either UVB absorbers (10% octocrylene and 2% phenyl-benzimidazole sulfonic acid) or UVB plus UVA absorbers (9% octocrylene, 0.3% phenyl-benzimidazole sulfonic acid, 3% butyl methoxydibenzoylmethane and 0.7% terephthalylidene dicamphor sulfonic acid) have been shown to protect C3H mouse skin against *p53* mutations induced by UVB plus UVA from Kodacel-filtered FS40 sunlamps or a solar simulator (Ananthaswamy *et al.*, 1997, 1999). By using a highly sensitive technique of allele-specific polymerase chain reaction, these investigators demonstrated that application of UVB or UVB plus UVA sunscreens onto the shaved dorsal skin of C3H mice 30 min before each exposure to radiation for 12–16 weeks resulted in a 80–100% reduction in CC→TT *p53* mutations when compared with the frequency in unprotected mouse skin.

The reduction of *p53* mutations and skin cancer induction by sunscreens can be attributed to their ability to protect the

skin against UVR-induced DNA damage. The UVB sunscreens used in studies of Ananthaswamy *et al.* (1997, 1999) appeared to be as effective as the UVB plus UVA sunscreens in inhibiting *p53* mutation. This finding is not unexpected because only UVB-induced mutations (CC→TT) were assayed; UVA-induced mutations, which are predominantly G→T transversions, were not assessed (Drobetsky *et al.*, 1995; Sage *et al.*, 1996). However, it is unlikely that UVA-type mutations play a role in UVR-induced skin carcinogenesis because they are seldom present in human or mouse UVR-induced skin cancers. In support of this contention, it was shown that even the mouse skin tumours induced by massive doses of UVA did not contain G→T transversions in the *p53* gene (van Kranen *et al.*, 1997). UVA therefore probably plays a minor role in the initiation of squamous-cell carcinoma.

Protection against p53 mutations in skin cancers arising in routine users of sunscreens

Although numerous epidemiological studies have been performed to assess the protective effects of sunscreens against melanoma and other skin cancers, none have addressed the mechanistic aspects. However, a recent study addressed the important question of whether basal-cell carcinomas arising in routine users of sunscreens are similar to or different from those arising in non-users (Rosenstein *et al.*, 1999). The findings suggest that the commercial sunscreens tested were quite effective in preventing UVB-induced mutations in basal-cell carcinomas.

Inhibition of UVR-induced non-melanoma skin cancer in mice

In several studies in mice, almost all the sunscreens tested protected against UVR-induced skin cancer (Kligman *et al.*, 1980; Wulf *et al.*, 1982; Forbes *et al.*, 1989; Flindt-Hansen *et al.* 1990a,b; Fourtanier, 1996). It was also shown *in*

vitro that UVR-irradiated PABA solution was still effective in protecting mice against UVR-induced skin cancer (Flindt-Hansen *et al.*, 1989). This suggests that, although irradiated PABA solution containing degradative photoproducts can enhance pyrimidine dimer formation and is potentially mutagenic, it can still protect mice against UVR-induced skin cancer. A second implication of this study is that the activity of a sunscreen *in vitro* has little relevance *in vivo*, and caution should be exercised in extrapolating data obtained *in vitro* to the situation *in vivo*.

Nonetheless, sunscreen formulations containing UVB absorbers or UVB plus UVA absorbers with SPFs of 15–22 were effective in protecting mice against skin cancers induced by a solar simulator. In this study, 100% of mice that received a cumulative dose of 1000 kJ/m^2 of UVB only or vehicle plus UVB developed skin tumours, whereas the probability of tumour development was 2% in mice treated with the sunscreens and 1000 kJ/m^2 of UVB and 15% in mice treated with sunscreens plus 1500 kJ/m^2 of UVB. The sunscreen formulations containing only UVB absorbers were as effective as those containing both UVB and UVA absorbers in inhibiting UVR-induced *p53* mutations and skin cancer. This suggests that, under the experimental conditions used, attenuating UVA with sunscreens containing UVA absorbers does not provide a detectable increase in photoprotection against *p53* mutations or skin cancer above that provided by sunscreen formulations containing only UVB absorbers. The added protective effect of UVA sunscreens is difficult to estimate, however, because of the small numbers of animals affected. These results suggest that the mutagenic and carcinogenic effects of solar-simulated UVR are due mainly to UVB and not UVA wavelengths. The sunscreens used in this study protected the mice against not only UVR-induced *p53* mutations but also skin cancers. The authors therefore concluded that inhibition of *p53* mutations is a useful early marker of photoprotection against an important initiating event in UVR-induced carcinogenesis (Ananthaswamy *et al.*, 1999). Additional markers of promotional events in the multistep process of photocarcinogenesis are needed to assess the role of sunscreens in protecting against skin cancer induction.

Protection against UVR-induced immune suppression

UVR is known to suppress various types of immune response (see section 4.2.2 (b)). In particular, irradiation before immunization suppresses the induction of contact hypersensitivity (Noonan *et al.*, 1981) and delayed-type hypersensitivity responses (Ullrich, 1986). UVR-induced DNA damage has been shown to play a role in some types of immune suppression (Applegate *et al.*, 1989; Kripke *et al.*, 1992; Vink *et al.*, 1996, 1997). In studies of the effects of enhanced repair of UVR-induced pyrimidine dimers on UVR-induced immune suppression, it was found that topical application of liposomes containing T4N5 endonuclease or DNA photolyase to mouse skin following UV irradiation abrogated UVR-induced suppression of contact hypersensitivity (Kripke *et al.*, 1992; Vink *et al.*, 1996, 1997). In addition to DNA damage, UVR can also isomerize urocanic acid present in the stratum corneum from the native *trans* to the *cis* form, which in turn causes immune suppression in mice (De Fabo & Noonan, 1983; Noonan & De Fabo, 1992). However, although sunscreens can block UV-induced isomerization of *trans-* to *the cis*-urocanic acid, there was no apparent correlation between the formation of *cis*-urocanic acid and suppression of the induction of contact hypersensitivity (Reeve *et al.*, 1994).

Most published results suggest that sunscreens do afford protection against UVR-induced immune suppression. Some of the early failures to demonstrate such protection can be attributed to use

of non-solar UVR sources (Gurish *et al.*, 1981; Lynch *et al.*, 1981) or use of a sunscreen designed to absorb one wavelength of light (e.g. UVB) when immune suppression was induced by a different wavelength (e.g. UVA; Hersey *et al.*, 1988). Roberts *et al.* (1996) found that considerable immune suppressive energy was contained in wavelengths below 295 nm emitted from an FS40 sunlamp. Transmission of 'non-solar' UVR (UVC and short-wave UVB) through a sunscreen was 15 times greater when the sunlamp was used than when a solar-simulated source was employed. These findings illustrate the limitations of using non-solar UVR sources to determine the efficacy of a sunscreen.

A second issue is the immunological end-point chosen and the wavelengths of UVR responsible for suppressing that end-point. Roberts *et al.* (1996) found that UVB-absorbing sunscreens were effective in preventing contact hypersensitivity induced by solar-simulated UVR. Sunscreens were reported to be ineffective in protecting against UVR-induced inhibition of NK cell function in humans (Hersey *et al.*, 1987). This may have been due to the design of the study (see p. 90), or the wavelengths involved in suppressing NK function may lie within the UVA region of the solar spectrum (Hersey *et al.*, 1988). Since the formulation used in this study absorbs primarily UVB and would not have provided substantial protection against UVA, it is not surprising that it did not block immune suppression. The absorptive qualities of the sunscreen being tested, the UVR wavelengths responsible for the biological effect measured and the spectral output of the artificial UVR source used in any particular study are important in determining the efficacy of a sunscreen.

As exposure to UVR before immunization suppresses the induction of contact hypersensitivity, many investigators have examined the protective effect of sunscreens against these reactions. Although some failed to find any protec-

tion (Fisher *et al.*, 1989; Ho *et al.*, 1992), in most studies sunscreens protected against immune suppression. The degree of protection, however, varied greatly. While some authors reported total protection (Reeve *et al.*, 1991; Wolf *et al.*, 1993b; Beasley *et al.*, 1996; Roberts *et al.*, 1996; Roberts & Beasley, 1997b), others found that the degree of immune protection was less than the degree of protection against erythema and/or oedema (Wolf *et al.*, 1993a; Bestak *et al.*, 1995; Whitmore & Morison, 1995; Hayag *et al.*, 1997; see pp. 87 and 102). The reasons for these discrepancies are not entirely clear. As solar-simulated light was not used in all the studies mentioned above, the complication of irrelevant wavebands and incomplete absorption of UVC and short-wave UVB may be a contributing factor. Walker and Young (1997) compared protection from oedema and suppression of contact hypersensitivity induced by monochromatic UVB, in order to eliminate confounding due to differences in action spectra for these end-points. Under these conditions, the protection factors for ethylhexyl methoxycinnamate were the same but the mice were more sensitive to immune suppression than to the induction of oedema. Similar results were obtained when sunscreens were applied to the mice and on Transpore tape above the mice. These data suggest that reports of lack of immune protection are not due to interactions between sunscreens and the skin.

Bestak *et al.* (1995) found better protection with broad-spectrum sunscreens (UVA plus UVB absorbers). Roberts and Beasley (1997b) reported that the SPF was equal to or exceeded the immune protection factor when a minimal immune suppressive dose (i.e. the amount of UVR required to induce 50% immune suppression) calculated from UVR dose–response curves (with solar-simulated light) was used in studies of protection by sunscreens. Fourtanier *et al.* (2000) conducted a study in mice to compare two sunscreens with the same SPF but different levels of UVA protection. The sunscreen with the higher UVA protection factor provided better protection against suppression of induction of contact hypersensitivity, but the immune protection factor was lower than the SPF. Three methods for the determination of the immune protection factor gave comparable results. Despite the reported discrepancies in the degree of immune protection, sunscreens do appear to afford protection against immune suppression of contact hypersensitivity and delayed-type hypersensitivity to varying degrees.

Effect on the immune response to recall antigens or contact hypersensitivity in humans

In the studies summarized above, normal mice or unsensitized volunteers were exposed to UVR and then immunized with an antigen or a contact allergen. Measurement of the immune response to recall antigens such as diphtheria, tetanus toxoid and tuberculin—antigens that most people encounter during childhood immunizations—offers a unique advantage in that no active immunization is required. Rather, the effect of exposure to UVR on the elicitation of the delayed-type hypersensitivity reaction is measured. Using a UVB-absorbing sunscreen, Hersey et al. (1987) found no protection against UVR-induced immune suppression of delayed-type hypersensitivity to recall antigens. Immune protection was observed, however, in two studies with broad-spectrum sunscreens (Moyal et al., 1997; Moyal, 1998; see p. 87). The degree of immune protection to recall antigens may depend on the total UVR-absorbing properties of the sunscreen. Volunteers exposed chronically to natural sunlight were treated with two sunscreen preparations, one with a SPF of 15 and a UVA protection factor of 6 and the second with a SPF of 30 and a UVA protection factor of 12. While both

blocked sunlight-induced erythema, only the SPF-30 sunscreen blocked immune suppression (Moyal, 1998).

The effect of sunscreen application on UVR-induced suppression of the elicitation of contact hypersensitivity to dinitrochlorobenzene or nickel has been examined. High-SPF sunscreens protected against UVB-induced suppression of contact hypersensitivity (Whitmore & Morison, 1995; Hayag et al., 1997). Damian et al. (1997) found that application of a broad-spectrum sunscreen protected against immune suppression; no protection was seen with a UVB-absorbing sunscreen alone, but addition of a UVA absorber to the sunscreen preparation made it effective. A similar result was obtained by Serre et al. (1997), who examined UVR-induced (solar-simulated light) suppression of induction of contact hypersensitivity in humans. Complete protection was achieved only when the sunscreen formulation absorbed both UVB and UVA. Nonetheless, Damian et al. (1999) generated linear dose–response curves for suppression of nickel contact hypersensitivity and demonstrated that the immune protection factor of a sunscreen can be determined in humans in vivo.

Effect on UVR-induced suppression of tumour rejection

UVR-induced murine skin tumours are highly antigenic and are immunologically rejected when transplanted into normal mice (Kripke, 1974). Exposure of mice to a sub-carcinogenic dose of UVR suppresses tumour rejection and allows the antigenic tumours to grow progressively (Kripke & Fisher, 1976; Fisher & Kripke, 1977). A series of studies was performed in mice to determine whether sunscreens can protect mice against the UVR-induced suppression of skin cancer rejection. Most of the studies showed sunscreens to be effective (Morison & Kelley, 1985; Reeve et al., 1991; Roberts & Beasley, 1997a), although two

exceptions were noted (Gurish et al., 1981; Morison, 1984).

In studies of the effect of sunscreens on the growth of transplanted melanoma cells in UVR-irradiated mouse skin, Wolf et al. (1994) took advantage of the fact that irradiation of the skin promotes the growth of melanoma cells transplanted into the irradiated site and is an immunologically mediated phenomenon (Donawho & Kripke, 1991). Although sunscreen preparations containing UVB only or both UVB and UVA absorbers blocked UVR-induced inflammation and the accumulation of sunburn cells in the skin, they failed to prevent the UVR-induced enhancement of melanoma growth. These results may have a number of explanations. The design of the study may not have been suitable for detecting a protective effect, as the dose–response relationship was not analysed (see p. 112). As unfiltered FS40 lamps were used as a source of UVR, the failure of the sunscreens to absorb UVC and incomplete absorption of short-wave UVB may play a role. The mechanism by which UVR enhances melanoma growth is not entirely clear, but it has been suggested (Donawho et al., 1998) that UVR-induced photoisomerization of urocanic acid is involved. Because wavelengths in the UVA region of the solar spectrum efficiently convert trans-urocanic acid into the cis isoform (Gibbs et al., 1993), use of a sunscreen with a higher absorbancy of UVA could block UVR-enhanced melanoma growth, as in the situation described above (Moyal, 1998).

Other immunological end-points

Other immunological end-points have been used to determine the efficacy of sunscreens. Studies have addressed the ability of sunscreens to block the depletion of epidermal Langerhans cells (Miyagi et al., 1994; Walker et al., 1994; Hayag et al., 1997; Neale et al., 1997; Beasley et al., 1998; Hochberg & Enk, 1999), UVR-induced suppression of allostimulatory activity in the mixed epidermal cell–lymphocyte reaction (van Praag *et al.*, 1991; Walker *et al.*, 1994; Davenport *et al.,* 1997; Hurks *et al.*, 1997), depression of antigen-presenting cells function in a conventional mixed lymphocyte reaction *in vitro* (Mommaas *et al.*, 1990), induction of IL-10 in mouse serum (Guéniche & Fourtanier, 1997) and in human skin (Hochberg & Enk, 1999) or suppression of NK function (Hersey *et al.*, 1987, 1988). For the most part, sunscreen application has been shown to afford some degree of protection. The most notable exception is the inability of sunscreens to block UVR-induced suppression of NK function, but, as mentioned above, this phenomenon is UVA-dependent and the sunscreens available when this study was performed were UVB absorbers.

Possible reasons for differences between the immune protection factor and SPF

The studies summarized above show a general lack of agreement between the immune protection factor and SPF. The possible reasons for this lack of agreement are:

- Use of non-solar sources, especially those containing UVC;
- Lack of assessment of the SPF (or erythemal protection factor) with the experimental source and in the same experimental model, and therefore reliance on the labelled SPF;
- Lack of dose–response relationships for immune suppression and inflammation (in humans and mice), and drawing of conclusions for various end-points from 'arbitrary' doses of UVR without reference to dose–response curves;
- Possible differences in action spectra for erythema and immune suppression;
- Comparison of an acute end-point (SPF) with the results of studies of repeated exposure;
- Lack of standard protocols for determining the immune protection factor.

Chapter 6
Other beneficial effects of sunscreens

Other potential beneficial effects of sunscreens that are not related to the prevention of skin cancer are prevention of painful sunburns, photodamage and photoageing, UVR-induced provocation of certain cutaneous diseases and photoimmune suppression. Use of sunscreens can prevent skin diseases from progressing acutely after exposure to the sun; these diseases include cutaneous lupus erythematosus (Taylor & Sober, 1996) and reactivation of herpes labialis (Rooney *et al.*, 1991). The other potential benefits of sunscreens are related to the type and duration of exposure to UVR. Prevention of photodamage and photoageing, which are related to cumulative exposure to UVR, in countries where solar irradiance is intense throughout the year requires daily, long-term sun protection (Fig. 40). Prevention of acute flares of cutaneous diseases, which may be related to episodic exposure to UVR, requires anticipatory use of sun protection. As an episode of exposure that will provoke a flare is difficult to predict reliably, people with skin diseases that are highly sensitive to the sun, such as chronic actinic dermatitis, are advised to protect themselves from the sun daily, with measures that include a broad-spectrum sunscreen.

Prevention of non-carcinogenic dermal effects of the sun
The type of protection required to prevent chronic photodamage may differ from that for preventing acute sunburn, as cutaneous injury as defined by histological changes is different from acute sunburn and photodamage. In acute sunburn, the most obvious change is epidermal, the dermal changes being subtle and transient. The changes seen with chronic photodamage are alterations to the epidermis and dermis.

Exposure to sunlight and blistering sunburns may occur more frequently during childhood and adolescence than later in life (Robinson *et al.*, 1997b). Sporadic or incomplete use of sun protection leads to episodic burning. In a study in the USA, although more adults claimed to use sunscreens in 1996 than in 1986, the proportion who reported having a sunburn was higher in 1996 (Robinson *et al.*, 1997a). Use of sunscreens with a high SPF has been associated with longer recreational exposure to the sun (Robinson, 1992; Autier *et al.*, 1999). Other examples of sunburn due to non-compliance with the recommended use of sunscreen include applying sunscreen after exposure has begun or when the first symptoms of sunburn are recognized or expected; failure to reapply sunscreen after swimming; and applying inadequate amounts and missing certain areas of the body, especially the ears, neck, feet and legs.

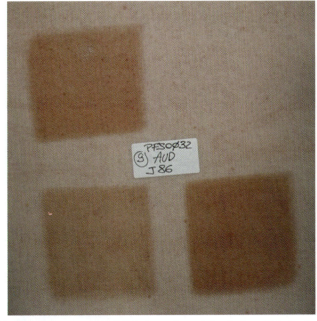

Figure 40 Repeated exposure to UVR induces pigmentation (bottom right). Application of a sunscreen before each exposure (bottom left) reduces this pigmentation, whereas application of a placebo with no UVR absorbers has no effect (top left).

Another reason that burning might occur even with use of sunscreen is that acclimitization (tanning and hyperplasia) is largely inhibited when sunscreens are initially applied effectively. Therefore, if on a subsequent occasion sunscreen is not applied, the skin remains vulnerable to burning.

Prevention of cumulative effects of exposure to the sun

Excessive exposure to UVR leads to premature ageing of the skin, with excessive wrinkles. Photo-damaged skin may have a rough, leathery appearance. The cumulative effects of the exposure weaken the skin's elasticity and tensile strength, resulting in sagging of the skin of the cheeks, deeper facial wrinkles and skin discolouration later in life (Gilmore, 1989). The skin becomes yellowish, with mottled hyperpigmentation, telengiactasia (Fig. 41) and purpura. The epidermis is thinned and lacks downward protuberance of rete ridges. Basophilic degeneration of the uppermost reticular dermis, which is common in sun-damaged skin, consists of swelling, coarsening and late homogenization of connective tissue in the upper dermis. Fibroblasts produce abnormal elastin and collagens. Matrix metalloproteins are also altered during repeated exposure, leading to photoageing, and this occurs at very low doses of UVR (Fisher et al., 1996).

There is no established action spectrum for photoageing and it is not known whether the action spectrum is different from that for erythema. Repeated sub-erythemagenic doses of UVA induce stratum corneum thickening and epidermal hyperplasia in humans and an increased number of inflammatory cells in the dermis (Lavker et al., 1995a). A persistent dermal infiltrate may lead to connective tissue damage and perhaps even to elastosis (Lavker & Kligman, 1988). This persistent dermal inflammation resulting from repeated sub-erythemagenic doses of UVR may adversely affect dermal cellular components, with

fibrosis as one of the end-points. Cytokines released by lymphocytes and mast cells can alter collagen and elastin production and vascular reactivity. Increased release of lysozyme during the initial phases of dermal inflammation (Kajiki et al., 1988) may be related to the increased staining of lysozyme seen in UVA-irradiated elastic fibres. Boyd et al. (1995) reported that solar elastosis was at least partly repaired over 2 years in people who used sunscreens with an SPF of 2–9 every day but not in those who applied a placebo. In a study of 10 people irradiated once daily for 28 days

with 11 MED of solar-simulated UVR through an SPF-22 sunscreen, epidermal hyperplasia, stratum corneum thickening, inflammation of the dermis and deposition of lysozyme in the dermis occurred more frequently than on an unirradiated site (Lavker et al., 1995b). Another study showed that sunscreens can reduce acute changes associated with exposure to UVR which may be related to photoageing, including deposition of lysozyme and α-1-antitrypsin on dermal collagen fibres, with up-regulation of matrix metalloproteinase-2 (Seité et al., 2000b). Studies in experi-

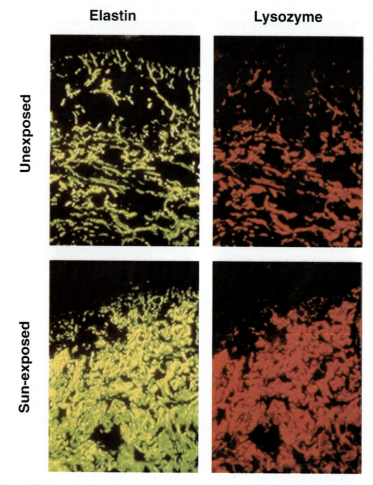

Figure 41 Telangiectasia, a lesion induced in blood vessels by chronic exposure to UVR

mental animals suggest that sunscreens can prevent or allow repair of many of these changes (Kligman *et al.*, 1982, 1983; Kligman, 1989).

Since no single action spectrum defines long-term photodamage, sunscreens that provide protection against a broad spectrum are recommended to prevent such damage (Bergfeld *et al.*, 1997). As it has been estimated that at least 24–48 h are required for skin to recover from a single, sub-threshold exposure, small, repeated doses of UVR within this interval result in cumulative damage (Arbabi *et al.*, 1983). The recovery interval is often cited in recommending daily use of sunscreens by people who spend significant amounts of time outdoors in regions where there is intense sunlight. In areas with less sunlight, daily use of sunscreens may be less important.

Prevention of UVR-induced stimulation of cutaneous diseases

Idiopathic photodermatoses
Idiopathic photodermatoses develop only with exposure to light. Severely affected persons, such as those with chronic actinic dermatitis or hydroa vacciniforme, must use physical measures of protection, and sunscreens play a minor role in the management of these disorders. People who are less affected, such as patients with polymorphic light eruption or juvenile springtime eruption, can have controlled, gradual exposure to the sun which allows the build-up of natural defences (Moyal & Binet, 1997) and may permit nearly normal exposure during summer months.

Photoaggravated dermatoses
Under certain circumstances, diseases of various etiologies can be aggravated by sunlight in patients who on other occasions may react normally. These diseases include lupus erythematosus, lichen planus and herpes simplex. The disease most frequently recognized as requiring careful photoprotection from both UVB and UVA is lupus erythematosus in the discoid, systemic and subacute forms.

Exposure of patients with systemic lupus erythematosus or of mice susceptible to a similar disease results in both systemic and cutaneous manifestations (Sakane *et al.*, 1978; Strickland, 1984). Patients with systemic lupus erythematosus show decreased proliferation of T cells in the autologous mixed leukocyte reaction. This deficiency may be due to the impaired suppressor T-cell function seen in this disease. Hence, in patients with lupus erythematosus, unrestrained autoreactive T-cell and B-cell responses to UVR-induced antigens may lead to cutaneous inflammation, autoantibody production or both. Sunscreens with an SPF of at least 15, providing protection against both UVB and UVA, are required (Drake *et al.*, 1996). The available evidence suggests that regular use of sunscreens reduces morbidity from both cutaneous and systemic lupus erythematosus (Callen *et al.*, 1991; Vila *et al.*, 1999).

Photodermatoses related to congenital abnormalities
Patients with xeroderma pigmentosum, Bloom syndrome, Cockayne syndrome, Rothmund-Thomson syndrome or Smith-Lemli-Optiz syndrome (Anstey *et al.*, 1999) can develop an erythematous, papular, exaggerated sunburn or other symptoms of photosensitivity. Treatment depends on avoidance of UVR by wearing photoprotective clothing, sunglasses and a broad-spectrum sunscreen (Schaefer *et al.*, 2000).

Chapter 7
Carcinogenicity

Human studies

Cohort and case–control studies relevant to evaluating associations between sunscreen use and the prevention of human cancer are summarized on pp. 69–85. The results with respect to carcinogenicity are summarized below.

Fifteen case–control studies were available to evaluate the association between sunscreen use and cutaneous melanoma. Eight of these studies showed statistically significantly higher risks for cutaneous melanoma among users of sunscreens than among non-users, the relative risks for the higher categories of use ranging up to 2.6. When adjustment was made in five studies for exposure and sensitivity to the sun, the relative risk fell in two studies and changed little in three. However, none of the adjusted relative risks fell much, if at all, below 1.0. Four of the case–control studies provided little evidence of an effect of sunscreen use on the risk for cutaneous melanoma among all subjects, and three showed statistically significantly lower risks in users of sunscreens than in non-users.

Most of these studies could be taken to support a positive association between sunscreen use and risk for cutaneous melanoma (Fig. 42); however, it was not possible exclude positive confounding between sunscreen use and sun exposure, sun sensitivity and a history of sun-related neoplasia, or negative confounding with other sun-protective behaviour such as use of protective clothing, wearing a hat or staying in the shade as an explanation for this finding. In none of the analyses was adjustment made for measures of history of sun-related neoplasia or other sun protective behaviour. When sun exposure and sun sensitivity were measured and controlled in the analysis, the control was judged to be insufficient to permit full control of confounding.

Two of the case–control studies of cutaneous melanoma that showed significantly increased risks among sunscreen users, however, provide evidence that use of sunscreens in relation to recreational sun exposure might be associated with a particularly high risk for cutaneous melanoma in subgroups of subjects. Autier et al. (1995) found that, when the risk for cutaneous melanoma was related to sunbathing during the hottest hours of the day, use of sunscreen and hair colour, the relative risk of those with blonde or red hair who sunbathed during the middle of the day and used sunscreens was 6.3 (95% CI, 1.7–23) with reference to those with black or brown hair who neither sunbathed during the hottest hours nor used sunscreens. These results were consistent with an additive interaction between sunbathing in the hottest hours of the day and use of sunscreens. Similarly, Westerdahl et al. (2000) reported a relative risk for cutaneous melanoma of 8.7 (95% CI, 1.0–76) for users of sunscreens compared with non-users when the users stated that they used sunscreens to be able to spend more time in the sun. In addition, although Elwood and Gallagher (1999) did not find an overall effect of sunscreens on the risk for cutaneous melanoma (RR, 1.1; 95% CI, 0.75–1.6), the risk was increased for people who used sunscreens 'only in the first few hours' of solar exposure (RR, 1.6; 95% CI, 1.0–2.5). Two of these studies thus suggest that use of sunscreens leads to spending more time in the sun, particularly during sunbathing, which may increase the risk for cutaneous melanoma.

One cohort study and one case–control study showed increased risks for

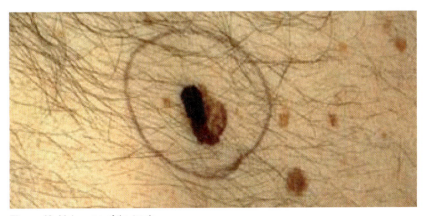

Figure 42 Melanoma of the trunk

basal-cell carcinoma in sunscreen users. No significant association between sunscreen use and cancer risk was observed in one cohort and one case–control study of squamous-cell carcinoma, one of squamous- and basal-cell carcinoma of the skin or one case–control study of squamous-cell carcinoma of the vermilion border of the lip. The same difficulties in control of confounding of sun sensitivity and exposure were present in these studies as in the case-control studies of cutaneous melanoma.

In seeking to explain the increased incidences of cutaneous melanoma and non-melanocytic skin cancer seen in most white populations, Garland et al. (1992, 1993) suggested that the advent of effective UVB sunscreens in the 1960s allowed individuals to remain outdoors in sunny climates for long periods without sunburn. Since these sunscreens did not, however, absorb UVA to any great extent, individuals who used them were probably exposed to substantially more UVA than before. While this is a theoretical possibility, there is no direct support for it in the epidemiological studies.

A further hypothesis was advanced, implicating sunscreens in the increasing incidence of cutaneous melanoma in white populations. It was suggested that sunscreens interfere with the role of UVB in the photosynthesis of vitamin D in human skin (Garland et al., 1990). As 1,25-dihydroxyvitamin D has been shown to inhibit the growth of cutaneous melanoma cells in vitro (Frampton et al., 1983), lowered serum levels of this hormone might place sunscreen users at higher risk for this cancer. Weinstock et al. (1992), however, found no difference in vitamin D intake from dietary sources among 165 cutaneous melanoma patients and 209 controls, suggesting that vitamin D intake is not associated with the incidence of this cancer. This study does not, however, address the issue of vitamin D synthesis in the skin as a result of exposure to UVR.

Several reviews (Ainsleigh, 1993; Studzinski & Moore, 1995) have suggested that sunlight may protect against a number of cancers, including those of the colon (Garland & Garland, 1980; Garland et al., 1989), prostate (Hanchette & Schwartz, 1992; Gann et al., 1996) and breast (Gorham et al., 1990; Janowsky et al., 1997; John et al., 1999). Most of these studies are descriptive or, if analytical, involved relatively few subjects. In addition, control for confounding in the analytical studies was incomplete.

At present, there is no convincing evidence that broad-spectrum sunscreens increase the risk for cutaneous or internal cancers by decreasing the levels of vitamin D.

Experimental models

Assessment of the carcinogenic risk of sunscreens in experimental animals requires long-term experiments with appropriate models, depending on whether internal organs are targeted or whether the risk is limited to a particular type of skin cancer. At present, the only adequate models for this purpose appear to be for squamous-cell carcinoma.

Carcinogenicity of UVR filters

Because some batches of ethylhexyl methoxycinnamate were found to cause reverse mutation in bacteria (see p. 137), Gallagher et al. (1984) assessed the carcinogenicity of mutagenic and non-mutagenic samples. The design of the study and the results with regard to protection are described on p. 93. In the various groups of 20–22 HRA/Skh-1 hairless mice, skin tumours developed in only 4/146 (2.7%) surviving protected mice but in 40–100% of unprotected mice, confirming the protective effect of ethylhexyl methoxycinnamate against UVR-induced skin carcinomas. In order to detect latent tumour initiation, the tumour promoter croton oil was applied to the dorsal skin of sunscreen-treated mice, sunscreen-treated UVR-irradiated mice and untreated mice. While croton oil

alone did not promote skin tumours in control mice, ethylhexyl methoxycinnamate may have initiated the skin tumours in 3/16 surviving unirradiated mice. No distinction could be made between the 'mutagenic' and the 'non-mutagenic' samples, since the numbers of mice were too small. Application of croton oil revealed latent skin tumours in 15–46% of mice previously exposed to UVR through ethylhexyl methoxycinnamate, but the two preparations did not differ significantly.

In a follow-up study (Forbes et al., 1989; see also p. 94), the protective effect of both the mutagenic and the non-mutagenic ethylhexyl methoxycinnamate was found to be dose-related, but consistently more tumours appeared in mice given the mutagenic preparation. Total protection was obtained with 7.5% non-mutagenic and 50% mutagenic samples. The reason for the reduced protection by the mutagenic sample was not apparent. Some of the skin tumours in unirradiated mice were found to be initiated after promotion with TPA. Whereas the prevalence of skin tumours in control mice treated only with TPA was 8.9%, the mutagenic sample of 7.5% ethylhexyl methoxycinnamate induced four times more tumours (17% prevalence) than the non-mutagenic sample (4.2%). With 50% ethylhexyl methoxycinnamate, however, only 4.2 and 4.3% of the mice responded to each sample, respectively. This experiment therefore provides inconsistent results with regard to the enhancement of carcinogenicity by this agent. [The Working Group noted that the SPF values of the two samples were not measured; a difference might have accounted for the difference in the effective UVR initiating doses.]

A working group convened by IARC (IARC, 1989) evaluated studies of the carcinogenicity of TiO_2 administered to rodents orally, subcutaneously, intraperitoneally, intratracheally or by inhalation. The group concluded that there was limited evidence of carcinogenicity in experimental animals exposed to high doses by inhalation (lung tumours) or to 90 mg given as five weekly intra-peritoneal injections (abdominal tumours). Studies of the co-carcinogenicity of TiO_2 in hamsters showed that intratracheal administration of 3 mg weekly for 15 weeks augmented the numbers of benzo[a]pyrene-induced benign and malignant tumours of the larynx (papil-loma and squamous-cell carcinoma), trachea (papilloma, squamous-cell carci-noma and adenocarcinoma) and lungs (adenoma, adenocarcinoma, squamous-cell carcinoma and anaplastic carcinoma).

Photocarcinogenicity of UVR filters
Relatively little information is available in the open scientific literature on possible enhancement of the carcinogenicity of UVR by sunscreens. Most sunscreen products have been tested primarily to assess their protective effect against the induction of squamous-cell carcinoma when applied before exposure to UVR. All the published studies (see p. 90) showed that UVR-induced skin tumour formation in rodents is inhibited by topical treatment with individual or combinations of sunscreens (Gasparro et al., 1998).

In studies designed to test the long-term safety of these products, the source of UVR used was a solar simulator and the sunscreen was applied after expo-sure to see whether it had a negative effect on the skin's protective responses to UV irradiation (Sambuco et al., 1991). Terephthalylidene dicamphor sulfonic acid and ethylhexyl methoxycinnamate did not enhance the carcinogenicity of UVR (Fourtanier, 1996). The study was not designed to ascertain protection factors, but a protection factor was cal-culated as the ratio of the dose required to attain a defined tumour response with the dose that is required to attain the same response under 'protected' conditions. It was calculated that a 5% preparation of ethylhexyl methoxycinna-mate offered a protection factor of only 1.3, and the 5 and 10% preparations of terephthalylidene dicamphor sulfonic acid

had a protection factor of 2.4. These low factors and the lack of difference between the 5 and 10% preparations may be explained by the design of the study, which limits the ability to detect small differences in protection. To avoid acute or subchronic damage in animals, only small doses of UVR were given through the sunscreens, making it difficult to detect a dose–effect relationship with two concentrations of the same UVR absorber with a difference of no more than 1.5 in the SPF or protection factor.

Carcinogenicity of sunscreens containing photosensitizing tanning agents
The photocarcinogenicity mediated by the furocoumarins has been well docu-mented (IARC, 1987), and there is suffi-cient evidence that 8- and 5-methoxy-psoralen increase the carcinogenic effects of UVA in mouse skin (Fig. 43). Addition of 5-methoxypsoralen to a sun-screen was intended to provide a rapid tan by UVA-driven photosensitization, while the sunscreen offered protection against UVB damage. It was thought that the acquired tan would subsequently protect the skin against solar UVR.

Two studies have addressed the inter-action of 5-methoxypsoralen and sun-screens in mice. The protocols and the effects of the sunscreens alone are des-cribed on p. 94, whereas the effects of 5-methoxypsoralen are described here.

Both 5- and 8-methoxypsoralen have phototumorigenic potential in hairless

mice (Young et al., 1983). A study was conducted in groups of 20 male and 20 female hairless albino mice (outbred St John's strain) to test the capacity of a sunscreen which contained two UVB absorbers, 12.5 µL/mL (1.25%) ethylhexyl methoxycinnamate and 10 mg/mL (1%) 3-benzylidene camphor, with and without 5-methoxypsoralen at 25 or 50 µg/mL, to protect against photocarcinogenesis. The effect of 5-methoxypsoralen alone was tested in irradiated and unirradiated mice. The treatments were continued on 5 days/week for 44–46 weeks. Tumour growth was monitored, the tumours were classified histologically, and the data were analysed statistically. 5-Methoxy-psoralen was clearly carcinogenic at both doses, and the sunscreen gave pro-tection against the tumorigenic effect up to week 40. After that time, however, the mean tumour multiplicity was increased by 25 µg/mL 5-methoxypsoralen in the presence of the sunscreen, from 0.81 to 4.5 tumours per mouse, and the number at 60 weeks (4.5) was similar to that in mice irradiated through the vehicle (6.0). This was significantly greater than the 1.09 tumours per mouse found in sun-screen-protected mice. Thus, solar-simu-lated UVR-induced photocarcinogenesis was clearly inhibited by the sunscreen alone, and the sunscreen was found to suppress the increased risk incurred by addition of 5-methoxypsoralen to the pre-paration during the first 40 weeks of treat-ment. The later increase in tumour inci-dence due to 5-methoxypsoralen after

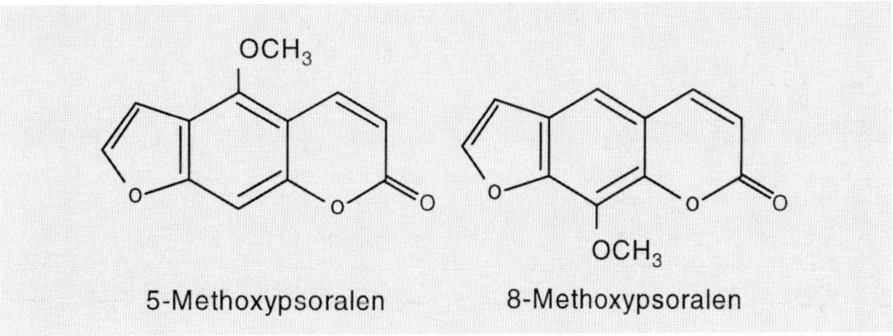

Figure 43 Formulae of 5-methoxypsoralen and 8-methoxypsoralen

irradiation was not, however, prevented by the sunscreen (Young et al., 1987).

In a further study, Young et al. (1990) treated groups of 30 female Skh-1 hairless albino mice with 100 μL of solutions containing 5-methoxypsoralen at 5, 15 or 50 μg/mL from bergamot oil, with and without added sunscreen consisting of the UVB absorber ethylhexyl methoxycinnamate at 0.5% and the UVA absorber butyl methoxydibenzoylmethane at 0.5% [SPF not determined]. Similar concentrations of 5-methoxypsoralen are found in cosmetics and perfumes. As described on p. 96, the mice were irradiated with solar-simulated UVR 20–40 min after the topical applications on 5 days/week for up to 73 weeks, the duration of treatment being determined by the severity of the tumour response. One group also received solar-simulated UVR 5–6 h after topical application, and a further group was treated and irradiated only every other 4-week period. The protection afforded by the sunscreen alone is described on p. 96. Treatment with 5-methoxy-psoralen and solar-simulated UVR did not induce tumours up to 57 weeks. Subsequently, an increase in the concentration of 5-methoxypsoralen decreased the average time to tumour onset from 62 weeks to 58, 49 and 28 weeks with 5, 15 and 50 μg/mL 5-methoxypsoralen, respectively. Irradiation 5–6 h after topical application of 50 μg/mL 5-methoxy-psoralen alone significantly reduced the time to tumour onset from 65 to 58 weeks. The intermittent treatments also appeared to be protective, but not when analysed in relation to the cumulative dose of solar-simulated UVR, in which case photocarcinogenesis with 50 μg/mL 5-methoxypsoralen alone was enhanced. This indicates that the 4-week 'rest' period did not result in repair of the damage caused by 5-methoxypsoralen and solar-simulated UVR.

As albino mice were used in these two studies, the results are indicative of the cancer risk in the absence of pigmentation. To assess whether psoralen-enhanced pigmentation would provide additional protection against photocarcinogenesis, experiments were conducted with the furocoumarin 6,6,4′-trimethylangelicin instead of 5-methoxypsoralen in pigmented female Skh hairless mice (HRA.HRII-c/+/Skh) (Kipp et al., 1998). 6,4,4′-Trimethylangelicin is more powerful in inducing pigmentation than 5-methoxypsoralen and causes mono-adducts in DNA but considerably fewer cross-links than 5-methoxypsoralen. The authors concluded that epidermal tanning with or without furocoumarin is not effective in preventing skin cancer in this mouse model.

Chapter 8
Toxic effects

Toxic and other adverse effects of sunscreens

In order for a sunscreen to have a toxic effect on living tissues, it must penetrate the skin. There is some evidence that this can occur (see p. 63 *et seq.*).

Human studies

No published studies of toxic effects in humans were available to the Working Group.

Contact sensitivity

There are numerous reports of cases of allergic reactions and photoreactivity to sunscreens, but the prevalence of this problem among sunscreen users is difficult to estimate. Since sunscreens are becoming more complex, with multiple active ingredients, fragances and other compounds, this problem could increase in the future. Reactions to sunscreens were found to be reasonably common among patients referred to a clinic because of suspected photosensitivity. Such patients are heavily exposed to sunscreen products and are thought to become more sensitive to chemicals than others (Green *et al.*, 1991; Bilsland & Ferguson, 1993; Stitt *et al.*, 1996; Berne & Ros, 1998).

The published reports of adverse effects range from case histories in one or several subjects (Schauder & Ippen, 1986; Knobler *et al.*, 1989; Motley & Reynolds, 1989; Murphy *et al.*, 1990; Torres & Correia, 1991; Buckley *et al.*, 1993; Collins & Ferguson, 1994; Kimura & Katoh, 1995; Parry *et al.*, 1995; Silva *et al.*, 1995; Marguery *et al.*, 1996; Ricci *et al.*, 1997; Zhang *et al.*, 1998) to

studies of tens or hundreds of patients (Thune, 1984; English *et al.*, 1987; Lenique *et al.*, 1992; Szczurko *et al.*, 1994; Trevisi *et al.*, 1994; Gonçalo *et al.*, 1995; Ang *et al.*, 1998) and reviews (Dromgoole & Maibach, 1990; González & González, 1996; Schauder & Ippen, 1997). In the past, PABA and its esters were the most commonly reported contact and photoallergens in sunscreens (Funk *et al.*, 1997), and this finding contributed to a reduction in their use in sunscreens. The contact or photocontact allergen in sunscreens most frequently cited today is benzophenone-3, followed by dibenzoyl methanes. There have also been a few reports of contact allergy to excipients included in the formulations (Jeanmougin *et al.*, 1988; Nishioka *et al.*, 1995; Silvestre *et al.*, 1996). In a longitudinal, population-based study to reactions to sunscreens carried out in Australia, of the 603 people tested with a commonly used sunscreen formulation, 114 developed an adverse reaction (e.g. skin irritation). When they were patch tested, however, none was allergic to the active ingredients. A higher than expected proportion of the subjects who developed an adverse reaction had a personal history consistent with atopy (Foley *et al.*, 1993).

Overexposure to UVA

An obvious but not readily recognized adverse effect of sunscreens is interference with accommodation by the skin to UVR. Because most sunscreens absorb primarily UVB and, in some cases, short-wavelength UVAII (315–340 nm), the use of sunscreens changes the UVR

spectrum to which the skin is exposed (Gasparro *et al.*, 1998). Since UVB is the primary stimulus for adaptation of the skin to sunlight, less adaptation might be expected to develop in individuals who use sunscreens regularly. The adaptive responses include thickening of the epidermis and transfer of melanin-containing granules to keratinocytes (tanning) (Fig. 44), which reduces the transparency of the skin to UVA and UVB (Fusaro *et al.*, 1966; Olson *et al.*, 1973). Several reports showed that UVR-induced injury, such as dermal connective tissue damage and sunburn cell formation, can occur in human epidermal cells in the absence of erythema and at doses that are far below the SPF of the sunscreen (Kaidbey, 1990; Kligman, 1997). Furthermore, prevention of sunburn by sunscreens may create a false sense of security, while allowing prolonged exposure to sunlight. An increasing number of studies indicate that, although UVB is the most damaging component of sunlight, UVA is responsible for numerous morphological, molecular and biochemical events which may contribute to photodamage of the skin (Kligman & Gebre, 1991; Scharffetter *et al.*, 1991; Wlaschek *et al.*, 1993; Lavker *et al.*, 1995b; Lavker & Kaidbey, 1997).

Vitamin D depletion

Vitamin D is produced when UVB absorbed by the epidermis causes 7-dehydroxycholesterol to form previtamin D_3, which isomerizes spontaneously to vitamin D_3 before entering the circulation, where it is metabolized by the liver into 25-hydroxyvitamin D_3 and by the

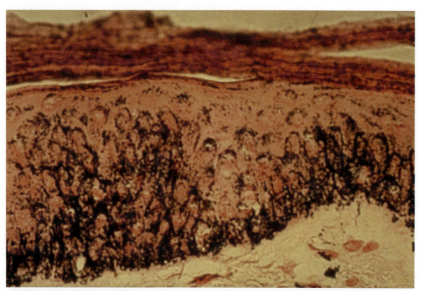

Figure 44 Increased melanin deposition induced by repeated exposure to the sun can be visualized throughout the epidermis by Fontana Masson staining

kidneys into 1,25-dihydroxyvitamin D_3. The latter is the most biologically active form. Vitamin D can also be supplied by the diet. With parathyroid hormone, it regulates calcium homeostasis. There has been concern that reduction of UVB absorption by the epidermis by sunscreen use could suppress vitamin D production, thus affecting calcium metabolism.

In one study, six women and two men received whole-body exposure to 1 MED UVR (Westinghouse sunlamps FS72T12, 260–360 nm) with or without protection from 5% PABA (SPF 8). The serum concentration of vitamin D in unprotected subjects increased from 1.5 ± 1.0 to 26 ± 6.7 ng/ml 24 h after exposure to UVR. In the sunscreen-protected volunteers, serum vitamin D was unaltered by exposure, with values of 5.6 ± 3.0 and 4.4 ± 2.4 ng/ml before and 24 h after exposure, respectively. PABA also completely inhibited previtamin D_3 production from 7-dehydroxycholesterol in triplicate samples of human skin exposed to UVR *in vitro* (Matsuoka *et al.*, 1987).

In a subsequent study, serum vitamin D was measured in groups of four healthy subjects 1 h before and 24 h after exposure to 0.8 MED from the same UVR source (Matsuoka *et al.*, 1990). The volunteers received either no sunscreen or sunscreen applied to increasing areas of the body. Whole-body protection completely prevented the UVR-induced increase in serum vitamin D, and selective protection of increasing skin areas correlated with the serum vitamin D concentration.

Twenty persons with a history of skin cancer (mean age, 64.6) who had been using PABA-based sunscreens for more than 1 year had a significantly lower serum vitamin D concentration (40 ± 3.2 nmol/L) than 20 healthy controls matched for age and exposure to sunlight (91 ± 6.2) (Matsuoka *et al.*, 1988).

In a study of eight patients with xeroderma pigmentosum who took extreme measures to protect themselves from light, including minimizing the time spent in sunlight, protective clothing and constant sunscreen use, the serum vitamin D concentration monitored over 6 years was found to be at the lower end of the

normal range. Nevertheless, the serum calcium concentration was within the normal range, as was that of parathyroid hormone, which might have been expected to be increased if the vitamin D level was low (Sollitto *et al.*, 1997).

A randomized double-blind controlled trial of 113 healthy adults over 40 years of age who used a sunscreen or a placebo cream included analyses of serum vitamin D concentrations over 7 months, including summer (Marks *et al.*, 1995). The broad-spectrum sunscreen had an SPF of 17 and contained 8% ethylhexyl methoxycinnamate and 2% butyl methoxydibenzoylmethane and was applied to the head and neck, forearms and dorsum of each hand at least once a day. The concentrations of 25-hydroxyvitamin D_3 rose to a similar extent in the groups given sunscreen and placebo over the summer period, whereas those of 1,25-dihydroxyvitamin D_3 increased in the group given the placebo but not in those given the sunscreen, although they did not fall below the normal range. This suggests that although vitamin D synthesis was reduced by the sunscreen it was not reduced sufficiently to cause deficiency.

This finding is in agreement with that of another study (Farrerons *et al.*, 1998) in which serum vitamin D, parathyroid hormone and bone biological markers were assessed in 24 users of a sunscreen (SPF 15) and compared with those in 19 controls over 2 years. Whereas significantly lower levels of vitamin D were observed in the sunscreen users, there were no changes in parathyroid hormone or bone biological markers.

Experimental studies
Whole animals and cells
All UVR filters used in over-the-counter sunscreen products are subjected to extensive testing for toxicity and safety, and the results are evaluated by regulatory bodies, including the Scientific Committee on Cosmetics and Non-food Products for the Commission of the

European Union (Loprieno, 1992) and the Food and Drug Administration in the USA (Food & Drug Administration, 1999). Only compounds proven to be safe and without significant toxicological effects receive approval for use in sunscreens. This information is supplied to the regulatory bodies by manufacturers but is not publicly available and could therefore not be reviewed by the Working Group.

A study of the safety of benzophenone-3 found that it was practically non-toxic when administered orally to rats and was not toxic when applied to the skin of rabbits at doses up to 16 g/kg bw, with no significant lesions at autopsy (Cosmetic Ingredient Review, 1983). It did not irritate the skin or eyes of rabbits and was not phototoxic in guinea-pigs and rabbits when applied five times per week for 2 weeks. When dissolved in petroleum jelly base and applied topically to the skin of male Sprague-Dawley rats twice daily for 4 weeks at 100 mg/kg bw per day, benzophenone-3 did not cause any observable toxicity. There was no effect on body weight, organ:body weight ratios or haematological, clinical chemical or histological parameters (Okereke et al., 1995). When fed to rats, it had an $LD_{50} > 13$ g/kg bw, and the no-effect level over 90 days of feeding was found to be 0.1%, corresponding to 0.33 g/kg bw per day (Lewerenz et al., 1972).

Groups of Hr/Hr pigmented female hairless mice treated with 0.1 ml of a commercial sunscreen containing ethylhexyl methoxycinnamate and benzophenone-3 on 4 days/week for 12 months developed some toxic side-effects, including amyloidosis, eczema-like oedema and ulceration and pigment deposition (Wulf et al., 1982). The specific component could not be identified. Application of the same sunscreen to the eyes of mice caused significant hyperplasia of the eyelid skin and acute inflammation of the cornea (Vangsted, 1985). A benzophenone-3-containing sunscreen was also reported to exacer-

bate dermal damage caused by chronic exposure to long-wavelength UVA (> 340 nm) (Kligman & Zheng, 1994).

Isoamyl-para-methoxycinnamate administered to pregnant Wistar rats on days 6–15 of gestation caused the death of 10% of the animals due to gastrointestinal erosion and haemorrhage when given at a dose of 2.25 but not 0.75 or 0.25 g/kg bw per day by intragastric instillation. The remainder of the animals at this dose lost weight and had reduced food and increased water consumption and hair loss. Mild hair loss and reduced food intake were observed in the group receiving 0.75 g/kg bw per day (Jekat et al., 1992).

Moderate skin irritation was caused by octocrylene applied topically at a dose of 264 mg/kg bw per day to New Zealand white rabbits, but not at lower doses (Odio et al., 1994). Reduced weight gain was also observed, but there were no macroscopic or histopathological abnormalities in blood cells, kidney or liver. Octocrylene did not induce mutation in lymphoma cells in vitro.

TiO_2-coated mica, 10–35 μm, added to the diet of Fischer 344 rats at up to 5% for 130 weeks did not cause consistent changes in any end-point studied, including survival, body-weight gain, haematological or clinical chemical parameters or histological appearance (Bernard et al., 1990). Intratracheal exposure of rats to 2 mg of ultrafine TiO_2 particles (< 30 nm), however, caused inflammation and cytotoxicity to pulmonary alveolar macrophages (Afaq et al., 1998).

In contrast, HeLa cells and T-24 human bladder cancer cells grown in vitro were killed by a suspension of TiO_2 particles and exposure to 300–400-nm UVR (Cai et al., 1992; Kubota et al., 1994). Furthermore, when TiO_2 was injected into the tumour and the animals were irradiated with the same UVR source, the growth of both tumour cell lines transplanted subcutaneously into athymic mice was inhibited.

PABA, ethylhexyl methoxycinnamate and benzophenone-3 inhibited cell

growth and DNA synthesis, retarding cell cycle progression from G_1 when added to cultured cell lines at doses of 50–100 μg/ml. As these doses could be achieved in vivo in sunscreen-treated skin, these effects may be of biological relevance (Xu & Parsons, 1999). PABA at a dose of 328 μmol/L was reported to inhibit platelet aggregation in vitro (Barbieri et al., 1999).

A mouse lymphoma cell line had decreased survival in a suspension of 0.1% PABA after exposure to 313 nm UVR (Osgood et al., 1982).

Production of reactive oxygen species by sunscreens

PABA has been reported to scavenge singlet molecular oxygen species (Fig. 45) (Allen et al., 1995). It also protected calf thymus DNA from damage by free radicals induced by exposure to UVR at 254 nm for 1 h at 1.9 mW/cm², due to either its sunscreening or its reactive oxygen quenching properties (Hu et al., 1995).

In contrast, irradiation of aqueous solutions of PABA, ethylhexyl PABA, octocrylene and ethylhexyl methoxycinnamate but not benzophenone-3 or benzophenone-8 with solar-simulated UVR (provided by a filtered 1000-W xenon arc lamp) generated singlet molecular oxygen (Allen et al., 1996a,b). In another study, benzophenone-3 interfered with antioxidant defence in the skin. Benzophenone-3 in a sunscreen (SPF 25) applied to human skin was photooxidized to benzophenone-3 semiquinone after 20 min of exposure to sunlight. The latter reacted with thiol groups on proteins, such as thioredoxin reductase and reduced glutathione, involved in antioxidant defence, causing their inactivation (Schallreuter et al., 1996).

Uncoated TiO_2 particles exposed to UVR can form reactive oxygen species (Sclafani et al., 1990), including hydroxyl radicals (Brezova & Stasko, 1994). TiO_2 particles extracted from commercial sunscreens and irradiated with UVR

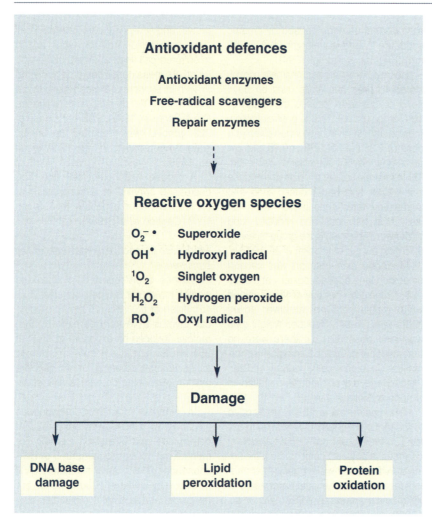

Antioxidant defences

Antioxidant enzymes

Free-radical scavengers

Repair enzymes

Reactive oxygen species

$O_2^- \cdot$	**Superoxide**
$OH^\bullet$	**Hydroxyl radical**
$^1O_2$	**Singlet oxygen**
H_2O_2	**Hydrogen peroxide**
$RO^\bullet$	**Oxyl radical**

Damage

DNA base damage	Lipid peroxidation	Protein oxidation

Figure 45 Reactive oxygen species: endogenous defences and damaging effects

(310–400 nm) oxidized organic substrates, indicating that sunlight-irradiated TiO$_2$ induces biological damage mediated by reactive oxygen species (Dunford *et al.*, 1997). When hydroxylation of guanine was used as a biomarker for reactive oxygen-mediated damage to nucleic acids, 0.45 µm of anatase TiO$_2$ particles irradiated with UVA (320–400 nm) induced oxidative damage to the RNA but not the DNA of cultured skin fibroblasts. The finding that these cells accumulated the TiO$_2$ particles in the cytoplasm but not the

nucleus suggests that reactive oxygen species generated by irradiated TiO$_2$ particles induce damage only at the site of their production (Wamer *et al.*, 1997).

Huang *et al.* (1997) found that uncoated, 10-nm TiO$_2$ particles exposed to 300–400 nm radiation induced oxidative damage to DNA, leading to cell death. This could be prevented by the addition of reactive oxygen scavengers.

Intratracheal exposure of rats to 2 mg of ultrafine, uncoated TiO$_2$ particles (< 30

nm) caused lipid peroxidation and hydrogen peroxide production associated with enhancement of antioxidant enzyme activity and cytotoxicity to pulmonary alveolar macrophages (Afaq *et al.*, 1998). This suggests that the TiO$_2$ particles kill the macrophages by increasing oxidative stress which cannot be overcome by the increase in anti-oxidant enzymes. Scavengers of reactive oxygen have also been shown to inhibit the killing of tumour cells by UV-irradiated uncoated TiO$_2$ (Cai *et al.*, 1992; Kubota *et al.*, 1994).

Immune system

Application of 8% ethylhexyl dimethyl PABA, 8% ethylhexyl methoxycinnamate or 7.2% microfine TiO$_2$ in an oil-in-water emulsion 5 days/week for 4 weeks suppressed the induction of contact sensitivity to trinitrochlorobenzene in female C3H/HeJ but not BALB/c mice, in the absence of UVR. This immune suppressive effect of the sunscreens could be overcome by supplementation with oxygen radical scavengers (Bestak *et al.*, 1995). A similar result was observed in a study in which three commercial sunscreens, applied topically to mice for 3 consecutive days suppressed the induction of contact sensitivity by about 50% (Reeve, 1997). It is not clear from either study whether the immune suppression was due to the UVR filter or another component of the sunscreen product. In contrast to the above findings, 0.2% 4-isopropyl-dibenzoylmethane, but not 5% PABA or 1% homosalate, induced contact sensitization and mild irritation in unirradiated Hartley outbred guinea-pigs after occlusion for 2 h. PABA, but not the other two agents, induced photoallergy when the guinea-pigs were irradiated with 100 kJ/m^2 UVA (320–400 nm) (Gerberick & Ryan, 1989). Thus, it appears that sunscreens can be immune suppressive, sensitizing or photoallergenic under some conditions.

Reproductive and developmental effects
Human studies
No epidemiological study has been conducted showing that sunscreen use has any reproductive or developmental effects.

Experimental studies
PABA injected intraperitoneally into pregnant rats on days 1–6, 6–16 or 1–16 of gestation at 5 mg/kg bw per day did not damage the fetuses (Stroeva & Popov, 1998). Benzophenone-3 dissolved in acetone and applied topically at doses ≤ 400 mg/kg bw per day had no toxic effects on the reproductive organs of male B6C3F$_1$ mice. Sperm concentration and motility, reproductive organ weight and histological appearance were normal (Daston et al., 1993). When benzophenone-3 was fed to Swiss CD-1 mice at 1.8, 4 or 9 g/kg bw per day, the two higher doses caused reduced body weight, a reduced number of live pups per litter, reduced pup weight and increased mortality among lactating dams (Chapin et al., 1997).

Isoamyl-*para*-methoxycinnamate given to pregnant Wistar rats on days 6–15 of gestation by intragastric instillation had a significant effect on reproduction or embryo development only at the highest dose tested, 2.25 g/kg bw per day (Jekat et al., 1992). The two lower doses, 0.75 and 0.25 g/kg bw per day, had no observable effect. The highest dose increased the rate of intrauterine deaths, decreased fetal weights and caused some signs of retarded development but no signs of teratogenicity.

Octocrylene at doses up to 267 mg/kg bw per day had no discernible reproductive or developmental effects when applied topically to New Zealand white does on days 6–18 of gestation, and no signs of toxicity were observed on the male reproductive system. In female CD-1 mice given octocrylene orally by gavage on days 8–12 of gestation, doses ≤ 1000 mg/kg bw per day had no

effect on pup survival or litter weight (Odio et al., 1994).

Genetic and related effects
Human studies
No data were available to the Working Group.

Experimental systems
Since sunscreens are exposed to UVR, it is important to consider the potential damaging effects of the compounds alone and in combination with UVR and visible light, including photosensitized damage and mutation. Consideration must be given to the wavelength distribution and energy of the source(s) employed. In all studies, it is crucial to define not only the exact chemical nature and concentration of the sunscreen ingredient(s) but also the precise nature of the test system.

Most sunscreens have now been tested for their ability to modify genetic material in a variety of test systems in the absence of UVR (Table 26). Those that have shown evidence of direct DNA damaging properties are ethylhexyl methoxycinnamate (or more likely an unidentified contaminant of the sunscreen preparation, Bonin et al., 1982) and a nitrosamine contaminant (2-ethylhexyl 4-*N*-methyl-*N*-nitrosamino-benzoate) of ethylhexyl dimethyl PABA, originally reported by Loeppky et al. (1991) but not confirmed by Dunkel et al. (1992). Benzophenone-3 was also shown to have some mutagenic properties (French, 1992), but the result was not confirmed in a further study (Robison et al., 1994). A review of data on the mutagenicity of ethylhexyl methoxycinnamate (Trueman & Schüpbach, 1982) shows that the results differ according to batch, even within a single laboratory. This finding lends credence to the idea that the clear positive results observed in certain studies are the result of a contaminant.

PABA has been shown to cause differential killing of repair-deficient bac-

teria (Hodges et al., 1977), and similar toxicity was later reported in mouse lymphoma (L5178Y) cells (Osgood et al., 1982). PABA also caused photosensitized formation of pyrimidine dimers in DNA (Sutherland & Griffin, 1984). Although PABA and UVR or visible light were not mutagenic in bacteria, a preliminary report showed that both conditions could lead to chromosomal aberrations in mammalian cells (Dean et al., 1991; Table 27). Ethylhexyl dimethyl PABA (Knowland et al., 1993) can cause genetic damage in combination with UVR or visible light. A classic example of genotoxicity in the presence of UVR is that of methoxypsoralens, which were previously used in sunscreens (Ashwood-Smith et al., 1980; Dean et al., 1991; Chételat et al., 1993a,b).

Phenylbenzimidazole sulfonic acid generated guanine-specific damage in DNA when a mixture of the compound and a synthetic oligodeoxyribonucleotide were irradiated with UVB (Stevenson & Davies, 1999), but studies have not yet been conducted in cells or in vivo.

TiO$_2$ was considered to be non-mutagenic (IARC, 1989), but an increased frequency of sister chromatid exchange in CHO-K1 cells and a slight increase in the frequency of micronuclei have since been shown after treatment with non-lethal doses of TiO$_2$ (Lu et al., 1998). Nakagawa et al. (1997) demonstrated that TiO$_2$ particles have no or weak genotoxicity in the absence of UVR or visible light, but significant DNA damage was found in the Comet assay and in the chromosomal aberration test after irradiation with a solar simulator.

Samples of a TiO$_2$ sunscreen catalysed the photooxidation of phenol, and sunlight-irradiated TiO$_2$ induced DNA damage in vitro and in human fibroblasts, as measured in the Comet assay (Dunford et al., 1997). Further information on the genotoxicity of TiO$_2$ can be found in The US Pharmacopeia of 1999.

Table 26. Genetic effects of sunscreen ingredients in the absence of UVR or visible light

Test substance	Test system[a]	Result	Metabolic activation	Concentration	Reference
Ethylhexyl methoxycinnamate	G SA8	+	−	?	Bonin et al. (1982)
	G DMX	+	−	?	
	S SIC[b]	+	−	0.18 mol/L	
Ethylhexyl dimethyl PABA contaminant: 2-ethylhexyl 4-N-methyl-N-nitrosaminobenzoate	G SA0	−	−	0–50 µmol/plate	Loeppky et al. (1991)
		+	+	0–50 µmol/plate	
	G SA5	−	−	0–50 µmol/plate	
		+	+	0–50 µmol/plate	
	G SA0	−	+/−	2.3–34.2 µmol/plate	Dunkel et al. (1992)
	G SA5	−	+/−	2.3–34.2 µmol/plate	
	G SA8	−	+/−	2.3–34.2 µmol/plate	
	G SA9	−	+/−	2.3–34.2 µmol/plate	
	G G5T	−	−	3.42×10^{-6} mol/L	
		−	+	1.06×10^{-4} mol/L	
Benzophenone-3	M MVR	−	−	$3–50 \times 10^3$ ppm in feed	French (1992)
	G SA0	−	+/−	0–1 mg/plate	
	G SA5	−	+/−	0–1 mg/plate	
	G SA7	−	+/−	0–1 mg/plate	
	G SA9	−	+/−	0–1 mg/plate	
	S SIC	−	−	1.7–17 µg/ml	
		+	+	5–50 µg/ml	
	C CIC	−	−	9.4–93 µg/ml	
		+	+	9.4–75 µg/ml	
	G DMM	−	−	$3.0–3.5 \times 10^3$ g/L	Robison et al. (1994)
	C CBA	−	−	0.5–5.0 g/kg bw	
PABA	C CIC	+	−	1900 µg/ml	Dean et al. (1991)

[a] See Appendix 2 for explanation of codes.

Table 27. Genetic effects of sunscreen ingredients in the presence of UVR or visible light

Test substance	Test system[a]	Result	Metabolic activation	UVR or visible light source	Concentration	Reference
PABA	C CIC	(+)	–	UVA/UVB	1500–1700 µg/ml (1900 µg/ml toxic)	Dean et al. (1991)
Ethylhexyl dimethyl PABA	D SSD	+	–	Solar simulator	50 µmol/L	Knowland et al. (1993)
	G SCR	+	–	Solar simulator	50 µmol/L	
	D DIH (human keratinocytes)	+	–	Solar simulator	50 µmol/L	Gulston & Knowland (1999
5-Methoxypsoralen	G ECW	+	–	UVA (320–380 nm) black light bulbs	40 µg/ml	Ashwood-Smith et al. (1980)
	S SIC	+	–	UVA (320–380 nm) black light bulbs	40 µg/ml	
8-Methoxypsoralen	G SA0	+	–	UVA and UVA/UVB UVA/UVB	6.25–5- µg/plate 50–1000 µg/plate	Dean et al. (1991)
	C CIC	+	–	UVA/UVB	50 µg/ml	
	G SA0	+	–	Solar simulator	0.3–3 µg/plate	Chétalat et al. (1993a)
	G SA2	+	–	Solar simulator	0.3–3 µg/plate	
	R SCG	+	–	Solar simulator	0.8–5 µg/ml	
	C CIC	+	–	Solar simulator	2 µg/ml (5 µg/ml phototoxic)	Chételat et al. (1993b)
TiO$_2$	R SCG	+	–	Solar simulator	0–3200 µg/ml	Nakagawa et al. (1997)
	G SA0	–	–	Solar simulator	0–40 mg/ml	
	G SA2	–	–	Solar simulator	0–40 mg/ml	
	G SA9	–	–	Solar simulator	0–40 mg/ml	
	G G51	–	–	Solar simulator	0–2000 µg/ml	
	C CIC	+	–	Solar simulator	0–50 µg/ml	

[a] See Appendix 2 for explanation of codes.

Chapter 9

Summary of Data

Chemistry, occurrence and human exposure

Chemical and physical characteristics of constituents of sunscreens

The term 'sunscreens' is used in this volume to refer to formulated products that are ready for use to protect the skin against solar ultraviolet radiation (UVR), including those commercially available and formulations under test. 'Active' ingredients of sunscreens are the chemicals included in sunscreen formulations for the purpose of reducing the amount of UVR that reaches the viable cells of the skin. The active ingredients can be classified as organic or inorganic chemical absorbers. The seven major groups of organic chemical absorbers currently used in sunscreen formulations are derivatives of cinnamates, salicylates, *para*-aminobenzoates, camphor derivatives, anthranilates, benzophenones and dibenzoylmethanes. The inorganic chemical absorbers are titanium dioxide and zinc oxide. Approximately 42 of these major groups or their derivatives are currently used as ingredients in hundreds of branded products. Although each ingredient has several names, each is associated with a unique Chemical Abstract Services (CAS) number. Sunscreen formulations are complex mixtures of solvents, wetting and suspending agents, preservatives, fragrance materials and other additives. The active ingredients are subject to analytical evaluation and quality control.

A major characteristic of sunscreen ingredients is photostability. Decay rates have been reported under conditions of exaggerated exposure and realistic use. In general, marketed sunscreen formulations are of acceptable stability but some ingredients have been reported to induce photoproducts, the biological and photobiological significance of which are under investigation.

Sunscreens are marketed as pharmaceuticals (drugs) in some countries (such as Australia, Canada and the USA) and as cosmetics in others (such as the countries of the European Union and Japan). The regional lists of approved ingredients are not identical but overlap broadly.

Measurement of UVR and human exposure

The solar UVR to which an individual is exposed depends on the following factors:

- intensity of ambient solar UVR,
- fraction of ambient exposure received on different anatomical sites,
- type of behaviour and time spent outdoors.

The dose of UVR absorbed by the skin is further modified by the use of photoprotective agents such as hats, clothing and sunscreens.

A number of studies indicate that adult indoor workers in northern Europe receive about 70% of their annual exposure to UVR during weekends and holidays and principally on the hands, forearms and face. Annual exposure is approximately 5% of the total ambient UVR available. As children and adolescents have more opportunities for exposure to the sun, they receive about 7% of ambient UVR. Studies of children in Australia and England showed that behaviour can be as important as ambient UVR on the exposure of an individual to the sun.

Increased frequency of holidays in sunny climates and of outdoor leisure activities are resulting in increasing exposure of populations, especially those in temperate latitudes.

The sun protection factor (SPF) is popularly interpreted as a measure of how much longer skin covered with sunscreen takes to burn compared with unprotected skin. This interpretation can encourage users to prolong their exposure accordingly. Nevertheless, there is ample evidence that the numerical measure of protection indicated on a package is generally higher than that achieved in practice. Because the typical thickness applied is considerably less than that used by manufacturers (2 mg/cm^2) during determination of SPF in the laboratory, consumers can expect to be protected to a degree closer to one-third of the value.

Behavioural aspects

Since 1950, an increasing number of white people have used sunscreens, principally in Australia, Europe and North America. Sunscreen use has also become common in Japan. Use of these products is one of the actions described as 'sun-related behaviour', i.e. any behaviour that increases or decreases exposure of skin or eyes to solar UVR. Other such behaviour includes wearing protective clothing, hats or sunglasses, remaining in the shade, staying indoors around solar noon and minimizing the time spent outdoors at high altitude and low latitudes and in sunny seasons. It is often difficult to separate the protection attributable to sunscreens from that afforded by other forms of sun protection.

Two types of exposure can be distinguished during which sunscreen may be applied to uncovered parts of the skin: intentional and unintentional sun exposure. Intentional exposure is that with the primary purpose of achieving a biological response from the sun, such as acquisition of a tan. During intentional exposure, significant portions of the trunk and limbs are frequently uncovered. Sunbathing is the most typical such behaviour. In children and in adults, most sunburns occur during intentional sun exposure. Unintentional sun exposure is that which occurs during usual daily life, without the specific intention of acquiring a tan or staying in the sun for its own sake. During this type of behaviour, the parts of the body that are uncovered are generally the face, ears, neck and hands. The forearms and legs especially of women may also be uncovered, but the trunk is rarely uncovered. The randomized trials of the ability of sunscreens to prevent non-melanocytic sun-induced lesions generally addressed unintentional exposure.

The results of a large number of studies on sunscreen use in various populations have been published. Geographic, racial and cultural characteristics account for much of the variation in sunscreen use, but some consistent features of use are that women are more likely than men to use sunscreens; children and adults are more likely to use them than are adolescents; sunscreen use is most common on the beach or during sunbathing; white-skinned people from high latitudes, particularly in 'sunny' situations, are heavy users of sunscreens. The limited published data on

how people actually use sunscreens strongly suggest that the products are often, probably usually, not used as recommended. While behavioural studies confirm that sunscreens are used to prevent sunburn, the other underlying reasons vary considerably, from motivation to stay in the sun as long as possible without burning to deliberately seeking maximum protection against skin cancer. Educational strategies, particularly in schools and communities, can increase sun protection behaviour and increase sunscreen use, but at a population level it is probably sunscreen advertising that is most influential and most likely to promote intentional sun exposure.

Sunscreens are designed primarily to prevent sunburn. Use of sunscreens during unintentional exposure appears to reduce the occurrence of sunburn, but use of sunscreens or of higher-SPF sunscreen during intentional exposure appears to have little effect. One study of intentional exposure indicated that subjects who use high-SPF sunscreens stay in the sun longer than those who use lower-SPF products and that at least 'sun-seeking' populations use sunscreen to avoid sunburn rather than total UVR exposure; guarding against skin cancer is at best a secondary motive.

In a study of persons aged 40 or more who were randomized to apply sunscreens of SPF 15 or more or a placebo moisturizer, those given sunscreens reported a similar frequency of other sun-protection behaviour, including time spent outdoors, to those not given sunscreen. This suggests that the way in which different sun protection behaviours are 'balanced' by individuals depends on personal characteristics and motivations.

Metabolism and kinetics

The percutaneous absorption of the active ingredients of sunscreens has been assessed in human skin *in situ* and in excised skin in various animal models.

Very few studies have been done with the inorganic active ingredients of sunscreens, but there is some, limited evidence that they reach the epidermis. More extensive research has been conducted with the organic active ingredients of sunscreens. Studies in humans and animals have consistently shown percutaneous absorption of PABA and benzophenone-3. In the case of PABA, 1.6–9.6% of an applied dose was recovered in urine within 48 h, mostly in the acetylated form. In humans, 1–2% of benzophenone-3 applied at high concentrations over a 10-h period was absorbed systemically. Studies of excised skin from micro-Yucatan pigs showed percutaneous absorption of ethylhexyl methoxycinnamate. In the most extensive studies of the pharmacokinetics of sunscreens, conducted by oral administration of benzophenone-3 to rats, three metabolites were identified, and urine was found to be the main route of excretion.

Some studies have shown that the vehicle can markedly affect the percutaneous absorption of sunscreens.

Cancer-preventive effects
Humans
Cutaneous melanoma
The results of 15 case–control studies were available to evaluate the potential preventive effect of sunscreens against cutaneous melanoma. No results were available from randomized controlled trials or cohort studies.

Four case–control studies provided little evidence of an effect of sunscreen use on the risk for melanoma among all subjects.

Three case–control studies showed significantly lower risks for melanoma in users of sunscreens than in non-users. Two of these were relatively small, hospital-based studies conducted in populations in Spain with both a low prevalence of sun-sensitive subjects and a low prevalence of sunscreen use. The third was conducted among white women 25–59 years of age in California, USA.

This study was unusual in showing the highest levels of risk for melanoma among women with the least solar exposure, but all of the relative risks were close to 1.0.

Eight case–control studies, in Australia, Europe and North America, showed significantly higher risks for melanoma in users of sunscreens than in non-users, with relative risks for the highest category of use ranging up to 2.6. When adjustment was made for sun exposure and sun sensitivity variables in five studies, the relative risk fell in two studies and changed little in three studies. However, none of the adjusted relative risks fell much, if at all, below 1.0.

In two of the studies that showed significantly increased risks for melanoma among sunscreen users, analysis of subgroups suggested that use of sunscreens during heavy intentional sun exposure was associated with a particularly high risk. One of these studies provided specific evidence that sunscreen use in such a group may have led them to prolong their sun exposure. In addition, one of the studies that showed little overall effect of sunscreens found a significantly increased risk for melanoma among people who used sunscreens only during the first hours of sun exposure.

All the studies of sunscreen use and melanoma are difficult to interpret because of problems of positive confounding of sunscreen use with sun exposure, sun sensitivity and history of sun-related neoplasia and negative confounding with other sun-protective behaviour (e.g. use of protective clothing, wearing a hat or staying in the shade). None of the studies adjusted for measures of sun-related neoplasia or other sun-protective behaviour, nor was it known whether this confounding was important. Where measurement and control of sun exposure and sun sensitivity were included in the analysis, there is serious concern that they were insufficient to control confounding.

Acquired melanocytic naevi are considered to be precursors of some cutaneous melanomas. One randomized trial of the ability of sunscreens to inhibit the formation of melanocytic naevi has been published and suggests a protective effect. Other evidence on this issue comes from four cross-sectional or cohort studies among children carried out in Australia and Europe. Two of these studies reported no reduction in naevus counts among children who used sunscreens when compared with children not using them. The two other studies reported higher naevus counts on children who used sunscreens, but the first presented no data to support this contention. In the other, the relationship persisted after attempts to control for sun sensitivity and sun exposure.

Two cross-sectional studies of melanocytic naevi have been conducted among adults. One report did not provide quantitative information on sunscreen use or the number of naevi. The other study showed a modest elevation in the prevalence of naevi among subjects who used ordinary sunscreens and a greater elevation among subjects who used psoralen-containing sunscreens. The studies in adults are difficult to interpret as it is not clear whether the naevi appeared before or after use of sunscreens.

The studies of melanocytic naevi, like those of cutaneous melanoma, suffer from possible confounding of sunscreen use with sun exposure, sun sensitivity and use of other sun-protective measures and from problems of accuracy of measurement.

Basal-cell carcinoma
One randomized trial of the effectiveness of sunscreens in reducing the risk for basal-cell carcinoma was conducted in an appropriate population with appropriate measures. No protective effect on sun-exposed body sites was seen in the 4–5 years of follow-up. A single cohort study conducted among female nurses in the USA showed a small but non-significant increased risk for basal-cell carcinoma. Two case–control studies gave contrasting results. An Australian study showed a modest increase in risk among subjects using sunscreens in the 10 years prior to diagnosis. The other case–control study, conducted in a Spanish population, showed a lower risk among subjects using sunscreens, but data on basal- and squamous-cell carcinomas were combined in the analysis. These studies faced the same difficulties in control of confounding of sun-sensitivity factors and sun exposure as the case–control studies of melanoma.

Squamous-cell carcinoma
A single randomized trial has been conducted to evaluate use of sunscreens in preventing squamous-cell carcinoma. Fewer participants in the sunscreen group developed new squamous-cell carcinomas than those in the comparison group, and the total number of squamous-cell carcinomas among participants given sunscreen was lower than that in the comparison group. Only the latter difference was statistically significant.

The single cohort study showed no decrease in risk for squamous-cell carcinomas with use of sunscreens. Two case–control studies have been conducted of sunscreen use and squamous-cell carcinoma. The Australian study showed no consistent pattern of decreased risk among subjects of three different age groups using sunscreens. The Spanish study showed a decrease in risk among sunscreen users, but data on basal- and squamous-cell carcinomas were combined in the analysis. One case–control study of lip cancer appeared to show a reduced risk with use of lip coverings; however, it is unclear whether the lip coverings were sunscreen preparations. Control for sun sensitivity and sun exposure was probably not complete in either the cohort or case–control studies.

Actinic keratoses are a recognized precursor lesion for squamous-cell carcinomas. Two randomized trials showed a significant protective effect of use of sunscreens against actinic keratoses. A cross-sectional study conducted in the United Kingdom was uninformative.

Experimental systems

Of the 20 reported studies of protection against photocarcinogenesis by sunscreens in experimental animals, 18 were performed in hairless mouse strains and two in haired mice. In most of the studies, suboptimal UVR sources were used. Solar-simulated UVR was used in only seven of 17 studies on the induction of skin carcinogenesis, and in two of three studies of co-carcinogenesis with 7,12-dimethylbenz[a]anthracene. Furthermore, in 10/20 studies, UVR was administered in various incremental regimens, in contrast to the constant daily exposure used in the other studies. The resulting tumours ranged from benign papillomas to malignant squamous-cell carcinomas. The carcinogenic effect was measured either as the median increase in latency for skin tumour development or as the tumour load per mouse. Sunscreens were shown to prevent UVR-induced carcinogenesis in all studies.

Inorganic sunscreens were tested in mice exposed only to solar-simulated UVR in two of the 20 reported studies, but not adequately. In one study of the co-carcinogenicity of solar-simulated UVR and 7,12-dimethylbenz[a]anthracene, a titanium dioxide-containing sunscreen was protective.

Formulations containing multiple UVR absorbers were tested with solar-simulated UVR in only three studies and with non-solar UVR in six of 20 studies. Single agents were tested in all other studies. Dose–response relationships were not established for UVR in any of the studies, and different sunscreen formulations could not be compared.

Mechanisms of cancer prevention

In studies of DNA damage induced by UVB and solar-simulated UVR in human skin, sunscreens reduced the number of adducts. The degree of protection against DNA damage provided by sunscreens varied among individuals. The relationship between DNA damage and the erythemal response remains uncertain. DNA damage is considered to be a transient early biomarker of photocarcinogenesis. Several additional studies in animals showed that sunscreens prevented DNA damage.

The protein TP53 plays an important role in the cellular response to DNA damage. Four experimental studies in humans have shown that topical sunscreen application decreases the accumulation of wild-type TP53 in epidermal keratinocytes, which represents the physiological response to UVR-induced DNA damage. Mutation of the p53 gene is considered to be a biomarker for the development of squamous-cell carcinoma of the skin. One study in mice showed that sunscreens protect against p53 mutations induced by solar-simulated UVR, and another showed protection against p53 mutations induced by a filtered FS40 sunlamp (UVB/UVA). In humans, UVR-induced DNA damage and p53 mutations appear to be involved in the development of squamous-cell carcinoma and basal-cell carcinoma. Use of sunscreens reduced the level of UVR-induced DNA damage, but only a single, small study showed a reduction in p53 mutations in basal-cell carcinoma.

Thirty-three studies in experimental animals have been published on protection by sunscreens against immune suppression, 18 of which were conducted with solar-simulated UVR. Ten of the latter showed a dose-related effect, and five of these were conducted with hairless mice. From these results, it was concluded that sunscreens provide some protection against various end-points in UVR-induced immune suppression.

In humans, sunscreens have been shown to provide at least some protection against several immunological end-points, including the induction of primary immune suppression, the suppression of elicitation of recall responses and suppression of allostimulation of T cells with epidermal dendritic cells. Most of these studies were defective with respect to the source of UVR used or the experimental design, and it is still not known whether these immunological end-points are predictive of skin cancer prevention.

There are no adequate experimental data to establish quantitative relationships between biomarkers and the risk for skin cancer.

Other beneficial effects

Sunscreens can prevent sunburn and have proven effectiveness in the prevention of UVR-induced provocation of certain cutaneous diseases. They may reduce the development of photoageing. Photosensitive cutaneous disorders consist of the idiopathic photodermatoses, which do not develop in the absence of light, and the photoaggravated dermatoses, which are sometimes provoked by exposure to light.

Carcinogenic effects
Humans

Eight case–control studies on cutaneous melanoma showed significantly higher risks among sunscreen users. While these studies could be taken to suggest an increase in the risk for melanoma due to use of sunscreens, they are difficult to interpret because of problems of positive confounding; that is, people who have fair, sun-sensitive skin, heavy sun exposure or a history of skin cancer are also the most likely to use sunscreens and the most likely to develop melanoma. Negative confounding with protective behaviour, such as use of clothing and hats, can also occur.

Two of the case–control studies showed significantly increased risks for melanoma in relation to intentional sun exposure among sunscreen users, suggesting that use of these products to extend time in the sun may increase the risk for melanoma.

One cohort and one case–control study showed increased risks for basal-cell carcinomas among sunscreen users. None of the studies of squamous-cell carcinoma indicated an increased risk among sunscreen users. The results of these studies are difficult to interpret because of the probable confounding noted above.

Experimental animals
No studies were available in which the carcinogenicity of sunscreens was adequately tested. However, numerous studies of the protective effect of sunscreens have not raised suspicion of a carcinogenic effect.

Other toxic effects
Humans
Few published reports are available of contact or photocontact sensitization to sunscreening agents. Case reports suggest a greater frequency of photocontact dermatitis among patients with photodermatoses such as polymorphic light eruption, who frequently use sunscreens.

Although there is evidence that sunscreen use reduces vitamin D production, the levels of vitamin D in sunscreen users appear to be within the normal range, and there have been no reports of biological responses suggesting reduced vitamin D levels.

Experimental systems
Topical application of sunscreen ingredients has not been shown to cause adverse effects on reproduction or fetal development, although some effects have been observed with high oral doses of sunscreen ingredients. Topically applied sunscreen preparations (in the absence of UVR) can have deleterious effects on the immune system under some experimental conditions. Most of the studies of the toxicity of the active ingredients of sunscreens have shown them to be relatively safe when applied topically at the concentrations normally found in sunscreens, and there have been no reports of gross or anatomical effects.

The active ingredients of sunscreens, with and without UVR, can cause cellular toxicity, including DNA damage, inhibition of normal cellular function and cell death. In one study, ethylhexyl dimethyl PABA was genotoxic in the presence of UVR or visible light, and phenylbenzimidazole sulfonic acid in the presence of UVR or visible light caused DNA damage.

Chapter 10

Recommendations

Recommendations for research

A prerequisite for determining the role of sunscreens in the prevention of cancers of the skin is an understanding of the role of UVR in the causation of these diseases. In particular, it is important to understand the nature of the dose–response relationship, the influence of dose rate and pattern of dose delivery on risk and the action spectrum for each effect. Therefore, the Working Group recommends that:

- Studies should be conducted to determine whether there is a direct link between skin cancer and exposure to quantifiable doses of UVR in a defined spectrum. One example would be a prospective study of patients receiving phototherapy from TL01 UVB lamps. Such a study should be designed to evaluate fully the role of potential confounders of any association.

- Prospective studies should be conducted on the relationship between exposure to the sun and skin cancer and precursor lesions, in which the measurement techniques used are capable of differentiating between UVA,

UVB and other wavelengths and show how solar radiation is distributed to skin cells.

- Randomized controlled trials, should be conducted among adults to evaluate whether a reduction in late-stage exposure to UVR can reduce the incidence of cutaneous melanoma and its precursor lesions, clinically atypical naevi, and among children to evaluate whether a reduction in early-stage exposure to UVR can reduce the prevalence of acquired naevi, which are precursors of cutaneous melanoma.

- Randomized controls trials should be conducted among adults to evaluate

whether a reduction in late-stage exposure to UVR can reduce the incidence of basal-cell carcinoma. Randomized controlled trials should be conducted among adults to evaluate whether a reduction in late-stage exposure to UVR can reduce the incidence of squamous-cell carcinoma.

- To the extent possible, such randomized controlled trials should include quantitative assessment of solar exposure and evaluation of the various methods for reducing solar exposure, which include sunscreens, clothing and sun avoidance.

A better understanding will be gained of the mechanisms of skin cancer induction and the way in which sunscreens can effect them if intermediate end-points, such as naevi, or biochemical markers of carcinogenesis, such as DNA damage and *p53* mutations, are studied in relation to sunscreen use. To this end, the Working Group recommends that:

- Adequate controlled trials in humans and studies on appropriate animal models should be conducted to evaluate the relationship of intermediate biomarkers of sun exposure with the development particularly of cutaneous melanoma and the role of sunscreens in influencing such markers.

- The relationship between expression of such biomarkers and carcinogenic risk must be established, and the role

of sunscreens in protecting against the appearance of biomarkers predictive of risk should be investigated.

- Studies should be conducted on the influence of photoinstability on the biomarkers.

- Studies should be conducted to determine whether there is a direct link between UVR-induced erythema (not necessarily from sunlight) and non-melanoma skin cancer.

- Studies should be conducted to establish the chromophore for erythema.

- Studies should be conducted to determine the importance of UVR-induced immunosuppresion in the causation and progression of human skin cancers.

- Biomarkers of UVA-induced oxidative stress should be developed.

The mechanisms of carcinogenesis by UVR and the role of sunscreens in inhibiting the process are still not fully understood. The Working Group therefore recommends that:

- Studies should be conducted in animal models for various skin tumours to determine the carcinogenic protection factors based on ratios of the doses of UVR required to reach

identical end-points. Squamous-cell carcinomas can be studied in existing models, but models are required for basal-cell carcinomas and cutaneous melanoma.

- Studies should be conducted on the effects of exposure to UVA in causing both photageing and skin cancer.

If it is assumed that sunscreens have some role in preventing skin cancer, the efficiency of sunscreen delivery should be increased and evaluated, and the effectiveness and safety of sunscreens should be increased. Therefore the Working Group recommends that:

- Sunscreens should be developed that by virtue of their content, consistency and ease of application achieve adequate protection against UVR when in common use.

- The most effect formulations of sunscreens should be determined by conducting research into optimal active ingredients, their distribution on the skin and the best spectral profile in terms of spectra and wavelength interactions.

- Studies should be conducted to determine whether sunscreens that provide much greater protection against UVR are required.

- Methods should be developed to discriminate between phototoxicity and photoprotection when these occur simultaneously with sunscreen use, for example, by use of a carrier that prevents skin contact, to assess the effect of UVR absorption alone.

- Studies should be conducted (or published if already conducted) to determine the carcinogenic risk of inorganic sunscreen ingredients.

- Studies should be conducted not only of single UVR filters but also of combinations of active ingredients in complete formulations. Such studies should include relevant controls,

such as exposure to UVR through the vehicle.

- Studies should be conducted to define the role of free radicals and active oxygen intermediates in solar UVR-induced damage, mutation, photageing and carcinogenesis, and the usefulness of adding free-radical scavengers to sunscreens should be assessed.

- Studies should be conducted to investigate the nature of endogenous antioxidant defence systems relevant to exposure to solar radiation, including genetic determinants, to provide a rationale for selection of sunscreen components.

The theoretical potential of sunscreens against skin cancer is probably reduced by failure to use them effectively. Further evaluation of the behavioural aspects of sunscreen use is therefore desirable. The Working Group recommends that:

- The place of sunscreens in the context of overall protection against the sun should be defined, and studies should be conducted to define the best ways of conveying this understanding to the public.

- Educational strategies should be devised to train people who expose themselves intentionally to the sun to use sunscreens as only one part of a sun protection strategy.

- Studies should be conducted to evaluate whether qualitative rating

of the potential protective function of sunscreens against UVR, such as low, medium, high and ultra-high, rather than SPF, would improve use of sunscreens.

Many of the studies recommended above cannot be conducted effectively unless qualitative and quantitative methods are developed for measuring sunscreen use and the major variables confounded with it, namely sun sensitivity and sun exposure. Therefore, the Working Group recommends that:

- Methods should be developed to increase the accuracy of measures of use of sunscreens and of individual cutaneous sun sensitivity and sun exposure.

- Portable instrumentation should be developed to measure, in the field, how much protection is provided by sunscreens at various sites on the skin.

Recommendations for public health action

- Protection of the skin from solar damage ideally involves a number of actions which include wearing tightly woven protective clothing that adequately covers the arms, trunk and legs, a hat that provides adequate shade to the whole of the head, seeking shade whenever possible, avoiding outdoor activities during periods of peak insolation and use of sunscreens. Sunscreens should not be the first choice for skin cancer prevention and should not be used as the sole agent for protection against the sun.

- Sunscreens should not be used as a means of extending the duration of solar exposure, such as prolonging sunbathing, and should not be used as a substitute for clothing on usually unexposed sites, such as the trunk and buttocks.

- Daily use of a sunscreen with a high SPF (greater than 15) on usually exposed skin is recommended for residents of areas of high insolation who work outdoors or enjoy regular outdoor recreation. Daily use of a sunscreen can reduce the cumulative solar exposure that causes actinic keratoses and squamous-cell carcinoma.

- Adequate solar protection is more important during childhood than at any other time in life, and the first two recommendations should be assiduously applied by parents and school managers.

- In view of the widespread use of sunscreens, even on children, stringent evaluation of their safety is necessary, particularly with regard to long-term effects. Data on the safety evaluation of sunscreens must be in the public domain so that they are available for independent scientific evaluation.

- Sunscreens should be subject to the same regulatory safety requirements as medicines.

- Once the optimal method for specifying protection against broad-spectrum UVA has been agreed, a labelling method should be introduced that is internationally congruent and understandable to the public.

- Advertising for sunscreens should promote a global sun protection strategy (see first recommendation). Advertising should avoid promoting sunscreen use for intentional exposure to the sun (e.g. acquisition of a tan), and avoid messages likely to provide a false sense of security for people using sunscreens.

- Health promotion interventions should be designed to increase the appropriate and effective use of sunscreens by the general public and subgroups at particular risk for skin cancer because of their phenotype or a predisposition to intentional solar exposure.

- A warning should be displayed on bottles of sunscreens informing consumers of the second recommendation.

Chapter 11
Evaluation

Cancer-preventive activity

Humans

There is *inadequate evidence* in humans for a cancer-preventive effect of topical use of sunscreen formulations against cutaneous malignant melanoma.

There is *inadequate evidence* in humans for a cancer-preventive effect of topical use of sunscreen formulations against basal-cell carcinoma of the skin.

There is *limited evidence* in humans for a cancer-preventive effect of topical use of sunscreen formulations against squamous-cell carcinoma of the skin.

Experimental animals

There is *sufficient evidence* in experimental animals for a cancer-preventive effect of sunscreen formulations. This evaluation is based on prevention of squamous-cell carcinoma of the skin induced in mice by solar-simulated radiation.

Overall evaluation

- Topical use of sunscreens reduces the risk for sunburn in humans.

- Sunscreens probably prevent squamous-cell carcinoma of the skin when used mainly during unintentional sun exposure.

- No conclusion can be drawn about the cancer-preventive activity of topical use of sunscreens against basal-cell carcinoma and cutaneous melanoma.

- Use of sunscreens can extend the duration of intentional sun exposure, such as sun-bathing. Such an extension may increase the risk for cutaneous melanoma.

References

Afaq, F., Abidi, P., Matin, R. & Rahman, Q. (1998) Cytotoxicity, pro-oxidant effects and antioxidant depletion in rat lung alveolar macrophages exposed to ultrafine titanium dioxide. *J. Appl. Toxicol.*, **18**, 307–312

Agin, P., Anthony, F.A. & Hermansky, S. (1998) Oxybenzone in sunscreen products. *Lancet*, **351**, 525

Agren, M.S. (1990) Percutaneous absorption of zinc from zinc oxide applied topically to intact skin in man. *Dermatologica*, **180**, 36–39

Ainsleigh H.G. (1993) Beneficial effects of sun exposure on cancer mortality. *Prev. Med.*, **22**, 132–140

Airey, D.K., Wong, J.C.F. & Fleming, R.A. (1995) A comparison of human- and head-form based measurements of solar ultraviolet B dose. *Photodermatol. Photoimmunol. Photomed.*, **11**, 155–158

Alberts, D.S., Goldman, R., Xu, M.J., Dorr, R.T., Quinn, J., Welch, K., Guillen-Rodriguez, J., Aickin, M., Peng, Y.M., Loescher, L. & Gensler, H. (1996) Disposition and metabolism of topically administered α-tocopherol acetate: A common ingredient of commercially available sunscreens and cosmetics. *Nutr. Cancer*, **26**, 193–201

Allen, J.M., Engenolf, S. & Allen, S.K. (1995) Rapid reaction of singlet molecular oxygen ($^1O_2$) with *p*-aminobenzoic acid (PABA) in aqueous solution. *Biochem. Biophys. Res. Commun.*, **212**, 1145–1151

Allen, J.M., Gossett, C.J. & Allen, S.F. (1996a) Photochemical formation of singlet molecular oxygen ($^1O_2$) in illuminated aqueous solutions of *p*-aminobenzoic acid (PABA). *J. Photochem. Photobiol. B*, **32**, 33–37

Allen, J.M., Gossett, C.J. & Allen, S.K. (1996b) Photochemical formation of singlet molecular oxygen in illuminated aqueous solutions of several commercially available sunscreen active ingredients. *Chem. Res. Toxicol.*, **9**, 605–609

Ananthaswamy, H.N., Loughlin, S.M., Cox, P., Evans, R.L., Ullrich, S.E. & Kripke, M.L. (1997) Sunlight and skin cancer: Inhibition of *p53* mutations in UV-irradiated mouse skin by sunscreens. *Nature Med.*, **3**, 510–514

Ananthaswamy, H.N., Fourtanier, A., Evans, R.L., Tison, S., Medaisko, C., Ullrich, S.E. & Kripke, M.L. (1998) *p53* mutations in hairless skh-hr1 mouse skin tumors induced by a solar simulator. *Photochem. Photobiol.*, **67**, 227–232

Ananthaswamy, H.N., Ullrich, S.E., Mascotto, R.E., Fourtanier, A., Loughlin, S.M., Khaskina, P., Bucana, C.D. & Kripke, M.L. (1999) Inhibition of solar simulator-induced *p53* mutations and protection against skin cancer development in mice by sunscreens. *J. Invest. Dermatol.*, **112**, 763–768

Anderson, M.W., Hewitt, J.P. & Spruce, S.R. (1997) Broad-spectrum physical sunscreens: Titanium dioxide and zinc oxide. In: Lowe, N.J., Shaath, N.A. & Pathak, M.A., eds, *Sunscreens, Development, Evaluation, and Regulatory Aspects,* New York, Marcel Dekker, pp. 353–397

Ang, P., Ng, S.K. & Goh, C.L. (1998) Sunscreen allergy in Singapore. *Am. J. Contact Dermatol.*, **9**, 42–44

Anstey, A.V., Ryan, A., Rhodes, L.E., Charman, C.R., Arlett, C.F., Tyrrell, R.M., Taylor, C.R. & Pearse, A.D. (1999) Characterization of photosensitivity in the Smith-Lemli-Opitz syndrome: a new congenital photosensitivity syndrome. *Br. J. Dermatol.*, **141**, 406–414

Applegate, L.A., Ley, R.D., Alcalay, J. & Kripke, M. L. (1989) Identification of the molecular target for the suppression of contact hypersensitivity by UVR. *J. Exp. Med.*, **170**, 1117–1131

Aragane, Y., Kulms, D., Luger, T.A. & Schwarz, T. (1997) Down-regulation of interferon gamma-activated STAT1 by UV light. *Proc. Natl Acad. Sci. USA*, **94**, 11490–11495

Arancibia, A., Borie, G., Cornwell, E. & Medrano, C. (1981) Pharmacokinetic study on the percutaneous absorption of *p*-aminobenzoic acid from three sunscreen preparations. *Farm. Ed. Prat.*, **36**, 357–365

Arase, S. & Jung, E.G. (1986) *In vitro* evaluation of the photoprotective efficacy of sunscreens against DNA damage by UVB. *Photodermatology*, **3**, 56–59

Arbabi, L., Gange, R.W. & Parrish, J.A. (1983) Recovery of skin from a single suberythemal dose of ultraviolet radiation. *J. Invest. Dermatol.*, **81**, 78–82

Arlett, C.F. & Lehmann, A.R. (1996) Xeroderma pigmentosum, Cockayne syndrome and trichothiodystrophy: Sun sensitivity, DNA repair defects and skin cancer. In: Eeles, R.A., Ponder, B.A., Easton, D.F. & Horwich, E.A., eds, *Genetic Predisposition to Cancer*, London, Chapman & Hall, pp. 185–206

Armstrong, B.K. (1997) Melanoma: Childhood or lifelong sun exposure. In: Grob, J.J., Stern, R.S., MacKie, R.M. & Weinstock, W.A., eds, *Epidemiology, Causes and Prevention of Skin Diseases*, Oxford, Blackwell Science, pp. 63–66

Armstrong, B.K. & Kricker, A. (1993) How much melanoma is caused by sun exposure? *Melanoma Res.*, **3**, 395–401

Armstrong, B.K. & Kricker, A. (1994) Cutaneous melanoma. *Cancer Surv.*, **19**, 219–2405

Armstrong, B.K. & Kricker, A. (1995) Skin cancer. *Dermatol. Clinics*, 13, 583–594

Armstrong, B.K., Kricker, A. & English, D.R. (1997) Sun exposure and skin cancer. *Australas, J. Dermatol.*, **38**, S1-S6

Ashwood-Smith, M.J., Poulton, G.A., Barker, M. & Mildenberger, M. (1980) 5-Methoxypsoralen, an ingredient in several suntan preparations, has lethal, mutatenic and clastogenic properties. *Nature,* **285**, 407–409

Aszterbaum, M., Epstein, J., Oro, A., Douglas, V., LeBoit, P.E., Scott, M.P. & Epstein, E.H., Jr (1999) Ultraviolet and ionizing radiation enhance the growth of BCCs and trichoblastomas in patched heterozygous knockout mice. *Nature Med.*, **5**, 1285–1291

Atillasoy, E.S., Seykora, J.T., Soballe, P.W., Elenitsas, R., Nesbit, M., Elder, D.E., Montone, K.T., Sauter, E. & Herlyn, M. (1998) UVB induces atypical melanocytic lesions and melanoma in human skin. *Am. J. Pathol.*, **152**, 1179–1186

Augustin, C., Collombel, C. & Damour, O. (1997a) Use of dermal equivalent and skin equivalent models for identifying phototoxic compounds in vitro. *Photodermatol. Photoimmunol. Photomed.*, **13**, 27–36

Augustin, C., Collombel, C. & Damour, O. (1997b) Measurements of the protective effect of topically applied sunscreens using *in vitro* three-dimensional dermal and skin equivalents. *Photochem. Photobiol.*, **66**, 853–859

Australian/New Zealand Standards (1998) *Sunscreen products – Evaluation and Classification,* Homebush, Standards Australia. Wellington. Standards, New Zealand

Autier, P., Doré, J.-F., Schifflers, E., Cesarini, J-P., Bollaerts, A., Koelmel, K., Gefeller, O., Liabeuf, A., Lejeune, F., Lienard, D., Joarlette, M., Chemaly, P. & Kleeberg, U.R. (1995) Melanoma and use of sunscreens: An EORTC case-control study in Germany, Belgium and France. *Int. J. Cancer*, **61**, 749–755

Autier, P., Doré, J.-F., Cesarini, J.P. & Boyle, P. (1997a) Should subjects who used psoralen suntan activators be screened for melanoma? Epidemiology and Prevention Subgroup, EORTC Melanoma Cooperative Group EORTC Prevention Research Division. *Ann. Oncol.*, **8**, 435–437

Autier, P., Doré, J.-F., Renard, F., Heike, L., Cattaruzza, M.S., Gefeller, O. & Grivegnée, A. (1997b) Melanoma and sunscreen use: Need for studies representative of actual behaviors. *Melanoma Res.*, **7** (Suppl. 2), S115–S120

Autier, P., Doré, J.-F., Cattaruzza, M.S., Renard, F., Luther, H., Gentiloni-Silverj, F., Zantedeschi, E., Mezzetti, M., Monjaud, I., Andry, M., Osborn, J. & Grivegnée, A.R. (1998) Sunscreen use, wearing clothes, and number of nevi in 6- to 7-year-old European children. *J. Natl Cancer Inst.*, **90**, 1873–1880

Autier, P., Doré, J.-F., Négrier, S., Liénard, D., Panizzon, R., Lejeune, F., Guggisberg, D. & Eggermont, A.M.M. (1999) Sunscreen use and duration of sun exposure: A double-blind, randomized trial. *J. Natl Cancer Inst.*, **91**, 1304–1309

Azurdia, R.M., Pagliaro, J.A., Diffey, B.L. & Rhodes, L.E. (1999) Sunscreen application by photosensitive patients is inadequate for protection. *Br. J. Dermatol.*, **140**, 255–258

Baade, P.D., Balanda, K.P. & Lowe, J.B. (1996) Changes in skin protection behaviours, attitudes and sunburn in a population with the highest incidence of skin cancer in the world. *Cancer Detect. Prev.*, **20**, 566–575

Banks, B.A., Silverman, R.A., Schwartz, R.H. & Tunnessen, W.W., Jr (1992) Attitudes of teenagers toward sun exposure and sunscreen use. *Pediatrics*, **89**, 40–42

Barbieri, B., Stain-Malmgren, R. & Papadogiannakis, N. (1999) p-Aminobenzoic acid and its metabolite p-acetamidobenzoic acid inhibit agonist-induced aggregation and arachidonic acid-induced $[Ca^{2+}]_i$ transients in human platelets. *Thrombosis Res.*, **95**, 235–243

Barr, R.M., Walker, S.L., Tsang, W., Harrison, G.I., Ettehadi, P., Greaves, M.W. & Young, A.R. (1999) Suppressed alloantigen presentation, increased TNF-α, IL-1, IL-1Ra, IL-10, and modulation of TNF-R in UV-irradiated human skin. *J. Invest. Dermatol.*, **112**, 692–698

Beasley, D.G., Beard, J., Stanfield, J.W. & Roberts, L.K. (1996) Evaluation of an economical sunlamp that emits a near solar UV power spectrum for conducting photoimmunological and sunscreen immune protection studies. *Photochem. Photobiol.*, **64**, 303–309

Beasley, D.G., Montgomery, M.A., Moloney, S.J., Edmonds, S. & Roberts, L.K. (1998) Commercial sunscreen lotions prevent ultraviolet radiation-induced depletion of epidermal Langerhans cells in Skh-1 and C3H mice. *Photodermatol. Photoimmunol. Photomed.*, **14**, 90–99

Bech-Thomsen, N. & Wulf, H.C. (1992) Sunbathers' application of sunscreen is probably inadequate to obtain the sun protection factor assigned to the preparation. *Photodermatol. Photoimmunol. Photomed.*, **9**, 242–244

Beitner, H., Norell, S.E., Ringborg, U., Wennersten, G. & Mattson, B. (1990) Malignant melanoma: Aetiological importance of individual pigmentation and sun exposure. *Br. J. Dermatol.*, **122**, 43–51

Bennetts, K., Borland, R. & Swerissen, H. (1991) Sun protection behaviour of children and their parents at the beach. *Psychol. Health*, **5**, 279–287

Berg, R.J.W., van Kranen, H.J., Rebel, H.G., de Vries, A., van Vloten, W.A., van Kreijl, C.F., van der Leun, J.C. & de Gruijl, F.R. (1996) Early p53 alterations in mouse skin carcinogenesis by UVB radiation: Immunohistochemical detection of mutant p53 protein in clusters of preneoplastic epidermal cells. *Proc. Natl Acad. Sci. USA*, **93**, 274–278

Bergfeld, W.F., Farris, P.K., Wyatt, S.W., Reilley, B., Bewerse, B.A. & Koh, H.K. (1997) Executive summary of the National Partners in Prevention Skin Care Conference. *Am. Acad. Dermatol. Centers Dis. Control Prev.*, **36**, 798–801

Bernard, B.K., Osheroff, M.R., Hofmann, A. & Mennear, J.H. (1990) Toxicology and carcinogenesis studies of dietary titanium dioxide-coated mica in male and female Fischer 344 rats. *J. Toxicol. Environ. Health*, **29**, 417–429

Berne, B. & Ros, A.-M. (1998) 7 years experience of photopatch testing with sunscreen allergens in Sweden. *Contact Derm.*, **38**, 61–64

Berne, B., Ponten, J. & Ponten, F. (1998) Decreased p53 expression in chronically sun-exposed human skin after topical photoprotection. *Photoderm. Photoimmunol. Photomed.*, **14**, 148–153

Berset, G., Gonzenbach, H., Christ, R., Martin, R., DeFlandre, A., Mascotto, R.E., Jolley, J.D.R., Lowell, W., Pelzer, R. & Stiehm, T. (1996) Proposed protocol for determination of photostability Part I: Cosmetic UV filters. *Int. J. Cosmet. Sci.*, **18**, 167–177

Berwick, M., Fine, J.A. & Bolognia, J.L. (1992) Sun exposure and sunscreen use following a community skin cancer screening. *Prev. Med.*, **21**, 302–310

Bestak, R. & Halliday, G.M. (1996) Sunscreens protect from UV-promoted squamous cell carcinoma in mice chronically irradiated with doses of UV radiation insufficient to cause edema. *Photochem. Photobiol.*, **64**, 188–193

Bestak, R., Barnetson, R.S., Nearn, M.R. & Halliday, G.M. (1995) Sunscreen protection of contact hypersensitivity responses from chronic solar-simulated ultraviolet irradiation correlates with the absorption spectrum of the sunscreen. *J. Invest. Dermatol.*, **105**, 345–351

Bilsland, D. & Ferguson, J. (1993) Contact allergy to sunscreen chemicals in photosensitiviy dermatitis/actinic reticuloid syndrome (PD/AR) and polymorphic light eruption (PLE). *Contact Derm.*, **29**, 70–73

Bissett, D.L. & McBride, J.F. (1996) Synergistic topical photoprotection by a combination of the iron chelator 2-furildioxime and sunscreen. *J. Am. Acad. Dermatol.*, **35**, 546–549

Bissett, D.L., McBride, J.F., Hannon, D.P. & Patrick, L.F. (1991) Time-dependent decrease in sunscreen protection against chronic photodamage in UVB-irradiated hairless mouse skin. *J. Photochem. Photobiol. B*, **9**, 323–334

Blum, H.F. (1959) *Carcinogenesis by Ultraviolet Light*, Princeton, New Jersey, Princeton University Press

Blum, H.F., Kirby-Smith, S. & Grady, H.G. (1941) Quantitative induction of tumours in mice with ultraviolet radiation. *J. Natl Cancer Inst.*, **2**, 259–268

Boiteux, S. (1993) Properties and biological functions of the NTH and FPG proteins in *Escherichia coli*: Two DNA glycosylases that repair oxidative damage in DNA. *J. Photochem. Photobiol. B*, **19**, 87–96

Boiteux, S., Gajewski, E., Laval, J. & Dizdaroglu, M. (1992) Substrate specificity of the *Escherichia coli* Fpg protein (formamidopyrimidine-DNA glycosylase): Excision of purine lesions in DNA produced by ionizing radiation or photosensitization. *Biochemistry*, **31**, 106–110

Boldeman, C., Beitner, H., Jansson, B., Nilsson, B. & Ullen, H. (1996) Sunbed use in relation to phenotype, erythema, sunscreen use and skin diseases. A questionnaire survey among Swedish adolescents. *Br. J. Dermatol.*, **135**, 712–716

Bonin, A.M., Arlauskas, A.P., Angus, D.S., Baker, R.S.U., Gallagher, C.H., Greenoak, G., Lane Brown, M.M., Meher-Homji, K.M. & Reeve, V. (1982) UV-absorbing and other sun-protecting substances: Genotoxicity of 2 ethylhexyl *p*-methoxycinnamate. *Mutat. Res.*, **105**, 303–308

Bootsma, D., Kraemer, K.H., Cleaver, J.E. & Hoeijmakers, J.H.J. (1998) Nucleotide excision repair syndromes: *Xeroderma pigmentosum*, Cockayne syndrome, and trichothiodystrophy. In: Vogelstein, B. & Kinzler, K.W., eds, *The Genetic Basis of Human Cancer*, New York, McGraw-Hill, pp. 245–274

Borland, R., Hill, D. & Noy, S. (1990) Being SunSmart: Changes in community awareness and reported behaviour following a primary prevention program for skin cancer control. *Behav. Change*, **7**, 126–135

Bose, B., Soriani, M. & Tyrrell, R.M. (1999) Activation of expression of the c-fos oncogene by UVA irradiation in cultured human skin fibroblasts. *Photo-chem. Photobiol.*, **69**, 489–493

Bourke, J.F. & Graham-Brown, R.A. (1995) Protection of children against sunburn: A survey of parental practice in Leicester. *Br. J. Dermatol.*, **133**, 264–266

Bourke, J.F., Healsmith, M.F. & Graham-Brown, R.A.C. (1995) Melanoma awareness and sun exposure in Leicester. *Br. J. Dermatol.*, **132**, 251–256

Boyd, A.S., Naylor, M., Cameron, G.S., Pearse, A.D., Gaskell, S.A. & Neldner, K.H. (1995) The effects of chronic sunscreen use on the histologic changes of dermatoheliosis. *J. Am. Acad. Dermatol.*, **33**, 941–946

Boyle, P., Maisonneuve, P. & Doré, J.-F. (1995) Epidemiology of malignant melanoma. *Br. Med. Bull.*, **51**, 523–547

Brash, D.E., Rudolph, J.A., Simon, J.A., Lin, A., McKenna, G.J., Baden, H.P., Halperin, A.J. & Pontén, J. (1991) A role for sunlight in skin cancer: UV-induced p53 mutations in squamous cell carcinoma. *Proc. Natl Acad. Sci. USA*, **88**, 10124–10128

Brezová, V. & Stasko, A. (1994) Spin trap study of hydroxyl radicals formed in the photocatalytic system TiO_2-water-*p*-cresol-oxygen. *J. Catalysis*, **147**, 156–162

Broadstock, M., Borland, R. & Hill, D. (1996) Knowledge, attitudes and reported behaviours relevant to sun protection and suntanning in adolescents. *Psychol. Health*, **11**, 527–539

Brown, S. & Diffey, B.L. (1986) The effect of applied thickness on sunscreen protection: *In vivo* and *in vitro* studies. *Photochem Photobiol.*, **44**, 509–513

Buckley, D.A., O'Sullivan, D. & Murphy, G.M. (1993) Contact and photocontact allergy to dibenzoylmethans and contact allergy to methylbenzylidene camphor. *Contact Derm.*, **28**, 47

Buller, D.B. & Borland, R. (1999) Skin cancer prevention for children: A critical review. *Health Educ. Behav.*, **26**, 317–343

Buller, D.B., Callister, M. & Reichert, T. (1995) Skin cancer prevention by parents of young children: Health information sources, skin cancer knowledge, and sun protection practices. *Oncol. Nurs. Forum*, **22**, 1559–1566

Buller, M.K., Goldberg, G. & Buller, D.B. (1997) Sun Smart Day: A pilot program for photoprotection education. *Pediatr. Dermatol.*, **14**, 257–263

Buller, D.B., Andersen, P.A. & Walkosz, B. (1998) Sun safety behaviours of alpine skiers and snowboarders in the western United States. *Cancer Prev. Control*, **2**, 133–139

Bykov, V.J., Jansen, C.T. & Hemminki, K. (1998a) High levels of dipyrimidine dimers are induced in human skin by solar-simulating UV radiation. *Cancer Epidemiol. Biomarkers Prev.*, **7**, 199–202

Bykov, V.J., Marcusson, J.A. & Hemminki, K. (1998b) Ultraviolet B-induced DNA damage in human skin and its modulation by a sunscreen. *Cancer Res.*, **58**, 2961–2964

Bykov, V.J., Sheehan, J.M., Hemminki, K. & Young, A.R. (1999) In situ repair of cyclobutane pyrimidine dimers and 6-4 photoproducts in human skin exposed to solar simulating radiation. *J. Invest. Dermatol.*, **112**, 326–331

Cadet, J. & Vigny, P. (1990) Bioorganic photochemistry. In: Morrison, H., ed., *The Photochemistry and Photobiology of Nucleic Acids*, New York, John Wiley & Sons, Vol. 1, pp. 1–273

Cadet, J., Berger, M., Douki, T., Morin, B., Raoul, S., Ravanat, J.L. & Spinelli, S. (1997) Effects of UV and visible radiation on DNA-final base damage. *Biol. Chem.*, **378**, 1275–1286

Cai, R., Kubota, Y., Shuin, T., Sakai, H., Hashimoto, K. & Fujishima, A. (1992) Induction of cytotoxity by photoexcited TiO_2 particles. *Cancer Res.*, **52**, 2346–2348

Callen, J.P., Roth, D.E., McGrath, C. & Dromgoole, S.H. (1991) Safety and efficacy of a broad-spectrum sunscreen in patients with discoid or subacute cutaneous lupus erythematosus. *Cutis*, **47**, 130–132, 135–136

Campbell, H.S. & Birdsell, J.M. (1994) Knowledge, beliefs, and sun protection behaviours of Alberta adults. *Prev. Med.*, **23**, 160–166

Campbell, C., Quinn, A.G., Angus, B., Farr, P.M. & Rees, J.L. (1993) Wavelength specific patterns of *p53* induction in human skin following exposure to UV radiation. *Cancer Res.*, **53**, 2697–2699

Challoner, A.V.J., Corless, D., Davis, A., Deane, G.H.W., Diffey, B.L., Gupta, S.P. & Magnus, I.A. (1976) Personnel monitoring of exposure to ultraviolet radiation. *Clin. Exp. Dermatol.*, **1**, 175–179

Chapin, R., Gulati, D. & Mounce, R. (1997) 2-Hydroxy-4-methoxybenzophenone. *Environ. Health Perspect.*, **105**, 313–314

Chedekel, M.R. & Zeise, L. (1997) Melanins. In: Lowe, N.J., Shaath, N.A. & Pathak, M.A., eds, *Sunscreens, Development, Evaluation, and Regulatory Aspects,* New York, Marcel Dekker, pp. 421–443

Chételat, A., Albertini, S., Dresp, J.H., Strobel, R. & Gocke, E. (1993a) Photo-mutagenesis test development: I. 8-Methoxypsoralen, chlorpromazine and sunscreen compounds in bacterial and yeast assays. *Mutat. Res.*, **292**, 241–250

Chételat, A., Dresp, J.H. & Gocke, E. (1993b) Photomutagenesis test development: I. 8-Methoxypsoralen, chlorpromazine and sunscreen compounds in chromosomal aberration assays using CHO cells. *Mutat. Res.*, **292**, 251–258

Chin, L., Pomerantz, J., Polsky, D., Jacobson, M., Cohen, C., Cordon-Cardo, C., Horner, J.W., II & DePinho, R.A (1997) Cooperative effects of *INK4a* and *ras* in melanoma susceptibility in vivo. *Genes Dev.*, **11**, 2822–2834

Cockburn, J., Thompson, S., Marks, R., Jolley, D., Schofield, D. & Hill, D. (1997) Behavioural dynamics of a clinical trial of sunscreens for reducing solar keratoses in Victoria, Australia. *J. Epidemiol. Community Health*, **51**, 716–721

Cole, C. & van Fossen, R. (1988) Rapid *in vitro* evaluation of sunscreens: SPF and PFA, *Photochem Photobiol. B*, **47**, 73S

Cole, C. & van Fossen, R. (1990) *In vitro* models for UVB and UVA photoprotection. In: Lowe, N.J. & Shaath, N.A., eds, *Sunscreens: Development, Evaluation, and Regulatory Aspects*, New York, Marcel Dekker, pp. 395–404

COLIPA (European Cosmetic Toiletry, and Perfumery Association) (1994) *Sun Protection Factor Method*, Brussels

Collins, P. & Ferguson, J. (1994) Photoallergic contact dermatitis to oxybenzone. *Br. J. Dermatol.*, **131**, 124–129

Commission Internationale de l'Éclairage (1998) *CIE Standard. Erythema Reference Action Spectrum and Standard Erythema Dose* (CIE S 007/E-1998), Vienna

Commonwealth Department of Human Services and Health (1995) *Guidelines for Applicants. Listing Drug Products in the Australian Register of Therapeutic Goods for Supply in Australia*, Woden, ACT

Connor, M.J. & Wheeler, L.A. (1987) Depletion of cutaneous glutathione by ultraviolet radiation. *Photochem. Photobiol.*, **46**, 239–245

Cosmetic Ingredient Review (1983) Final report on the safety assessment of benzophenones-1, -3, -4, -5, -9 and -11. *J. Am. Coll. Toxicol.*, **2**, 35–77

Council on Scientific Affairs (1989) Harmful effects of ultraviolet radiation. *J. Am. Med. Assoc.*, **262**, 380–384

Cox, N.H., Diffey, B.L. & Farr, P.M. (1992) The relationship between chronological age and the erythemal response to ultraviolet B radiation. *Br. J. Dermatol.*, **126**, 315–319

Cristofolini, M., Bianchi, R., Boi, S., Decarli, A., Micciolo, R., Cristofolini, P. & Zumiani, G. (1993) Effectiveness of the health campaign for the early diagnosis of cutaneous melanoma in Trentino, Italy. *J. Dermatol. Surg. Oncol.*, **19**, 117–120

Damian, D.L., Halliday, G.M. & Barnetson, R.StC. (1997) Broad-spectrum sunscreens provide greater protection against ultraviolet-radiation-induced suppression of contact hypersensitivity to a recall antigen in humans. *J. Invest. Dermatol.*, **109**, 146–151

Damian, D.L., Barnetson, R.StC. & Halliday, G.M. (1999) Measurement of *in vivo* sunscreen immune protection factors in humans. *Photochem. Photobiol.*, **70**, 910–915

Darr, D., Dunston, S., Faust, H. & Pinnell, S. (1996) Effectiveness of antioxidants (vitamin C and E) with and without sunscreens as topical photoprotectants. *Acta Dermatol. Venereol.*, **76**, 264–268

Daston, G.P., Gettings, S.D., Carlton, B.D., Chudkowski, M., Davis, R.A., Kraus, A.L., Luke, C.F., Ouellette, R.E., Re, T.A., Hoberman, A.M. & Sambuco, C.P. (1993) Assessment of the reproductive toxic potential of dermally applied 2-hydroxy-4-methoxy-benzophenone to male B6C3F1 mice. *Fundam. Appl. Toxicol.*, **20**, 120–124

Davenport, V., Morris, J.F. & Chu, A.C. (1997) Immunologic protection afforded by sunscreens *in vitro*. *J. Invest. Dermatol.*, **108**, 859–863

Dean, S.W., Lane, M., Dunmore, R.H., Ruddock S.P., Martin, C.N., Kirkland, D.J. & Loprieno, N. (1991) Development of assays for the detection of photomutagenicity of chemicals during exposure to UV light. I. Assay development. *Mutagenesis*, **6**, 335–341

De Fabo, E.C. & Noonan, F.P. (1983) Mechanism of immune suppression by ultraviolet irradiation *in vivo*. I. Evidence for the existence of a unique photoreceptor in skin and its role in photoimmunology. *J. Exp. Med.*, **157**, 84–98

DeFlandre, A. & Lang, G. (1988) Photostability assessment of sunscreens. Benzylidene camphor and dibenzoylmethane derivatives. *Int. J. Cosmet. Sci.*, **10**, 53–62

Dennis, L.K., White, E., Lee, J.A.H., Kristal, A., McKnight, B. & Odland, P. (1996) Constitutional factors and sun exposure in relation to nevi: A population-based cross-sectional study. *Am. J. Epidemiol.*, **143**, 248–256

D'Errico, M., Calcagnile, A., Iavarone, I., Sera, F., Baliva, G., Chinni, L.M., Corona, R., Pasquini, P. & Dogliotti, E. (1999) Factors that influence the DNA repair capacity of normal and skin cancer-affected individuals. *Cancer Epidemiol. Biomarkers Prev.*, **8**, 553–559

Derry, J.E., McLean, W.M. & Freeman, J.B. (1983) A study of the percutaneous absorption from topically applied zinc oxide ointment. *J. Parent. Ent. Nutr.*, **7**, 131–135

Detweiler, J.B., Bedell, B.T., Salovey, P., Pronin, E. & Rothman, A.J. (1999) Message framing and sunscreen use: Gain-framed messages motivate beachgoers. *Health Psychol.*, **18**, 189–196

Dietrich, A.J., Olson, A.L., Sox, C.H., Stevens, M., Tosteson, T.D., Ahles, T., Winchell, C.W., Grant-Petersson, J., Collison, D.W. & Sanson-Fisher, R. (1998) A community-based randomized trial encouraging sun protection for children. *Pediatrics,* **102**, E64–E71

Diffey, B.L. (1989a) Ultraviolet radiation dosimetry with polysulphone film. In: Diffey, B.L., ed., *Radiation Measurement in Photobiology,* London, Academic Press, pp. 135–139

Diffey, B.L. (1989b) Pitfalls in the in vitro determination of sunscreen protection factors using broad band ultraviolet radiation detectors and solar simulating radiation. *Int. J. Cosmet. Sci.,* **11**, 245–249

Diffey, B.L. (1996) Population exposure to solar UVA radiation. *Eur. J. Dermatol.,* **6**, 221–222

Diffey, B.L. (1998) Human exposure to ultraviolet radiation. In: Hawk, J.L.M., ed., *Photodermatology,* London, Chapman & Hall, pp. 5–24

Diffey, B.L. (1999) Sun protection. *Ned. Tijdschr. Dermatol. Venereol.,* **9**, 333–334

Diffey, B.L. (2000) Has the sun protection factor had its day? *Br. Med. J.,* **320**, 176–177

Diffey, B.L. & Cheeseman, J. (1992) Sun protection with hats. *Br. J. Dermatol.,* **127**, 10–12

Diffey, B.L. & Gies, H.P. (1998) The confounding influence of sun exposure in melanoma. *Lancet*, **351**, 1101–1102

Diffey, B.L. & Grice, J. (1997) The influence of sunscreen type on photoprotection. *Br. J. Dermatol.,* **137**, 103–105

Diffey, B.L. & Robson, J.A. (1989) A new substrate to measure sunscreen protection factors throughout the ultraviolet spectrum. *J. Soc. Cosmet. Chem.,* **40**, 127–133

Diffey, B.L. & Saunders, P.J. (1995) Behaviour outdoors and its effect on personal ultraviolet exposure rate measured using an ambulatory datalogging dosimeter. *Photochem. Photobiol.,* **61**, 615–618

Diffey, B.L., Kerwin, M. & Davis, A. (1977) The anatomical distribution of sunlight. *Br. J. Dermatol.,* **97**, 407–410

Diffey, B.L., Tate, T.J. & Davis, A. (1979) Solar dosimetry of the face: The relationship of natural ultraviolet radiation exposure to basal cell carcinoma localisation. *Phys. Med. Biol.,* **24**, 931–939

Diffey, B.L., Gibson, C.J., Haylock, R. & McKinlay, A.F. (1996) Outdoor ultraviolet exposure of children and adolescents. *Br. J. Dermatol.,* **134**, 1030–1034

Diffey, B.L., Stokes, R.P., Forestier, S., Mazilier, C. & Rougier, A. (1997) Sun-care product photostability: A key parameter for a more realistic *in vitro* efficacy evaluation. *Eur. J. Dermatol.,* **7**, 226–228

Dixon, H., Shatten, R. & Borland, R. (1997) Reaction to the 1995/1996 SunSmart Campaign: Results from a representative household survey of Victorians. In: *SunSmart Evaluation Studies No 5*, Melbourne, Anti-Cancer Council of Victoria, pp. 70–96

Dixon, H., Borland, R. & Hill, D. (1999) Sun protection and sunburn in primary school children: The influence of age, gender, and coloring. *Prev. Med.,* **28**, 119–130

Dobbinson, S., Borland, R. & Anderson, M. (1999) Sponsorship and sun protection practices in lifesavers. *Health Promot. Int.,* **14**, 167–175

Doetsch, P.W., Helland, D.E. & Lee, K. (1988) Wavelength dependence for human redoxyendonuclease-mediated DNA cleavage at sites of UV-induced photoproducts. *Radiat. Res.,* **113**, 543–549

Domanski, D., Bosnic, M. & Reeve, V.E. (1999) Does sunscreen protection from immunosuppression by solar UV radiation predict protection from photocarcinogenesis? *Redox Rep.,* **4**, 309–310

Donavan, D.T. & Singh, S.N. (1999) Sun-safety behavior among elementary school children: The role of knowledge, social norms, and parental involvement. *Psychol. Rep.,* **84**, 831–836

Donawho, C.K. & Kripke, M.L. (1991) Evidence that the local effect of ultraviolet radiation on the growth of murine melanoma is immunologically mediated. *Cancer Res.,* **51**, 4176–4181

Donawho, C.K., Norval, M. & Yarosh, D.B. (1998) Molecular target of UV-B radiation in the melanoma enhancing effect of UV irradiation in a murine model. *Photochem. Photobiol.,* **6**, 64S

Douki, T., Perdiz, D., Grof, P., Kuluncsics, Z., Moustacchi, E., Cadet, J. & Sage, E. (1999) Oxidation of guanine in cellular DNA by solar UV radiation: Biological role. *Photochem. Photobiol.,* **70**, 184–190

Drake, L.A., Dinehart, S.M., Farmer, E.R., Goltz, R.W., Graham, G.F., Hordinsky, M.K., Lewis, C.W., Pariser, D.M., Skouge, J.W., Webster, S.B., Whitaker, D.C., Butler, B., Lowery, B.J., Sontheimer, R.D., Callen, J.P., Camisa, C., Provost, T.T. & Tuffanelli, D.L. (1996) Guidelines of care for cutaneous lupus erythematosus. *J. Am. Acad. Dermatol.,* **34**, 830–836

Drobetsky, E.A., Turcotte, J. & Châteauneuf, A. (1995) A role for ultraviolet A in solar mutagenesis. *Proc. Natl Acad. Sci. USA,* **92**, 2350–2354

Dromgoole, S.H. & Maibach, H.I. (1990) Sunscreening agent intolerance: Contact and photocontact sensitization and contact urticaria. *J. Am. Acad. Dermatol.,* **22**, 1068–1078

Druckrey, H. (1967) Quantitative aspects in chemical carcinogenesis. In: Truhaut, E., ed., *Potential Carcinogenic Hazards from Drugs; Evaluation and Risks* (UICC Monograph Series 7), New York, Springer Verlag, pp. 60–78

Dumaz, N., Van Kranen, H.J., De Vries, A., Berg, R.J.W., Wester, P.W., Van Kreijl, C.F., Sarasin, A., Daya-Grosjean, L. & De Gruijl, F.R. (1997) The role of UVB light in skin carcinogenesis through the analysis of *p53* mutations in squamous cell carcinomas of hairless mice. *Carcinogenesis*, **18**, 897–904

Dundas, S.A.C. & Laing, R.W. (1988) Titanium balanitis with phimosis. *Dermatologica*, **176**, 305–307

Dunford, R., Salinaro, A., Cai, L.Z., Serpone, N., Horikoshi, S., Hidaka, H. & Knowland, J. (1997) Chemical oxidation and DNA damage catalysed by inorganic sunscreen ingredients. *FEBS Lett.,* **418**, 87–90

Dunkel, V.C., San, R.H.C., Harbell, J.W., Seifriend, H.E. & Cameron, T.P. (1992) Evaluation of the mutagenicity of an N-nitroso contaminant of the sunscreen Padimate O: N-Nitroso-N-methyl-p-aminobenzoic acid, 2-ethylhexyl ester (NPABAO). *Environ. Mol. Mutag.,* **20**, 188–198

Dupre, A., Touron, P., Daste, J., Lassere, J., Bonafe J.-L. & Viraben, R. (1985) Titanium pigmentation. An electron probe microanalysis study. *Arch. Dermatol.,* **121**, 656–658

Dussert, A.-S, Gooris, E. & Hemmerle, S. (1997) Characterization of the mineral content of a physical sunscreen emulsion and its distribution onto human stratum corneum. *Int. J. Cosmet. Sci.,* **19**, 119–129

Eiser, J.R., Eiser, C., Sani, F., Sell, L. & Casas, R.M. (1995) Skin cancer attitudes: A cross-national comparison. *Br. J. Soc. Psychol.*, **34**, 23–30

El Dareer, S.M., Kalin, J.R., Tillery, K.F. & Hill, D.L. (1986) Disposition of 2-hydroxy 4-methoxybenzophenone in rats dosed orally, intravenously, or topically. *J. Toxicol. environ. Health*, **19**, 491–502

El-Deiry, W.S., Tokino, T., Velculescu, V.E., Levy, D.B., Parsons, R., Trent, J.M., Lin, D., Mercer, W.E., Kinzler, K.W. & Vogelstein, B. (1993) *WAF1*, a potential mediator of p53 tumor suppression. *Cell*, **75**, 817–825

El-Deiry, W.S., Tokino, T., Waldman, T., Oliner, J.D., Velculescu, V.E., Burrell, M., Hill, D.E., Healy, E., Rees, J.L., Hamilton, S.R., Kinzler, K.W. & Vogelstein, B. (1995) Topological control of p21$^{WAF1/CIP1}$ expression in normal and neoplastic tissues. *Cancer Res.*, **55**, 2910–2919

Elwood, M. & Gallagher, R.P. (1999) More about: Sunscreen use, wearing clothes, and number of nevi in 6- to 7-year-old European children. *J. Natl Cancer Inst.*, **91**, 1164–1166

Elwood, J.M. & Jopson, J. (1997) Melanoma and sun exposure: An overview of published studies. *Int. J. Cancer*, **73**, 198–203

Elwood, J.M., Gallagher, R.P., Hill, G.B., Spinelli, J.J., Pearson, J.C. & Threlfall, W. (1984) Pigmentation and skin reaction to sun as risk factors for cutaneous melanoma: Western Canada Melanoma Study. *Br. Med. J. (Clin. Res. Ed.)*, **288**, 99–102

English, D.R. & Armstrong, B.K. (1994a) Melanocytic nevi in children. I. Anatomic sites and demographic and host factors. *Am. J. Epidemiol.*, **139**, 390–401

English, D.R. & Armstrong, B.K. (1994b) Melanocytic nevi in children. II. Observer variation in counting nevi. *Am. J. Epidemiol.*, **139**, 402–407

English, J.S.C., White, I.R. & Cronin, E. (1987) Sensitivity to sunscreens. *Contact Derm.*, **17**, 159–162

English, D.R., MacLennan, R., Rivers, J.K., Kelly, J. & Amstrong, B.K. (1990) *Epidemiological Studies of Melanocytic Naevi: Protocol for Identifying and Recording Naevi* (IARC Internal Report No. 90/002), Lyon, International Agency for Research on Cancer

English, D.R., Armstrong, B.K., Kricker, A. & Fleming, C. (1997) Sunlight and cancer. *Cancer Causes Control*, **8**, 271–283

English, D.R., Armstrong, B.K., Kricker, A., Winter, M.G., Heenan, P.J. & Randell, P.L. (1998a) Case–control study of sun exposure and squamous cell carcinoma of the skin. *Int. J. Cancer,* **77**, 347–353

English, D.R., Armstrong, B.K., Kricker, A., Winter, M.G., Heenan, P.J. & Randell, P.L. (1998b) Demographic characteristics, pigmentary and cutaneous risk factors for squamous cell carcinoma of the skin: A case–control study. *Int. J Cancer*, **76**, 628–634

Espinosa-Arranz, J., Sanchez-Hernandez, J.J., Bravo Fernandez, P., Gonzalez-Baron, M., Zamora Aunon, P., Espinosa Arranz, E., Jalon-Lopez, J.I. & Ordonez Gallego, A. (1999) Cutaneous malignant melanoma and sun exposure in Spain. *Melanoma Res.*, **9**, 199–205

European Commission (1976) *Directive 76/768. Guidelines for Testing of Cosmetic Ingredients* (SCCMFP 10321/00), Brussels

European Commission (2000) *24th Directive 2000/6/CE of the Commission, 29 February 2000, Annex VII, List of UV Sunscreens Which Cosmetic Products May Contain*, Luxembourg

Fairhurst, D. & Mitchnick, M.A. (1997) Particulate sun blocks: General principles. In: Lowe, N.J., Shaath, N.A. & Pathak, M.A., eds, *Sunscreens, Development, Evaluation, and Regulatory Aspects,* New York, Marcel Dekker, pp. 313–352

Fan, H., Oro, A.E., Scott, M.P. & Khavari, P.A. (1997) Induction of basal cell carcinoma features in transgenic human skin expressing *sonic hedgehog. Nature Med.*, **3**, 788–792

Farr, P.M. & Diffey, B.L. (1985) How reliable are sunscreen protection factors? *Br. J. Dermatol.*, **112**, 113–118

Farrerons, J., Barnadas, M., Rodriguez, J., Renau, A., Yoldi, B., Lopez-Navidad, A. & Moragas, J. (1998) Clinically prescribed sunscreen (sun protection factor 15) does not decrease serum vitamin D concentration sufficiently either to induce changes in parathyroid function or in metabolic markers. *Br. J. Dermatol.,* **139,** 422–427

Ferguson, J. (1997) European guidelines (COLIPA) for evaluation of sun protection factors. In: Lowe, N.J., Shaath, N.A. &

Pathak, M.A., eds, *Sunscreens: Development, Evaluation, and Regulatory Aspects*, 2nd Ed., New York, Marcel Dekker, pp. 513–525

Ferguson, J., Brown, M.W. Hubbard, A.W. & Shaw, M.I. (1988) Determination of sun protection factors. Correlation between *in vivo* human studies and an *in vitro* skin cast method. *Int. J. Cosmet. Sci.,* **10**, 117–129

Findlay, G.M. (1928) Ultraviolet light and skin cancer. *Lancet*, **ii**, 1070–1073

Fisher, G.J. & Johns, H.E. (1976) Pyrimidine photohydrates. In: Wang, S., ed., *Photochemistry and Photobiology of Nucleic Acids*, Vol. 1, New York, Academic Press, pp. 169–224

Fisher, M.S. & Kripke, M.L. (1977) Systemic alteration induced in mice by ultraviolet light irradiation and its relationship to ultraviolet carcinogenesis. *Proc. Natl Acad. Sci. USA*, **74**, 1688–1692

Fisher, M.S., Menter, J.M. & Willis, I. (1989) Ultraviolet radiation-induced suppression of contact hypersensitivity in relation to Padimate O and oxybenzone. *J. Invest. Dermatol.*, **92**, 337–341

Fisher, G.J., Datta, S.C., Talwar, H.S., Wang, Z.Q., Varani, J., Kang, S. & Voorhees, J.J. (1996) Molecular basis of sun-induced premature skin ageing and retinoid antagonism. *Nature*, **379**, 335–339

Flindt-Hansen, H., Thune, P. & Nielsen, C.J. (1989) Photocarcinogenesis is retarded by a partly photodegraded solution of *para*-aminobenzoic acid. *Photodermatology*, **6**, 263–267

Flindt-Hansen, H., Thune, P. & Eeg-Larsen, T. (1990a) The inhibiting effect of PABA on photocarcinogenesis. *Arch. Dermatol. Res.*, **282**, 38–41

Flindt-Hansen, H., Thune, P. & Eeg-Larsen, T. (1990b) The effect of short-term application of PABA on photocarcinogenesis. *Acta Dermatol. Venereol.*, **70**, 72–75

Foley, P., Nixon, R., Marks, R., Frowen, K. & Thompson, S. (1993) The frequency of reactions to sunscreens: Results of a longitudinal population-based study on the regular use of sunscreens in Australia. *Br. J. Dermatol.,* **128**, 512–518

Foltz, A.T. (1993) Parental knowledge and practices of skin cancer prevention: A pilot study. *J. Pediatr. Health Care*, **7**, 220–225

Food & Drug Administration (1978) Sunscreen drug products for over the counter use: Proposed safety, effectiveness and labelling conditions. *Fed. Regist.*, **43**, 38206–38269

Food & Drug Administration (1993) Sunscreen drug products for over-the-counter human use; tentative final monograph. *Fed. Regist.*, **58**, 28194–28302

Food & Drug Administration (1998) Sunscreen drug products for over-the-counter human use; Amendment to the tentative final monograph; Enforcement policy. *Fed. Regist.*, **63**, 56584–56589

Food & Drug Administration (1999) Sunscreen drug products for over-the-counter human use; Final monograph. *Fed. Regist.*, **64**, 27666–27693

Food & Drug Administration (2000) Draft guidance for Industry. Photosafety testing. *Fed. Regist.*, **10 Jan.**, 1–22

Foot, G., Girgis, A., Boyle, C.A. & Sanson-Fisher, R.W. (1993) Solar protection behaviours: A study of beachgoers. *Aust. J. Public Health*, **17**, 209–214

Forbes, P.D., Davies, R.E., Sambuco, C.P. & Urbach, F. (1989) Inhibition of ultraviolet radiation-induced skin tumors in hairless mice by topical application of the sunscreen 2-ethyl hexyl-*p*-methoxycinnamate. *J. Toxicol. Cut. Ocular Toxicol.*, **8**, 209–226

Fourtanier, A. (1996) Mexoryl® SX protects against solar-simulated UVR-induced photocarcinogenesis in mice. *Photochem. Photobiol.*, **64**, 688–693

Fourtanier, A., Labat-Robert, J., Kern, P., Berrebi, C., Gracia, A.M. & Boyer, B. (1992) *In vivo* evaluation of photoprotection against chronic ultraviolet-A irradiation by a new sunscreen Mexoryl® SX. *Photochem. Photobiol.*, **55**, 549–560

Fourtanier, A., Guéniche, A., Compan, D., Walker, S.L. & Young, A.R. (2000) Improved protection against solar-simulated radiation-induced immunosuppression by a sunscreen with enhanced ultraviolet A protection. *J. Invest. Dermatol.*, **114**, 620–627

Frampton, R.J., Omond, S.A. & Eisman, J.A. (1983) Inhibition of human cancer cell growth by 1,25-dihydrovitamin D_3 metabolites. *Cancer Res.*, **43**, 4443–4447

Freeman, S.E., Blackett, A.D., Monteleone, D.C., Setlow, R.B., Sutherland, B.M. & Sutherland, J.C. (1986) Quantitation of radiation-, chemical-, or enzyme-induced single strand breaks in nonradioactive DNA by alkaline gel electrophoresis: Application to pyrimidine dimers. *Anal. Biochem.*, **158**, 119–129

Freeman, S.E., Ley, R.D. & Ley, K.D. (1988) Sunscreen protection against UV-induced pyrimidine dimers in DNA of human skin *in situ*. *Photodermatology*, **5**, 243–247

Freeman, S.E., Hacham, H., Gange, R.W., Maytum, D.J., Sutherland, J.C. & Sutherland, B.M. (1989) Wavelength dependence of pyrimidine dimer formation in DNA of human skin irradiated *in situ* with ultraviolet light. *Proc. Natl Acad. Sci. USA*, **86**, 5605–5609

French, J.E. (1992) *Toxicity Studies of 2-Hydroxy-4-methoxybenzophenone* (NTP Report No. 21, NIH Publication No. 92-3344), Research Triangle Park, North Carolina, National Toxicology Program

Friedman, L.C., Webb, J.A., Bruce, S., Weinberg, A.D. & Cooper, H.P. (1995) Skin cancer prevention and early detection intentions and behavior. *Am. J. Prev. Med.*, **11**, 59–65

Fritschi, L., Green, A. & Solomon, P.J. (1992) Sun exposure in Australian adolescents. *J. Am. Acad. Dermatol.*, **27**, 25–28

Fuchs, J. & Packer, L. (1999) Antioxidant protection from solar-simulated radiation-induced suppression of contact hypersensitivity to the recall antigen nickel sulfate in human skin. *Free Radicals Biol. Med.*, **27**, 422–427

Fukuda, M. & Naganuma, M. (1997) The sunscreen industry in Japan: Past, present, and future. In: Lowe, N.J., Shaath, N.A. & Pathak, M.A., eds, *Sunscreens, Development, Evaluation, and Regulatory Aspects*, New York, Marcel Dekker, pp. 241–260

Fukuda, M. & Takata, S. (1997) The evolution of recent sunscreens. In: Altmeyer, P., Hoffmann, K. & Stücker, M., eds, *Skin Cancer and UV Radiation*, Berlin, Springer-Verlag, pp. 265–276

Funk, J.O., Dromgoole, S.H. & Maibach, H.I. (1997) Contact sensitization and photocontact sensitization of sunscreening agents. In: Lowe, N.J., Shaath, N.A. & Pathak, M.A., eds, *Sunscreens, Development, Evaluation and Regulatory Aspects*, New York, Marcel Dekker, pp. 631–653

Fusaro, R.M., Runge, W.J., Lynch, F.W. & Watson, C.J. (1966) Sunlight protection in normal skin. *Arch. Dermatol.*, **93**, 106–111

Gailani, M.R., Stahle-Bäckdahl, M., Leffell, D.J., Glynn, M., Zaphiropoulos, P.G., Pressman, C., Undén, A.B., Dean, M., Brash, D.E., Bale, A.E. & Toftgard, R. (1996) The role of the human homologue of *Drosophila patched* in sporadic basal cell carcinomas. *Nature Genet.*, **14**, 78–81

Gallagher, P.E. & Duker, N.J. (1989) Formation of purine photoproducts in a defined human DNA sequence. *Photochem. Photobiol.*, **49**, 599–605

Gallagher, C.H., Greenoak, G.E., Reeve, V.E., Canfield, P.J., Baker, R.S. & Bonin, A.M. (1984) Ultraviolet carcinogenesis in hairless mouse skin. Influence of the sunscreen 2-ethylhexyl-p-methoxycinnamate. *Aust. J. Exp. Biol. Med. Sci.*, **62**, 577–588

Gallagher, R.P., McLean, D.I., Yang, C.P., Coldman, A.J., Silver, H.K., Spinelli, J.J. & Beagrie, M. (1990) Suntan, sunburn, and pigmentation factors and the frequency of acquired melanocytic nevi in children. Similarities to melanoma: The Vancouver Mole Study. *Arch. Dermatol.*, **126**, 770–776

Gallagher, R.P., Rivers, J.K., Lee, T.K., Bajdik, C.D., McLean, D.I. & Coldman, A.J. (2000) Broad spectrum sunscreen use and the development of new nevi in white children: A randomized controlled trial. *JAMA*, **283**, 2955–2960

Gange, R.W. & Parrish, J.A. (1983) Acute effects of ultraviolet radiation upon the skin. In: Parrish, J.A., Kripke, M.L., & Morison, W.L., eds, *Photoimmunology*, New York, Plenum Press, pp. 77–94

Gann, P.H., Ma, J., Hennekens, C.H., Hollis, B.W., Haddad, J.G. & Stampfer, M.J. (1996) Circulating vitamin D metabolites in relation to subsequent development of prostate cancer. *Cancer Epidemiol. Biomarkers Prev.*, **5**, 121–126

Garland, C.F. & Garland, F.C. (1980) Do sunlight and vitamin D reduce the likelihood of colon cancer? *Int. J. Epidemiol.*, **9**, 227–231

Garland, C.F., Comstock, G.W., Garland, F.C., Helsing, K.J., Shaw, E.K. & Gorham, E.D. (1989) Serum 25-dihydroxyvitamin D and colon cancer: Eight-year prospective study. *Lancet*, **ii**, 1176–1178

Garland, F.C., White, M.R., Garland, C.F., Shaw, E. & Gorham, E.D. (1990) Occupational sunlight exposure and melanoma in the US Navy. *Arch. Environ. Health,* **45**, 261–267

Garland, C.F., Garland, F.C. & Gorham, E.D. (1992) Could sunscreens increase melanoma risk? *Am. J. Public Health,* **82**, 614–615

Garland, C.F., Garland, F.C. & Gorham, E.D. (1993) Rising trends in melanoma: An hypothesis concerning sunscreen effectiveness. *Ann. Epidemiol., 3,* 103–110

Gasparro, F.P., Mitchnick, M. & Nash, J.F. (1998) A review of sunscreen safety and efficacy. *Photochem. Photobiol.,* **68**, 243–256

Geller, A.C., Hufford, D., Miller, D.R., Sun, T., Wyatt, S.W., Reilley, B., Bewerse, B., Lisco, J., Brooks, D., Grupenhoff, J., Weary, P., Lew, R.A. & Koh, H.K. (1997) Evaluation of the ultraviolet index: Media reactions and public response. *J. Am. Acad. Dermatol.,* **37**, 935–941

Gerberick, G.F. & Ryan, C.A. (1989) Contact photoallergy testing of sunscreens in guinea pigs. *Contact Derm.,* **20,** 251–259

Gerbert, B., Johnston, K., Bleecker, T. & McPhee, S. (1996) Attitudes about skin cancer prevention: A qualitative study. *J. Cancer Educ.,* **11**, 96–101

Gibbs, N.K., Norval, M., Traynor, N.J., Wolf, M., Johnson, B.E. & Crosby, J. (1993) Action spectra for the *trans* to *cis* photoisomerisation of urocanic acid *in vitro* and in mouse skin. *Photochem. Photobiol.,* **57**, 584–590

Gies, P., Roy, C. & Elliott, G. (1988) The anatomical distribution of solar UVR with emphasis on the eye. In: *Proceedings of the Seventh International Congress of the International Radiation Protection Association*, Sydney, Pergamon Press, pp. 341–344

Gies, H.P., Roy, C.R., Herlihy, E. & Rivers, J. (1992) Personal dosimetry of solar UVB using polysulphone film. In: *Proceedings of the Eighth International Congress of the International Radiation Protection Association,* Montreal, pp. 791-794

Gies, H.P., Roy, C.R., Elliott, G. & Zongli, W. (1994) Ultraviolet radiation protection factors for clothing. *Health Phys.,* **67**, 131–139

Gies, H.P., Roy, C.R., Toomey, S., MacLennan, R. & Watson, M. (1995) Solar UVR exposures of three groups of outdoor workers on the Sunshine Coast, Queensland. *Photochem. Photobiol.,* **62**, 1015–1021

Gies, H.P., Roy, C.R. & McLennan, A. (1996) Textiles and sun protection. In: Volkmer, B. & Heller, H., eds, *Environmental UV-radiation, Risk of Skin Cancer and Primary Prevention*. Stuttgart, Gustav Fischer, pp. 213–234

Gies, H.P., Roy, C.R., Toomey, S., MacLennan R. & Watson, M. (1998) Solar UVR exposures of primary school children at three locations in Queensland. *Photochem. Photobiol.,* **68**, 78–83

Gilchrest, B.A. (1996) A review of skin ageing and its medical therapy. *Br. J. Dermatol.,* **135**, 867–875

Gilchrest, B.A. & Yaar, M. (1992) Ageing and photoageing of the skin: Observations at the cellular and molecular level. *Br. J. Dermatol.,* **127** (Suppl. 41), 25–30

Giles, G.G. & Thursfield, V. (1996) Trends in skin cancer in Australia. *Cancer Forum,* **20**, 188–191

Gillardon, F., Eschenfelder, C., Uhlmann, E., Hartschuh, W. & Zimmermann, M. (1994) Differential regulation of c-*fos, fosB,* c-*jun, junB, bcl-2* and *bax* expression in rat skin following single or chronic ultraviolet irradiation and *in vivo* modulation by antisense oligodeoxynucleotide superfusion.*Oncogene,* **9**, 3219–3225

Gilmore, G.D. (1989) Sunscreens: A review of the skin cancer protection value and educational opportunities. *J. Sch. Health,* **59**, 210–213

Girgis, A., Sanson-Fisher, R.W., Tripodi, D.A. & Golding, T. (1993) Evaluation of interventions to improve solar protection in primary schools. *Health Educ. Q.,* **20**, 275–287

Girgis, A., Sanson-Fisher, R.W. & Watson, A. (1994) A workplace intervention for increasing outdoor workers' use of solar protection. *Am. J. Public Health,* **84**, 77–81

Glanz, K., Silverio, R. & Farmer, A. (1997) Daily diary reveals sun protective practices. *Primary Care Cancer,* **17**, 21–23

Glanz, K., Carbone, E. & Song, V. (1998a) Formative research for developing targeted skin cancer prevention programs for children in multiethnic Hawaii. *Health Educ. Res.,* **14**, 155–166

Glanz, K., Chang, L., Song, V., Silverio, R. & Muneoka, L. (1998b) Skin cancer prevention for children, parents, and caregivers: A field test of Hawaii's SunSmart Program. *J. Am. Acad. Dermatol.,* **38**, 413–417

Glanz, K., Lew, R.A., Song, V. & Cook, V.A. (1999) Factors associated with skin cancer prevention practices in a multiethnic population. *Health Educ. Behav.,* **26**, 344–359

Gonçalo, M., Ruas, E., Figueiredo, A. & Gonçalo, S. (1995) Contact and photocontact sensitivity to sunscreens. *Contact Derm.,* **33**, 278–280

González, E. & González, S. (1996) Drug photosensitivity, idiopathic photodermatoses, and sunscreens. *J. Am. Acad. Dermatol.,* **35**, 871–885

Gooderham, M.J. & Guenther, L. (1999) Sun and the skin: Evaluation of a sun awareness program for elementary school students. *J. Cut. Med. Surg.,* **3**, 230–235

Goodman, G.J., Marks, R., Selwood, T.S., Ponsford, M.W. & Pakes, W. (1984) Nonmelanotic skin cancer and solar keratoses in Victoria—Clinical studies II. *Australas. J. Dermatol.,* **25**, 103–106

Gordon, V. (1992) SPF evaluation via *in vitro* methodology. *Drug Cosmet. Ind.,* 30–75

Gorham, E.D., Garland, F.C. & Garland, C.F. (1990) Sunlight and breast cancer incidence in the USSR. *Int. J. Epidemiol.,* **19**, 820–824

Gottlieb, A., Bourget, T.D. & Lowe, N.J. (1997) Sunscreens: Effects of amounts of application of sun protection factors. In: Lowe, N.J., Shaath, N.A. & Pathak, M.A., eds, *Sunscreens: Development, Evaluation, and Regulatory Aspects*, New York, Marcel Dekker, pp. 583–588

Graham, S., Marshall, J., Haughey, B., Stoll, H., Zielezny, M., Brasure, J. & West, D. (1985) An inquiry into the epidemiology of melanoma. *Am. J. Epidemiol.,* **122**, 606–619

Grant-Petersson, J., Dietrich, A.J., Sox, C.H., Winchell, C.W. & Stevens, M.M. (1999) Promoting sun protection in elementary schools and child care settings: The Sunsafe project. *J. School Health,* **69**, 100–107

Gray, D.T., Suman, V.J., Su, W.P., Clay, R.P., Harmsen, W.S. & Roenigk, R.K. (1997) Trends in the population-based incidence of squamous cell carcinoma of the skin first diagnosed between 1984 and 1992. *Arch. Dermatol.*, **133**, 735–740

Green, A.C. (1991) Premature ageing of the skin in a Queensland population. *Med. J. Aust.*, **155**, 473–478

Green, C., Norris, P.G. & Hawk, J.L.M. (1991) Photoallergic contact dermatitis from oxybenzone aggravating polymorphic light eruption. *Contact Derm.*, **24**, 62–63

Green, A., Williams, G., Neale, R., Hart, V., Leslie, D., Parsons, P., Marks, G.C., Gaffney, P., Battistutta, D., Frost, C., Lang, C. & Russell, A. (1999a) Daily sunscreen application and beta-carotene supplementation in prevention of basal-cell and squamous-cell carcinomas of the skin: A randomised controlled trial. *Lancet,* **354**, 723–729

Green, A., Williams, G., Neale, R. & Battistutta, D. (1999b) Betacarotene and sunscreen use (Author's reply). *Lancet*, **354**, 2163–2164

Greenoak, G.E., Torkamanzehi, A. & Nearn, M. (1993) Reduction in tumour incidence by a sunscreen containing microfine titanium dioxide. *Cosmet. Aerosols Toiletries Aust.*, **7**, 12–17

Greenoak, G.E., Nearn, M.R., Cope, R. & Xia-Yao, R. (1998) Sunscreen protects against photocarcinogenic promotion. *Cosmet. Aerosols Toiletries Aust.*, **12**, 21–28

Greiter, F. (1974) [Sun protection factor – Origin and methods.] *Sonderdr. Parfüm. Kosmet.*, **55**, 70–75 (in German)

Greiter, F. (1981) [What is light protection]? Sun protection factor and problems in determining it.] *Apotheker J.*, **4/5**, 58–61(in German)

Greiter, P., Bilek, P., Doskoczil, S., Washuttl, J. & Wurst, F. (1979) Methods for water resistance testing of sun protection products. *Int. J. Cosmet. Sci.*, **1**, 147–157

Grob, J.J., Gouvernet, J., Aymar, D., Mostaque, A., Romano, M.H., Collet, A.M., Noé, M.C., Diconstanzo, M.P. & Bonerandi, J.J. (1990) Count of benign melanocytic nevi as a major indicator of risk for nonfamilial nodular and superficial spreading melanoma. *Cancer*, **66**, 387–395

Grob, J.J., Guglielmina, C., Gouvernet, J., Zarour, H., Noé, C. & Bonerandi, J.J. (1993) Study of sunbathing habits in children and adolescents: Application to the prevention of melanoma. *Dermatology*, **186**, 94–98

Grodstein, F., Speizer, F.E. & Hunter, D.J. (1995) A prospective study of incident squamous cell carcinoma of the skin in the nurses' health study. *J. Natl. Cancer Inst.*, **87**, 1061–1066

Grove, G.L. & Kaidbey, K.H. (1980) Sunscreens prevent sunburn cell formation in human skin. *J. Invest. Dermatol.*, **75**, 363–364

de Gruijl, F.R. & Forbes, P.D. (1995) UV-induced skin cancer in a hairless mouse model. *BioEssays*, **17**, 651–660

de Gruijl, F.R., Sterenborg, H.J.C.M., Forbes, P.D., Davies, R.E., Cole, C., Kelfkens, G., Van Weelden, H., Slaper, H. & Van der Leun, J.C. (1993) Wave-length dependence of skin cancer induction by ultraviolet irradiation of albino hairless mice. *Cancer Res.*, **53**, 53–60

de Gruijl, F.R. & van der Leun, J.C. (1994) Estimate of the wavelength dependency of ultraviolet carcinogenesis in humans and its relevance to the risk assessment of a stratospheric ozone depletion. *Health Phys.*, **67**, 319–325

Guéniche, A. & Fourtanier, A. (1997) Mexoryl SX protects against photoimmunosuppression. In: Altmeyer, P., Hoffmann, K. & Stücker, M., eds, *Skin Cancer and UV Radiation*, Heidelberg, Springer-Verlag, pp. 249–262

Gulston, M. & Knowland, J. (1999) Illumination of human keratinocytes in the presence of the sunscreen ingredient Padimate-O and through an SPF-15 sunscreen reduces direct photodamage to DNA but increases strand breaks. *Mutat. Res.*, **444**, 49–60

Gupta, V.K., Zatz, J.L. & Rerek, M. (1999) Percutaneous absorption of sunscreens through micro-Yucatan pig skin *in vitro*. *Pharm. Res.*, **16**, 1602–1607

Gurish, M.F., Roberts, L.K., Krueger, G.G. & Daynes, R.A. (1981) The effect of various sunscreen agents on skin damage and the induction of tumor susceptibility in mice subjected to ultraviolet irradiation. *J. Invest. Dermatol.*, **76**, 246–251

Hagedorn-Leweke, U. & Lippold, B.C. (1995) Absorption of sunscreens and other compounds through human skin *in vivo*: Derivation of a method to predict maximum fluxes. *Pharm. Res.*, **12**, 1354–1360

Hall, P.A., McKee, P.H., Menage, H.D.P., Dover, R. & Lane, D.P. (1993) High levels of p53 protein in UV-irradiated normal human skin. *Oncogene*, **8**, 203–207

Hall, J., English, D.R., Artuso, M., Armstrong, B.K. & Winter, M. (1994) DNA repair capacity as a risk factor for non-melanocytic skin cancer—A molecular epidemiological study. *Int. J. Cancer*, **58**, 179–184

Hall, H.I., May, D.S., Lew, R.A., Koh, H.K. & Nadel, M. (1997) Sun protection behaviors of the US white population. *Prev. Med.*, **26**, 401–407

Hallmans, G. & Liden, S. (1979) Penetration of ^{65}Zn through the skin of rats. *Acta Dermatol. Venereol.*, **59**, 105–112

Hanchette, C.L. & Schwartz, G.G. (1992) Geographic patterns of prostate cancer mortality. Evidence for a protective effect of ultraviolet radiation. *Cancer*, **70**, 2861–2869

Hany, J. & Nagel, R. (1995) Detection of UV screens in breast milk. *Deutsche Lebensmittel Rundschau*, **91**, 341–345

Hariharan, P.V. & Cerutti, P.A. (1977) Formation of products of the 5,6-dihydroxydihydrothymine type by ultraviolet light in HeLa cells. *Biochemistry*, **16**, 2391–2395

Harper, J.W., Adami, G.R., Wei, N., Keyomarsi, K. & Elledge, S.J. (1993) The p21 Cdk-interacting protein Cip1 is a potent inhibitor of G1 cyclin-dependent kinases. *Cell*, **75**, 805–816

Harrison, J.A., Walker, S.L., Plastow, S.R., Batt, M.D., Hawk, J.L. & Young, A.R. (1991) Sunscreens with low sun protection factor inhibit ultraviolet B and A photoaging in the skin of the hairless albino mouse. *Photodermatol. Photoimmunol. Photomed.*, **8**, 12–20

Harrison, S.L., MacLennan, R., Speare, R. & Wronski, I. (1994) Sun exposure and melanocytic naevi in young Australian children. *Lancet*, **344**, 1529–1532

Harth, Y., Ulman, Y., Peled, I. & Friedman-Birnbaum, R. (1995) Sun protection and sunscreen use after surgical treatment of basal cell carcinoma. *Photodermatol. Photoimmunol. Photomed.,* **11**, 140–142

Harvey, I., Frankel, S., Marks, R., Shalom, D. & Nolan-Farrell, M. (1996a) Non-melanoma skin cancer and solar keratoses. I. Methods and descriptive results of the South Wales skin cancer study. *Br. J. Cancer*, **74**, 1302–1307

Harvey, I., Frankel, S., Marks, R., Shalom, D. & Nolan-Farrell, M. (1996b) Non-melanoma skin cancer and solar keratoses. II. Analytical results of the South Wales skin cancer study. *Br. J. Cancer*, **74**, 1308–1312

Hayag, M.V., Chartier, T., DeVoursney, J., Tie, C., Machler, R.B. & Taylor, J.R. (1997) A high SPF sunscreen's effects on UVB-induced immunosuppression of DNCB contact hypersensitivity. *J. Dermatol. Sci.*, **16**, 31–37

Hayden, C.G., Roberts, M.S. & Benson, H.A. (1997) Systemic absorption of sunscreen after topical application. *Lancet*, **350**, 863–864

Health Canada (1999) *Regulatory Strategy for Pharmaceutical Products with Photo Co-carcinogenic Potential*. Ottawa, Therapeutic Products Programme.

Health Education Authority (1996) *Sunscreens and the Consumer*, London, pp. 1–32

Healy, E., Sikkink, S. & Rees, J.L. (1996) Infrequent mutation of the p16^{INK4} in sporadic melanoma. *J. Invest. Dermatol.*, **107**, 318–321

Herlihy, E., Gies, P.H., Roy, C.R. & Jones, M. (1994) Personal dosimetry of solar UV radiation for different outdoor activities. *Photochem. Photobiol.*, **60**, 228–294

Hersey, P., MacDonald, M., Burns, C., Schibeci, S., Matthews, H. & Wilkinson, F.J. (1987) Analysis of the effect of a sunscreen agent on the suppression of natural killer cell activity induced in human subjects by radiation from solarium lamps. *J. Invest. Dermatol.*, **88**, 271–276

Hersey, P., MacDonald, M., Henderson, C., Schibeci, S., D'Alessandro, G., Pryor, M. & Wilkinson, F.J. (1988) Suppression of natural killer cell activity in humans by radiation from solarium lamps depleted of UVB. *J. Invest. Dermatol.*, **90**, 305–310

Herzfeld, P.M., Fitzgerald, E.F., Hwang, S.A. & Stark, A. (1993) A case–control study of malignant melanoma of the trunk among white males in upstate New York. *Cancer Detect. Prev.*, **17**, 601–608

Hill, J. & Boulter, J. (1996) Sun protection behaviour—Determinants and trends. *Cancer Forum*, **20**, 204–211

Hill, D., Rassaby, J. & Gardner, G. (1984) Determinants of intentions to take precautions against skin cancer. *Community Health Stud.*, **8**, 33–44

Hill, D., White, V., Marks, R., Theobald, T., Borland, R. & Roy, C. (1992) Melanoma prevention: Behavioural and nonbehavioural factors in sunburn among an Australian urban population. *Prev. Med.*, **21**, 654–669

Hill, D., White, V., Marks, R. & Borland, R. (1993) Changes in sun-related attitudes and behaviors, and reduced sunburn prevalence in a population at high risk of melanoma. *Eur. J. Cancer Prev.*, **2**, 447–456

Hill, L.L., Ouhtit, A., Loughlin, S.M., Kripke, M.L., Ananthaswamy, H.N. & Owen-Schaub, L.B. (1999) Fas ligand: A sensor for DNA damage critical in skin cancer etiology. *Science*, **285**, 898–900

Hillhouse, J.J., Stair, A.W., 3rd & Adler, C.M. (1996) Predictors of sunbathing and sunscreen use in college under-graduates. *J. Behav. Med.*, **19**, 543–561

Hillhouse, J.J., Adler, C.M., Drinnon, J. & Turrisi, R. (1997) Application of Azjen's theory of planned behavior to predict sunbathing, tanning salon use, and sunscreen use intentions and behaviors. *J. Behav. Med.*, **20**, 365–378

Ho, K.K., Halliday, G.M. & Barnetson, R.S. (1992) Sunscreens protect epidermal Langerhans cells and Thy-1$^+$ cells but not local contact sensitization from the effects of ultraviolet light. *J. Invest. Dermatol.*, **98**, 720–724

Hochberg, M. & Enk, C.D. (1999) Partial protection against epidermal IL-10 transcription and Langerhans cell depletion by sunscreens after exposure of human skin to UVB. *Photochem. Photobiol.*, **70**, 766–772

Hodges, N.D.M., Moss, S.H. & Davies, D.J.G. (1977) The sensitising effect of a sunscreening agent, p-aminobenzoic acid, on near UV-induced damage in a repair deficient strain of Escherichia coli. *Photochem. Photobiol.*, **26**, 493–498

Hoegh, H.J., Davis, B.D. & Manthe, A.F. (1999) Sun avoidance practices among non-Hispanic white Californians. *Health Educ. Behav.*, **26**, 360–368

Holly, E.A., Kelly, J.W., Shpall, S.N. & Chiu, S.H. (1987) Number of melanocytic nevi as a major risk factor for malignant melanoma. *J. Am. Acad. Dermatol.*, **17**, 459–468

Holly, E.A., Aston, D.A., Cress, R.D., Ahn, D.K. & Kristiansen, J.J. (1995) Cutaneous melanoma in women. I. Exposure to sunlight, ability to tan, and other risk factors related to ultraviolet light. *Am. J. Epidemiol.*, **141**, 923–933

Holman, C.D.J. & Armstrong, B.K. (1984) Pigmentary traits, ethnic origin, benign nevi, and family history as risk factors for cutaneous malignant melanoma. *J. Natl Cancer Inst.*, **72**, 257–266

Holman, C.D., Mulroney, C.D. & Armstrong, B.K. (1980) Epidemiology of pre-invasive and invasive malignant melanoma in Western Australia. *Int. J. Cancer*, **25**, 317–323

Holman, C.D.J., Gibson, I.M., Stephenson, M. & Armstrong, B.K. (1983) Ultraviolet irradiation of human body sites in relation to occupation and outdoor activity: Field studies using personal UVR dosimeters. *Clin. Exp. Dermatol.*, **8**, 269–277

Holman, C.D., Evans, P.R., Lumsden, G.J. & Armstrong, B.K. (1984) The determinants of actinic skin damage: Problems of confounding among environmental and constitutional variables. *Am. J. Epidemiol.*, **120**, 414–422

Holman, C.D.J., Armstrong, B.K. & Heenan, P.J. (1986) Relationship of cutaneous malignant melanoma to individual sunlight-exposure habits. *J. Natl Cancer Inst.*, **76**, 403–414

Hourani, L.L. & LaFleur, B. (1995) Predictors of gender differences in sunscreen use and screening outcome among skin cancer screening participants. *J. Behav. Med.*, **18**, 461–477

Hu, M.L., Chen, Y.K., Chen, L.C. & Sano, M. (1995) para-Aminobenzoic acid scavenges reactive oxygen species and protects DNA against UV and free radical damage. *J. Nutr. Biochem.*, **6**, 504–508

Huang, N.P., Xu, M.H., Yuan, C.W. & Yu, R.R. (1997) The study of the photokilling effect and mechanism of ultrafine Ti$_{O2}$ particles on U937 cells. *J. Photochem. Photobiol. A*, **108**, 229–233

Hughes, B.R., Altman, D.G. & Newton, J.A. (1993) Melanoma and skin cancer: Evaluation of a health education programme for secondary schools. *Br. J. Dermatol.*, **128**, 412–417

Hunter, D.J., Colditz, G.A., Strampfer, M.J., Rosner, B., Willett, W.C. & Speizer, F.E. (1990) Risk factors for basal cell carcinoma in a prospective cohort of women. *Ann. Epidemiol.*, **1**, 13–23

Hurks, H.M., van der Molen, R.G., Out-Luiting, C., Vermeer, B.J., Claas, F.H.J. & Mommaas, A.M. (1997) Differential effects of sunscreens on UVB-induced immunomodulation in humans. *J. Invest. Dermatol.*, **109**, 699–703

Hussussian, C.J., Struewing, J.P., Goldstein, A.M., Higgins, P.A., Ally, D.S., Sheahan, M.D., Clark, W.H., Jr, Tucker, M.A. & Dracopoli, N.C. (1994) Germline p16 mutations in familial melanoma. *Nature Genet.*, **8**, 15–21

IARC (1987) *IARC Monographs on the Evaluation of Carcinogenic Risks to Humans*, Suppl. 7, *Overall Evaluation of Carcinogenicity: An Updating of IARC Monographs Volumes 1 to 42*, Lyon, IARCPress, pp. 242–245

IARC (1989) *IARC Monographs on the Evaluation of Carcinogenic Risks to Humans*, Vol. 47, *Some Organic Solvents, Resin Monomers and Related Compounds, Pigments and Occupational Exposures in Paint Manufacture and Painting*, Lyon, IARCPress, pp. 307–327

IARC (1992) *IARC Monographs on the Evaluation of Carcinogenic Risks to Humans*, Vol. 55, *Solar and Ultraviolet Radiation*, Lyon, IARCPress, pp. 1–316

IARC (1998) *GLOBOCAN 1: Cancer Incidence and Mortality Worldwide*. IARC Cancer Bases No. 3. Lyon, IARCPress

Iscovich, J., Paltiel, O., Azizi, E., Kuten, A., Gat, A., Lifzchitz-Mercer, B., Zlotogorski, A. & Polliack, A. (1998) Cutaneous lymphoma in Israel, 1985–1993: A population-based incidence study. *Br. J. Cancer*, **77**, 170–173

Janousek, A. (1997) Regulatory aspects os sunscreens in Europe. In: Lowe, N.J., Shaath, N.A. & Pathak, M.A., eds, *Sunscreens, Development, Evaluation, and Regulatory Aspects*, New York, Marcel Dekker Inc., pp. 215–225

Janowsky, E.C., Lester, G. & Hulka, B. (1997) *Vitamin D and Breast Cancer*, Washington DC, Department of Defense, pp. 999–1000

Jeanmougin, M., Manciet, J.R., Moulin, J.P., Blanc, F., Pons, A. & Civatte, J. (1988) Contact allergy to dexpanthenol in sunscreens. *Contact Derm.*, **18**, 240

Jekat, F.W., Kemper, F.H. & Winterhoff, H. (1992) Embryotoxicity study of propenoic acid, 3-(4-methoxyphenyl)-3-methylbutylester in the Wistar rat. *Food Chem. Toxicol.*, **30**, 803–807

Jerkegren, E., Sandrieser, L., Brandberg, Y. & Rosdahl, I. (1999) Sun-related behaviour and melanoma awareness among Swedish university students. *Eur. J. Cancer Prev.*, **8**, 27–34

Jiang, R., Roberts, M.S., Collins, D.M. & Benson, H.A. (1999) Absorption of sunscreens across human skin: An evaluation of commercial products for children and adults. *Br. J. Clin. Pharmacol.*, **48**, 635–637

John, E.M., Schwartz, G.G., Dreon, D.M. & Koo, J. (1999) Vitamin D and breast cancer risk: The NHANES I epidemiologic follow-up study, 1971–1975 to 1992. *Cancer Epidemiol. Biomarkers Prev.*, **8**, 399–406

Jonason, A.S., Kunala, S., Price, G., Restifo, R.J., Spinelli, H.M., Persing, J.A., Leffell, D.J., Tarone, R.E. & Brash, D.E. (1996) Frequent clones of p53-mutated keratinocytes in normal human skin. *Proc. Natl Acad. Sci. USA*, **93**, 14025–14029

Kadry, A.M., Okereke, C.S., Abdel-Rahman, M.S., Friedman, M.A. & Davis, R.A. (1995) Pharmacokinetics of benzophenone-3 after oral exposure in male rats. *J. Appl. Toxicol.*, **15**, 97–102

Kaidbey, K.H. (1990) The photoprotective potential of the new superpotent sunscreens. *J. Am. Acad. Dermatol.*, **22**, 449–452

Kajiki, A., Higuchi, K., Nakamura, M., Liu, L.H., Pula, P.J. & Dannenberg, A.M., Jr (1988) Sources of extracellular lysosomal enzymes released in organ-culture by developing and healing inflammatory lesions. *J. Leukocyte Biol.*, **43**, 104–116

Kakourou, T., Bakoula, C., Kavadias, G., Gatos, A., Bilalis, L., Krikos, X. & Matsaniotis, N. (1995) Mothers' knowledge and practices related to sun protection in Greece. *Pediatr. Dermatol.*, **12**, 207–210

Kamb, A., Gruis, N.A., Weaver-Feldhaus, J., Liu, Q., Harshman, K., Tavtigian, S.V., Stockert, E., Day, R.S., Johnson, B.E. & Skolnick, M.H. (1994) A cell cycle regulator potentially involved in genesis of many tumor types. *Science*, **264**, 436–440

Kammeyer, A., Westerhof, W., Bolhuis, P.A, Ris, A.J & Hische, E.A. (1987) The spectral stability of several sunscreening agents on stratum corneum sheets. *Int. J. Cosmet. Sci.*, **9**, 125–136

Kanjilal, S., Pierceall, W.E., Cummings, K.K., Kripke, M.L. & Ananthaswamy, H.N. (1993) High frequency of p53 mutations in ultraviolet radiation-induced skin tumors: Evidence for strand bias and tumor heterogeneity. *Cancer Res.*, *53*, 2961–2964

Kanjilal, S., Strom, S.S., Clayman, G.L., Weber, R.S., El-Naggar, A.K., Kapur, V., Cummings, K.K., Hill, L.A., Spitz, M.R., Kripke, M.L. & Ananthaswamy, H.N. (1995) *p53* mutations in nonmelanoma skin cancer of the head and neck: Molecular evidence for field cancerization. *Cancer Res.*, **55**, 3604–3609

Kapur, S.P., Bhussry, B.R., Rao, S. & Harmuth-Hoene, E. (1974) Percutaneous uptake of zinc in rabbit skin. *Proc. Soc. Exp. Biol. Med.*, **145**, 932–937

Kastan, M.B., Onyekwere, O., Sidransky, D., Vogelstein, B. & Craig, R.W. (1991) Participation of p53 protein in the cellular response to DNA damage. *Cancer Res.*, **51**, 6304–6311

Kastan, M.B., Canman, C.E. & Leonard, C.J. (1995) P53, cell cycle control and apoptosis: Implications for cancer. *Cancer Metastasis Rev.*, **14**, 3–15

Kawada, A., Hiruma, M., Noda, T. & Kukita, A. (1989) Skin typing, sun exposure, and sunscreen use in a population of Japanese. *J. Dermatol.*, **16**, 187–190

Kazianis, S., Gutbrod, H., Nairn, R.S., McEntire, B.B., Della-Colletta, L., Walter, R.B., Borowsky, R.L., Woodhead, A.D., Setlow, R.B., Schartl, M. & Morizot, D.C. (1998) Localization of a *CDKN2* gene in linkage group V of *Xiphophorus* fishes defines it as a candidate for the *DIFF* tumor suppressor. *Genes Chromosomes Cancer*, **22**, 210–220

Keeley, K.A., Laskar, P.A., Ewing, G.D. Dromgoole, S.H. Lichtin, J.L. & Sakr, A.A. (1993) *In vitro* sun protection factor evaluation of sunscreen products. *J. Soc. Cosmet. Chem.*, **44**, 139–151

Keesling, B. & Friedman, H. S. (1987) Psychosocial factors in sunbathing and sunscreen use. *Health Psychol.*, **6**, 477–493

Keijzer, W., Mulder, M.P., Langeveld, J.C.M., Smit, E.M.E., Bos, J.L., Bootsma, D. & Hoeijmakers, J.H.J. (1989) Establishment and characterization of a melanoma cell line from a xeroderma pigmentosum patient: Activation of N-*ras* at a potential pyrimidine dimer site. *Cancer Res.*, **49**, 1229–1235

Kelly, J.W., Rivers, J.K., MacLennan, R., Harrison, S., Lewis, A.E. & Tate, B.J. (1994) Sunlight: A major factor associated with the development of melanocytic nevi in Australian schoolchildren. *J. Am. Acad. Dermatol.*, **30**, 40–48

Kibitel, J., Hejmadi, V., Alas, L., O'Connor, A., Sutherland, B.M. & Yarosh, D. (1998) UV-DNA damage in mouse and human cells induces the expression of tumor necrosis factor alpha. *Photochem. Photobiol.*, **67**, 541–546

Kielbassa, C., Roza, L. & Epe, B. (1997) Wavelength dependence of oxidative DNA damage induced by UV and visible light. *Carcinogenesis*, **18**, 811–816

Kimlin, M.G., Parisi, A.V. & Wong, J.C.F. (1998a) Quantification of personal solar UV exposure of outdoor workers, indoor workers and adolescents at two locations in Southeast Queensland. *Photodermatol. Photoimmunol. Photomed.*, **14**, 7–11

Kimlin, M.G., Parisi, A.V. & Wong, J.C.F. (1998b) The facial distribution of erythemal ultraviolet exposure in south-east Queensland. *Phys. Med. Biol.*, **43**, 231–240

Kimura, K. & Katoh, T. (1995) Photoallergic contact dermatitis from the sunscreen ethyl-hexyl-*p*-methoxycinnamate (Parsol® MCX). *Contact Derm.*, **32**, 304–305

Kipp, C., Lewis, E.J. & Young, A.R. (1998) Furocoumarin-induced epidermal melanogenesis does not protect against skin photocarcinogenesis in hairless mice. *Photochem. Photobiol.*, **67**, 126–132

Klein, K. (1992) Encyclopedia of UV absorbers for sunscreen products. *Cosmet. Toiletries*, **107**, 45–64

Klein, K. (1997) Sunscreen products: Formulation and regulatory considerations. In: Lowe, N.J., Shaath, N.A. & Pathak, M.A., eds, *Sunscreens, Development, Evaluation, and Regulatory Aspects,* New York, Marcel Dekker, pp. 285–311

Klepp, O. & Magnus, K. (1979) Some environmental and bodily characteristics of melanoma patients. A case–control study. *Int. J. Cancer,* **23**, 482–486

Kligman, A.M. (1966) The identification of contact allergens by human assay. 3. The maximization test: A procedure for screening and rating contact sensitizers. *J. Invest. Dermatol.*, **47**, 393–409

Kligman, A.M. (1969) Early destructive effect of sunlight on human skin. *JAMA*, **210**, 2377–2380

Kligman, A.M. (1979) Perspectives and problems in cutaneous gerontology. *J. Invest. Dermatol.*, **73**, 39–46

Kligman, L.H. (1989) Prevention and repair of photoaging: Sunscreens and retinoids. *Cutis*, **43**, 458–465

Kligman, L.H. (1997) Do broad spectrum sunscreens allow ultraviolet-induced photodamage in the absence of erythema? In: Gasparro, F.P., ed., *Sunscreen Photobiology: Molecular, Cellular and Physiological Aspects*, Berlin, Springer-Verlag, pp. 69–83

Kligman, L.H. & Gebre, M. (1991) Biochemical changes in hairless mouse skin collagen after chronic exposure to ultraviolet-A radiation. *Photochem. Photobiol.*, **54**, 233–237

Kligman, L.H. & Zheng, P. (1994) The protective effect of a broad-spectrum sunscreen against chronic UVA radiation in hairless mice: A histologic and ultrastructural assessment. *J. Soc. Cosmet. Chem.*, **45**, 21–33

Kligman, L.H., Akin, F.J. & Kligman, A.M. (1980) Sunscreens prevent ultraviolet carcinogenesis. *J. Am. Acad. Dermatol.*, **3**, 30–35

Kligman, L.H., Akin, F.J. & Kligman, A.M. (1982) Prevention of ultraviolet damage to the dermis of hairless mice by sunscreens. *J. Invest. Dermatol.*, **78**, 181–189

Kligman, L.H., Akin, F.J. & Kligman, A.M. (1983) Sunscreens promote repair of ultraviolet radiation-induced dermal damage. *J. Invest. Dermatol.*, **81**, 98–102

Kligman, L.H., Akin, F.J. & Kligman, A.M. (1985) The contributions of UVA and UVB to connective tissue damage in hairless mice. *J. Invest. Dermatol.*, **84**, 272–276

Kligman, L.H., Agin, P. & Sayre, R.M. (1996) Broad-spectrum sunscreens with UVA I and UVA II absorbers provide increased protection against solar-simulating radiation-induced dermal damage in hairless mice. *J. Soc. Cosmet. Chem.*, **47**, 129–155

Knobler, E., Almeida, L., Ruzkowski, A.M., Held, J., Harber, L. & DeLeo, V. (1989) Photoallergy to benzophenone. *Arch. Dermatol.*, **125**, 801–804

Knowland, J., McKenzie, E.A., McHugh, P.J. & Cridland, N.A. (1993) Sunlight-induced mutagenicity of a common sunscreen ingredient. *FEBS Lett.*, **324**, 309–313

Knox, J.M., Griffin, A.C. & Hakim, R.E. (1960) Protection from ultraviolet carcinogenesis. *J. Invest. Dermatol.*, **34**, 51–58

Knuschke, P. & Barth, J. (1996) Biologically weighted personal UV dosimetry. *J. Photochem. Photobiol. B*, **36**, 77–83

Koh, H.K., Bak, S.M., Geller, A.C., Mangione, T.W., Hingson, R.W., Levenson, S.M., Miller, D.R., Lew, R.A. & Howland, J. (1997) Sunbathing habits and sunscreen use among white adults: Results of a national survey. *Am. J. Public Health*, **87**, 1214–1217

Kondoh, M., Ueda, M., Nakagawa, K. & Ichihaski, M. (1994) Siblings with xeroderma pigmentosum complementation group A with different skin cancer development: Importance of sun protection at an early age. *J. Am. Acad. Dermatol.*, **31**, 993–996

van Kranen, H.J., de Laat, A., van de Ven, J., Wester, P.W., de Vries, A., Berg, R.J., Van Kreijl, C.F. & de Gruijl, F.R. (1997) Low incidence of *p53* mutations in UVA (365-nm)-induced skin tumors in hairless mice. *Cancer Res.*, **57**, 1238–1240

Krekels, G., Voorter, C., Kuik, F., Verhaegh, M., Ramaekers, F. & Neumann, M. (1997) DNA-protection by sunscreens: Using p53-immunostaining. *Eur. J. Dermatol.*, **7**, 259–262

Krekels, G.A.M., Lenders, M.H., Hoekzema, R., Neumann, H.A.M. & Ramaekers, F.C.S. (2000) Dissociation between SPF and p53 protection by sunscreens. PhD Thesis, University of Maastricht

Kress, S., Sutter, C., Strickland, P.T., Mukhtar, H., Schweizer, J. & Schwarz, M. (1992) Carcinogen-specific mutational pattern in the *p53* gene in ultraviolet B radiation-induced squamous cell carcinomas of mouse skin. *Cancer Res.*, **52**, 6400–6403

Kricker, A., Armstrong, B.K., English, D.R. & Heenan, P.J. (1995) Does intermittent sun exposure cause basal cell carcinoma? A case–control study in Western Australia. *Int. J. Cancer,* **60**, 489–494

Krien, P.M. & Moyal, D. (1994) Sunscreens with broad-spectrum absorption decrease the trans to cis photoisomerization of urocanic acid in the human stratum corneum after multiple UV light exposures. *Photochem. Photobiol.*, **60**, 280–287

Kripke, M.L. (1974) Antigenicity of murine skin tumors induced by ultraviolet light. *J. Natl Cancer Inst.*, **53**, 1333–1336

Kripke, M.L. & Fisher, M.S. (1976) Immunologic parameters of ultraviolet carcinogenesis. *J. Natl Cancer Inst.*, **57**, 211–215

Kripke, M.L., Cox, P.A., Alas, L.G. & Yarosh, D.B. (1992) Pyrimidine dimers in DNA initiate systemic immunosuppression in UV-irradiated mice. *Proc. Natl Acad. Sci. USA*, **89**, 7516–7520

Kubar, W.L., Rodrigue, J.R. & Hoffmann, R.G., 3rd (1995) Children and exposure to the sun: Relationships among attitudes, knowledge, intentions, and behaviour. *Psychol. Rep.*, **77**, 1136–1138

Kubota, Y., Shuin, T., Kawasaki, C., Hosaka, M., Kitamura, H., Cai, R., Sakai, H., Hashimoto, K. & Fujishima, A. (1994) Photokilling of T-24 human bladder cancer cells with titanium dioxide. *Br. J. Cancer,* **70**, 1107–1111

Kumar, R., Lundh Rozell, B., Louhelainen, J. & Hemminki, K. (1998) Mutations in the *CDKN2A* (*p16^{INK4}*) gene in microdissected sporadic primary melanomas. *Int. J. Cancer*, **75**, 193–198

Kumar, R., Smeds, J., Lundh Rozell, B. & Hemminki, K. (1999) Loss of heterozygosity at chromosome 9p21 (*INK4-p14^{ARF}* locus): Homozygous deletions and mutations in the *p16* and *p14^{ARF}* genes in sporadic primary melanomas. *Mela-noma Res.*, **9**, 138–147

Kvam, E. & Tyrrell, R.M (1997a) Artificial background and induced levels of oxidative base damage in DNA from human cells. *Carcinogenesis*, **18**, 2281–2283

Kvam, E. & Tyrrell, R.M. (1997b) Induction of oxidative DNA base damage in human skin cells by UV and near visible radiation. *Carcinogenesis*, **18**, 2379–2384

Larkö, O. & Diffey, B.L. (1983) Natural UV-B radiation received by people with outdoor, indoor and mixed occupations and UV-B treatment of psoriasis. *Clin. Exp. Dermatol.*, **8**, 279–285

Lavker, R. & Kaidbey, K. (1997) The spectral dependence for UVA-induced cumulative damage in human skin. *J. Invest. Dermatol.*, **108**, 17–21

Lavker, R.M. & Kligman, A.M. (1988) Chronic heliodermatitis: A morphologic evaluation of chronic actinic dermal damage with emphasis on the role of mast cells. *J. Invest. Dermatol.*, **90**, 325–330

Lavker, R.M., Gerberick, G.F., Veres, D., Irwin, C.J. & Kaidbey, K.H. (1995a) Cumulative effects from repeated exposures to suberythemal doses of UVB and UVA in human skin. *J. Am. Acad. Dermatol.*, **32**, 53–62

Lavker, R.M., Veres, D.A., Irwin, C.J. & Kaidbey, K.H. (1995b) Quantitative assessment of cumulative damage from repetitive exposures to suberythemogenic doses of UVA in human skin. *Photochem. Photobiol.*, **62**, 348–352

Lawler, P.E. (1989) Be sunsensible: Steps toward safety in the sun—An information handout. *Oncol. Nurs. Forum*, **16**, 424–427

Leach, J.F., McLeod, V.E., Pingstone, A.R., Davis, A. & Deane, G.H.W. (1978) Measurement of the ultraviolet doses received by office workers. *Clin. Exp. Dermatol.*, **3**, 77–79

Leary, M.R. & Jones, J.L. (1993) The social psychology of tanning and sunscreen use: Self-representation motives as a predictor of health risk. *J. Appl. Soc. Psychol.*, **23**, 1390–1406

Lenique, P., Machet, L., Vaillant, L., Bensaïd, P., Muller, C., Khallouf, R. & Lorette, G. (1992) Contact and photocontact allergy to oxybenzone. *Contact Derm.*, **26**, 177–181

Lewerenz, H.J., Lewerenz, G. & Plass, R. (1972) Acute and subacute toxicity studies of the UV absorber MOB in rats. *Food Cosmet. Toxicol.*, **10**, 41–50

Ley, R.D. (1997) Ultraviolet radiation A-induced precursors to cutaneous melanoma in *Monodelphis domestica. Cancer Res.*, **57**, 3682–3684

Ley, R.D. & Fourtanier, A. (1997) Sunscreen protection against ultraviolet radiation-induced pyrimidine dimers in mouse epidermal DNA. *Photochem. Photobiol.*, **65**, 1007–1011

Lindahl, T. & Wood, R.D. (1999) Quality control by DNA repair. *Science*, **286**, 1897–1905

Liu, Q., Neuhausen, S., McClure, M., Frye, C., Weaver-Feldhaus, J., Gruis, N.A., Eddington, K., Allalunis-Turner, M.J., Skolnick, M.H., Fujimura, F.K. & Kamb, A. (1995) CDKN2 (MTS1) tumor suppressor gene mutations in human tumor cell lines. *Oncogene*, **10**, 1061–1067

Lock-Andersen, J. & Wulf, H.C. (1996) Threshold level for measurement of UV sensitivity: Reproducibility of phototest. *Photodermatol. Photoimmunol. Photomed.*, **12**, 154–161

Lock-Andersen, J., Wulf, H.C. & Mortensen, N.N. (1998) Erythemally weighted radiometric dose and Standard Erythema Dose (SED). In: Hönigsmann, H., Knobler, R.M., Trautinger, F. & Jori, G., eds, *Landmarks in Photobiology*, Milan, Organizzazione Editoriale Medico Farmaceutica, pp. 315–317

Loeppky, R.N., Hastings, R., Sandbothe, J., Heller, D., Bao, Y. & Nagel, D. (1991) Nitrosation of tertiary aromatic amines related to sunscreen ingredients. In: *Relevance to Human Cancer of N-Nitroso Compounds, Tobacco Smoke and Mycotoxins* (IARC Scientific Publications No. 105), Lyon, IARCPress, pp. 244–252

Lombard, D., Neubauer, T.E., Canfield, D. & Winett, R.A. (1991) Behavioral community intervention to reduce the risk of skin cancer. *J. Appl. Behav.*, **24**, 677–686

Loprieno, N. (1992) Guidelines for safety evaluation of cosmetics ingredients in the EC countries. *Food Chem. Toxicol.*, **30**, 809–815

Lovato, C.Y., Shoveller, J.A., Peters, L. & Rivers, J.K. (1998) Canadian national survey on sun exposure and protective behaviours: Parents' reports on children. *Cancer Prev. Control*, **2**, 123–128

Lowe, J.B., Balanda, K.P., Gillespie, A.M., Del-Mar, C.B. & Gentle, A.F. (1993) Sun-related attitudes and beliefs among Queensland school children: The role of gender and age. *Aust. J. Public Health*, **17**, 202–208

Lu, X. & Lane, D.P. (1993) Differential induction of transcriptionally active p53 following UV or ionizing radiation: Defects in chromosome instability syndromes? *Cell*, **75**, 765–778

Lu, P.-J., Ho, I.-C. & Lee, T.-C. (1998) Induction of sister chromatid exchanges and micronuclei by titanium dioxide in Chinese hamster ovary-K1 cells. *Mutat. Res.*, **414**, 15–20

Luther, H., Altmeyer, P., Garbe, C., Ellwanger, U., Jahn, S., Hoffmann, K. & Segerling, M. (1996) Increase of melanocytic nevus counts in children during 5 years of follow-up and analysis of associated factors. *Arch. Dermatol.*, **132**, 1473–1478

Lynch, D.H., Gurish, M.F. & Daynes, R.A. (1981) Relationship between epidermal Langerhans cell density ATPase activity and the induction of contact hypersensitivity. *J. Immunol.*, **126**, 1892–1897

MacKie, R.M., Hole, D., Hunter, J.A., Rankin, R., Evans, A., McLaren, K., Fallowfield, M., Hutcheon, A. & Morris, A. (1997) Cutaneous malignant melanoma in Scotland: Incidence, survival, and mortality, 1979–94. The Scottish Melanoma Group. *Br. Med. J.*, **315**, 1117–1121

Madronich, S. (1993) The atmosphere and UV-B radiation at ground level. In: Young, A.R., Bjorn, L.O., Moan, J. & Nultsch, W., eds, *Environmental UV Photobiology*, New York, Plenum Press, pp. 1–39

Maducdoc, L.R., Wagner, R.F., Jr & Wagner, K.D. (1992) Parents' use of sunscreen on beach-going children. The burnt child dreads the fire. *Arch. Dermatol.*, **128**, 628–629

Maltzman, W. & Czyzyk, L. (1984) UV irradiation stimulates levels of p53 cellular tumor antigen in nontransformed mouse cells. *Mol. Cell. Biol.*, **4**, 1689–1694

Marginean Lazar, G., Fructus, A.E., Baillet, A., Bocquet, J.L., Thomas, P. & Marty, J.P. (1997) Sunscreens' photochemical behaviour: *In vivo* evaluation by the stripping method. *Int. J. Cosmet. Sci.*, **19**, 87–101

Marguery, M.C., Rakotondrazafy, J., El Sayed, F., Bayle-Lebey, P., Journe, F. & Bazex, J. (1996) Contact allergy to 3-(4'-methylbenzylidene) camphor and contact and photocontact allergy to 4-isopropyl dibenzoylmethane. *Photodermatol. Photoimmunol. Photomed.*, **11**, 209–212

Marks, R. (1996) The use of sunscreens in the prevention of skin cancer. *Cancer Forum*, **20**, 211–215

Marks, R., Ponsford, M.W., Selwood, T.S., Goodman, G. & Mason, G. (1983) Non-melanotic skin cancer and solar keratoses in Victoria. *Med. J. Aust*, **2**, 619–622

Marks, R., Foley, P., Goodman, G., Hage, B.H. & Selwood, T.S. (1986) Spon-taneous remission of solar keratoses: The case for conservative management. *Br. J. Dermatol.*, **115**, 649–655

Marks, R., Rennie, G. & Selwood, T.S. (1988) Malignant transformation of solar keratoses to squamous cell carcinoma. *Lancet*, **i**, 795–797

Marks, R., Foley, P.A., Jolley, D., Knight, K.R., Harrison, J. & Thompson, S.C. (1995) The effect of regular sunscreen use on vitamin D levels in an Australian population. Results of a randomized controlled trial. *Arch. Dermatol.*, **131**, 415–421

Marlenga, B. (1995) The health beliefs and skin cancer prevention practices of Wisconsin dairy farmers. *Oncol. Nurs. Forum*, **22**, 681–686

Marrot, L., Belaidi, J.-P., Meunier, J.-R., Perez, P. & Agapakis-Causse, C. (1999) The human melanocyte as a particular target for UVA radiation and an endpoint for photoprotection assessment. *Photochem. Photobiol.*, **69**, 686–693

Martin, R.H. (1995) Relationship between risk factors, knowledge and preventive behaviour relevant to skin cancer in general practice patients in South Australia. *Br. J. Gen. Pract.*, **45**, 365–367

Martin, S.C., Jacobsen, P.B., Lucas, D.J., Branch, K.A. & Ferron, J.M. (1999) Predicting children's sunscreen use: Application of the theories of reasoned action and planned behavior. *Prev. Med.*, **29**, 37–44

Martincigh, B.S., Allen, J.M. & Allen, S.K. (1997) Sunscreens: The molecules and their photochemistry. In: Gasparro, F.P., ed.,

Sunscreen Photobiology: Molecular, Cellular and Physiological Aspects, Berlin, Springer Verlag and Landes Biosciences, pp. 11–45

Masutani, C., Kusumoto, R., Yamada, A., Dohmae, N., Yokoi, M., Yuasa, M., Araki, M., Iwai, S., Takio, K. & Hanaoka, F. (1999) The XPV (*xeroderma pigmentosum* variant) gene encodes human DNA polymerase eta. *Nature*, **399**, 700–704

Mathers, C., Penm, R., Sanson-Fisher, R., Carter, R. & Campbell, E. (1998) *Health System Costs of Cancer in Australia 1993–94*, Canberra, Australian Institute of Health and Welfare

Matsuoka, L.Y., Ide, L., Wortsman, J., MacLaughlin, J.A. & Holick, M.F. (1987) Sunscreens suppress cutaneous vitamin D_3 synthesis. *J. Clin. Endocrinol. Metab.*, **64**, 1165–1168

Matsuoka, L.Y., Wortsman, J., Hanifan, N. & Holick, M.F. (1988) Chronic sunscreen use decreases circulating concentrations of 25-hydroxyvitamin D. A preliminary study. *Arch. Dermatol.*, **124**, 1802–1804

Matsuoka, L.Y., Wortsman, J. & Hollis, B.W. (1990) Use of topical sunscreen for the evaluation of regional synthesis of vitamin D. *J. Am. Acad. Dermatol.*, **22**, 772–775

Mawn, V.B. & Fleischer, A.B., Jr (1993) A survey of attitudes, beliefs, and behavior regarding tanning bed use, sunbathing, and sunscreen use. *J. Am. Acad. Dermatol.*, **29**, 959–962

McCarthy, E.M., Ethridge, K.P. & Wagner, R.F., Jr (1999) Beach holiday sunburn: The sunscreen paradox and gender differences. *Cutis*, **64**, 37–42

McGee, R. & Williams, S. (1992) Adolescence and sun protection. *N. Z. Med. J.*, **105**, 401–403

McGee, R., Williams, S., Cox, B., Elwood, M. & Bulliard, J.L. (1995) A community survey of sun exposure, sunburn and sun protection. *N. Z. Med. J.*, **108**, 508–510

McGee, R., Williams, S. & Glasgow, H. (1997) Sunburn and sun protection among young children. *J. Paediatr. Child Health*, **33**, 234–237

McGregor, J.M. & Young, A.R. (1996) Sunscreens, suntans, and skin cancer. *Br. Med. J.*, **312**, 1621–1622

McGregor, J.M., Crook, T., Fraser-Andrews, E.A., Rozycka, M., Crossland, S., Brooks, L. & Whittaker, S.J. (1999) Spectrum of p53 gene mutations suggests a possible role for ultraviolet radiation in the pathogenesis of advanced cutaneous lymphomas. *J. Invest. Dermatol.*, **112**, 317–321

McKinlay, A.F. & Diffey, B.L. (1987) A reference action spectrum for ultraviolet induced erythema in human skin. *CIE J.*, **6**, 17–22

McVean, M. & Liebler, D.C. (1997) Inhibition of UVB induced DNA photodamage in mouse epidermis by topically applied α-tocopherol. *Carcinogenesis*, **18**, 1617–1622

McVean, M. & Liebler, D.C. (1999) Prevention of DNA photodamage by vitamin E compounds and sunscreens: Roles of ultraviolet absorbance and cellular uptake. *Mol. Carcinog.*, **24**, 169–176

Melia, J. & Bulman, A. (1995) Sunburn and tanning in a British population. *J. Public Health Med.*, **17**, 223–229

Melville, S.K., Rosenthal, F.S., Luckmann, R. & Lew, R.A. (1991) Quantitative ultraviolet skin exposure in children during selected outdoor activities. *Photodermatol. Photoimmunol. Photomed.*, **8**, 99–104

Mera, S.L., Lovell, C.R., Jones, R.R. & Davies, J.D. (1987) Elastic fibres in normal and sun-damaged skin: An immunohistochemical study. *Br. J. Dermatol.*, **117**, 21–27

Mermelstein, R.J. & Riesenberg, L.A. (1992) Changing knowledge and attitudes about skin cancer risk factors in adolescents. *Health Psychol.*, **11**, 371–376

Michielutte, R., Dignan, M.B., Sharp, P.C., Boxley, J. & Wells, H.B. (1996) Skin cancer prevention and early detection practices in a sample of rural women. *Prev. Med.*, **25**, 673–683

Miller, R.W. & Rabkin, C.S. (1999) Merkel cell carcinoma and melanoma: Etiological similarities and differences [Published erratum appears in *Cancer Epidemiol. Biomarkers Prev.*, 1999, **8**, 485]. *Cancer Epidemiol. Biomarkers Prev.*, **8**, 153–158

Miller, A.G., Ashton, W.A., McHoskey, J.W. & Gimbel, J. (1990) What price attractiveness? Stereotype and risk factors in suntanning behaviour. *J. Appl. Soc. Psychol.*, **20**, 1272–1300

Miller, D.R., Geller, A.C., Wood, M.C., Lew, R.A. & Koh, H.K. (1999) The Falmouth Safe Skin Project: Evaluation of a community program to promote sun protection in youth. *Health Educ. Behav.*, **26**, 369–384

Milne, E., English, D.R., Corti, B., Cross, D., Borland, R., Gies, P., Costa, C. & Johnston, R. (1999a) Direct measurement of sun protection in primary schools. *Prev. Med.*, **29**, 45–52

Milne, E., English, D.R., Cross, D., Corti, B., Costa, C. & Johnston, R. (1999b) Evaluation of an intervention to reduce sun exposure in children: Design and baseline results. *Am. J. Epidemiol.*, **150**, 164–173

Ministry of Health and Welfare (1999) *The Comprehensive Licencing Standards of Cosmetics by Category*, Tokyo

Mitchell, D.L. (1988) The relative cytotoxicity of (6-4) photoproducts and cyclobutane dimers in mammalian cells. *Photochem. Photobiol.*, **48**, 51–57

Mitchell, D.L. & Nairn, R.S. (1989) The biology of the (6–4) photoproduct. *Photochem. Photobiol.*, **49**, 805–819

Mitchell, D.L., Jen, J. & Cleaver, J.E. (1991) Relative induction of cyclobutane dimers and cytosine photohydrates in DNA irradiated in vivo and in vitro with ultraviolet-C and ultraviolet-B light. *Photochem. Photobiol.*, **54**, 741–746

Mitchell, D.L., Jen, J. & Cleaver, J.E. (1992) Sequence specificity of cyclobutane pyrimidine dimers in DNA treated with solar (ultraviolet B) radiation. *Nucl. Acids Res.*, **20**, 225–229

Miyagi, T., Bhutto, A.M. & Nonaka, S. (1994) The effects of sunscreens on UVB erythema and Langerhans cell depression. *J. Dermatol.*, **21**, 645–651

Miyashita, T. & Reed, J.C. (1995) Tumor suppressor p53 is a direct transcriptional activator of the human *bax* gene. *Cell*, **80**, 293–299

Miyashita, T., Krajewski, S., Krajewska, M., Wang, H.G., Lin, H.K., Liebermann, D.A., Hoffman, B. & Reed, J.C. (1994) Tumor suppressor p53 is a regulator of *bcl-2* and *bax* gene expression *in vitro* and *in vivo*. *Oncogene*, **9**, 1799–1805

Moise, A.F., Gies, H.P. & Harrison, S.L. (1999a) Estimation of the annual solar UVR exposure dose of infants and small children in tropical Queensland, Australia. *Photochem. Photobiol.*, **69**, 457–463

Moise, A.F., Harrison, S.L. & Gies, H.P. (1999b) Solar ultraviolet radiation exposure of infants and small children. *Photodermatol. Photoimmunol. Photo-med.*, **15**, 109–114

Moise, A.F., Büttner, P.G. & Harrison, S.L. (1999c) Sun exposure at school. *Photochem. Photobiol.*, **70**, 269–274

van der Molen, R.G., Spies, F., van't Noordende, J.M., Boelsma, E., Mommaas, A.M. & Koerten, H.K. (1997) Tape stripping of human stratum corneum yields cell layers that originate from various depths because of furrows in the skin. *Arch. Dermatol. Res.*, **289**, 514–518

van der Molen, R.G., Driller, H., van't Noordende, J.M., Mommaas, A.M. & Koerten, H.K. (1999) Determination of the stability of titanium dioxide particles in a sunscreen after application on the skin. *J. Invest. Dermatol.*, **113**, 703

Mommaas, A.M., van Praag, M.C., Bouwes-Bavinck, J.N., Out-Luiting, C., Vermeer, B.J. & Claas, F.H. (1990) Analysis of the protective effect of topical sunscreens on the UVB-radiation-induced suppression of the mixed-lymphocyte reaction. *J. Invest. Dermatol.*, **95**, 313–316

Mondon, P. & Shahin, M.M. (1992) Protective effect of two sunscreens against lethal and genotoxic effects of UVB in V79 Chinese hamster cells and *Saccharomyces cerevisiae* strains XV185-14C and D5. *Mutat. Res.*, **279**, 121–128

Montagna, W., Kirchner, S. & Carlisle, K. (1989) Histology of sun-damaged human skin. *J. Am. Acad. Dermatol.*, **21**, 907–918

Moran, C.A., Mullick, F.G., Ishak, K.G., Johnson, F.B. & Hummer, W.B. (1991) Identification of titanium in human tissues: Probable role in pathologic processes. *Hum. Pathol.*, **22**, 450–454

Morison, W.L. (1984) The effect of a sunscreen containing *para*-aminobenzoic acid on the systemic immunologic alterations induced in mice by exposure to UVB radiation. *J. Invest. Dermatol.*, **83**, 405–408

Morison, W.L. & Kelley, S.P. (1985) Sunlight suppressing rejection of 280 to 320-nm UV-radiation induced skin tumors in mice. *J. Natl Cancer Inst.*, **74**, 525–527

Morison, W.L. & Stern, R.S. (1982) Polymorphous light eruption: A common reaction uncommonly recognized. *Acta Dermatol. Venereol.*, **62**, 237–240

Morison, W.L., Pike, R.A. & Kripke, M.L. (1985) Effect of sunlight and its component wavebands on contact hypersensitivity in mice and guinea pigs. *Photodermatology*, **2**, 195–204

Morlière, P., Moysan, A., Santus, R., Huppe, G., Maziere, J.C. & Dubertret, L. (1991) UVA-induced lipid peroxidation in cultured human fibroblasts. *Biochim. Biophys. Acta*, **1084**, 261–268

Motley, R.J. & Reynolds, A.J. (1989) Photocontact dermatitis due to isopropyl and butyl methoxy dibenzoylmethans (Eusolex 8020 and Parsol 1789). *Contact Derm.*, **21**, 109–110

Moyal, D. (1998) Immunosuppression induced by chronic ultraviolet irradiation in humans and its prevention by sunscreens. *Eur. J. Dermatol.*, **8**, 209–211

Moyal, D. & Binet, O. (1997) Polymorphic light eruption: Its reproduction and prevention by sunscreens. In: Lowe, N.J., Shaath, N.A. & Pathak, M.A., eds, *Sunscreens, Development, Evaluation, and Regulatory Aspects*, New York, Marcel Dekker, pp. 611–617

Moyal, D., Coubière, C., Le Corre, Y., de Lacharrière, O. & Hourseau, C. (1997) Immunosuppression induced by chronic solar-simulated irradiation in humans and its prevention by sunscreens. *Eur. J. Dermatol.*, **7**, 223–225

Murphy, E.G. (1997) Regulatory aspects of sunscreens in the United States. In: Lowe, N.J., Shaath, N.A., & Pathak, M.A., eds, *Sunscreens, Development, Evaluation, and Regulatory Aspects*, New York, Marcel Dekker Inc., pp. 201–213

Murphy, G.M., White, I.R. & Cronin, E. (1990) Immediate and delayed photocontact dermatitis from isopropyl dibenzoylmethane. *Contact Derm.*, **22**, 129–131

Nakagawa, Y., Wakuri, S., Sakamoto, K. & Tanaka, N. (1997) The photogenotoxicity of titanium dioxide particles. *Mutat. Res.*, **394**, 125–132

Nakazawa, H., English, D., Randell, P.L., Nakazawa, K., Martel, N., Armstrong, B.K. & Yamasaki, H. (1994) UV and skin cancer: Specific p53 gene mutation in normal skin as

a biologically relevant exposure measurement. *Proc. Natl Acad. Sci. USA*, **91**, 360–364

Nathan, D., Sakr, A., Lichtin, J.L. & Bronaugh, R.L. (1990) *In vitro* skin absorption and metabolism of benzoic acid, p-aminobenzoic acid, and benzocaine in the hairless guinea pig. *Pharm. Res.*, **7**, 1147–1151

Naylor, M.F., Boyd, A., Smith, D.W., Cameron, G.S., Hubbard, D. & Neldner, K.H. (1995) High sun protection factor sunscreens in the suppression of actinic neoplasia. *Arch. Dermatol.*, **131**, 170–175

Neale, R., Russell, A., Muller, H.K. & Green, A. (1997) Sun exposure, sunscreen and their effects on epidermal Langerhans cells. *Photochem. Photo-biol.*, **66**, 260–264

Nelson, D. & Gay, R.J. (1993) Effects of UV irradiation on a living skin equivalent. *Photochem. Photobiol.*, **57**, 830–837

Nelson, M.A., Einspahr, J.G., Alberts, D.S., Balfour, C.A., Wymer, J.A., Welch, K.L., Salasche, S.J., Bangert, J.L., Grogan, T.M. & Bozzo, P.O. (1994) Analysis of the *p53* gene in human precancerous actinic keratosis lesions and squamous cell cancers. *Cancer Lett.*, **85**, 23–29

Newman, W.G., Agro, A.D., Woodruff, S.I. & Mayer, J.A. (1996) A survey of recreational sun exposure of residents of San Diego, California. *Am. J. Prev. Med.*, **12**, 186–194

Nguyen, G.T., Topilow, A.A. & Frank, E. (1994) Protection from the sun: A survey of area beachgoers. *N. J. Med.*, **91**, 321–324

Nishigori, C., Yarosh, D.B., Ullrich, S.E., Vink, A.A., Bucana, C.D., Roza, L. & Kripke, M.L. (1996) Evidence that DNA damage triggers interleukin 10 cytokine production in UV-irradiated murine keratinocytes. *Proc. Natl Acad. Sci. USA*, **93**, 10354–10359

Nishioka, K., Murata, M. & Ishikawa, T. (1995) Contact allergy to neopentyl glycol diisooctanoate. *Contact Derm.*, **33**, 208–209

Noonan, F.P. & De Fabo, E.C. (1992) Immunosuppression by ultraviolet B radiation: Initiation by urocanic acid. *Immunol. Today*, **13**, 250–254

Noonan, F.P., De Fabo, E.C. & Kripke, M.L. (1981) Suppression of contact hypersensitivity by ultraviolet radiation and its relationship to UV-induced suppression of tumor immunity. *Photochem. Photobiol.*, **34**, 683–689

Novick, M. (1997) To burn or not to burn: Use of computer-enhanced stimuli to encourage application of sunscreens. *Cutis*, **60**, 105–108

Odio, M.R., Azri-Meehan, S., Robison, S.H. & Kraus, A.L. (1994) Evaluation of subchronic (13 week), reproductive, and *in vitro* genetic toxicity potential of 2-ethylhexyl-2-cyano-3,3-diphenyl acrylate (octocrylene). *Fundam. Appl. Toxicol.*, **22**, 355–368

Office of National Statistics (1998) *Travel Trends: A Report on the 1997 International Passenger Survey*, London, HMSO

Okamoto, H., Mizuno, K., Itoh, T., Tanaka, K. & Horio, T. (1999) Evaluation of apoptotic cells induced by ultraviolet light B radiation in epidermal sheets stained by the TUNEL technique. *J. Invest. Dermatol.*, **113**, 802–807

Okereke, C.S., Kadry, A.M., Abdel-Rahman, M.S., Davis, R.A. & Friedman, M.A. (1993) Metabolism of benzophenone-3 in rats. *Drug Metab. Disposition*, **21**, 788–791

Okereke, C.S., Abdel-Rhaman, M.S. & Friedman, M.A. (1994) Disposition of benzophenone-3 after dermal administration in male rats. *Toxicol. Lett.*, **73**, 113–122

Okereke, C.S., Barat, S.A. & Abdel-Rahman, M.S. (1995) Safety evaluation of benzophenone-3 after dermal administration in rats. *Toxicol. Lett.*, **80**, 61–67

Olson, R.L., Gaylor, J. & Everett, M.A. (1973) Skin color, melanin, and erythema. *Arch. Dermatol.*, **108**, 541–544

O'Riordan, D.L., Stanton, W.R., Eyeson-Annan, M., Gies, P. & Roy, C. (2000) Correlations between reported and measured ultraviolet radiation exposure of mothers and young children. *Photochem. Photobiol.*, **71**, 60–64

Oro, A.E., Higgins, K.M., Hu, Z., Bonifas, J.M., Epstein, E.H., Jr & Scott, M.P. (1997) Basal cell carcinomas in mice overexpressing *sonic hedgehog*. *Science*, **276**, 817–821

Osgood, P.J., Moss S.H. & Davies, D.J.G. (1982) The sensitization effect of near-ultraviolet radiation killing of mammalian cells by the sunscreen agent para-aminobenzoic acid. *J. Invest. Dermatol.*, **79**, 354–357

Osterlind, A., Tucker, M.A., Stone, B.J. & Jensen, O.M.. (1988) The Danish case–control study of cutaneous malignant melanoma. II. Importance of UV-light exposure. *Int. J. Cancer*, **42**, 319–324

Ouhtit, A., Ueda, M., Nakazawa, H., Ichihashi, M., Dumaz, N., Sarasin, A. & Yamasaki, H. (1997) Quantitative detection of ultraviolet-specific p53 mutations in normal skin from Japanese patients. *Cancer Epidemiol. Biomarkers Prev.*, **6**, 433–438

Ouhtit, A., Nakazawa, H., Armstrong, B.K., Kricker, A., Tan, E., Yamasaki, H. & English, D.R. (1998) UV-radiation-specific p53 mutation frequency in normal skin as a predictor of risk of basal cell carcinoma. *J. Natl Cancer Inst.*, **90**, 523–531

Padua, R.A., Barrass, N.C. & Currie, G.A. (1985) Activation of N-*ras* in a human melanoma cell line. *Mol. Cell Biol.*, **5**, 582–585

Parisi, A.V., Meldrum, L.R., Wong, J.C.F., Aitken, J. & Fleming, R.A. (2000) Effect of childhood and adolescent ultraviolet exposures on cumulative exposure in South East Queensland schools. *Photodermatol. Photoimmunol. Photomed.*, **16**, 19–24

Parkin, D.M., Pisani, P. & Ferlay, J. (1999) Estimates of the worldwide incidence of 25 major cancers in 1990. *Int. J. Cancer*, **80**, 827–841

Parrott, R., Duggan, A., Cremo, J., Eckles, A., Jones, K. & Steiner, C. (1999) Communicating about youth's sun exposure risk to soccer coaches and parents: A pilot study in Georgia. *Health Educ. Behav.*, **26**, 385–395

Parry, E.J., Bilsland, D. & Morley, W.N. (1995) Photocontact allergy to 4-tert-butyl-4'-methoxy-dibenzoylmethane (Parsol 1789). *Contact Derm.*, **32**, 251–252

Peak, M.J., Peak, J.G. & Carnes, B.A. (1987) Induction of direct and indirect single-strand breaks in human cell DNA by far- and near-ultraviolet radiations: Action spectrum and mechanisms. *Photochem. Photobiol.*, **45**, 381–387

Pearse, A.D. & Edwards, C. (1993) Human stratum corneum as a substrate for *in vitro* sunscreen testing. *Int. J. Cosmet. Sci.*, **15**, 234–244

Pearse, A.D., Gaskell, S.A. & Marks, R. (1987) Epidermal changes in human skin following irradiation with either UVB or UVA. *J. Invest. Dermatol.*, **88**, 83–87

Petit-Frère, C., Clingen, P.H., Grewe, M., Krutmann, J., Roza, L., Arlett, C.F. & Green, M.H.L. (1998) Induction of interleukin-6 production by ultraviolet radiation in normal human epidermal keratinocytes and in a human keratinocyte cell line is mediated by DNA damage. *J. Invest. Dermatol.*, **111**, 354–359

Pflaum, M., Boiteux, S. & Epe, B. (1994) Visible light generates oxidative DNA base modifications in high excess of strand breaks in mammalian cells. *Carcinogenesis*, **15**, 297–300

Piepkorn, M.W., Barnhill, R.L., Cannon-Albright, L.A., Elder, D.E., Goldgar, D.E., Lewis, C.M., Maize, J.C., Meyer, L.J., Rabkin, M.S., Sagebiel, R.W., Skolnick, M.H. & Zone, J.J. (1994) A multiobserver, population-based analysis of histologic dysplasia in melanocytic nevi. *J. Am. Acad. Dermatol.*, **30**, 707–714

Pincus, M.W., Rollings, P.K., Craft, A.B. & Green, A. (1991) Sunscreen use on Queensland beaches. *Australas. J. Dermatol.*, **32**, 21–25

Pogoda, J.M. & Preston-Martin, S. (1996) Solar radiation, lip protection, and lip cancer risk in Los Angeles County women (California, United States). *Cancer Causes Control*, **7**, 458–463

Pollock, P.M., Yu, F., Qiu, L., Parsons, P.G. & Hayward, N.K. (1995) Evidence for UV induction of *CDKN2* mutations in melanoma cell lines. *Oncogene*, **11**, 663–668

Pollock, P.M., Pearson, J.V. & Hayward, N.K. (1996) Compilation of somatic mutations of the *CDKN2* gene in human cancers: Non-random distribution of base substitutions. *Genes Chromosomes Cancer*, **15**, 77–88

Pontén, F., Berne, B., Ren, Z.P., Mister, M. & Pontén, J. (1995) Ultraviolet light induces expression of p53 and p21 in human skin: Effect of sunscreen and constitutive p21 expression in skin appendages. *J. Invest. Dermatol.*, **105**, 402–406

Pope, D.J., Sorahan, T., Marsden, J.R., Ball, P.M., Grimley, R.P. & Peck, I.M. (1992) Benign pigmented nevi in children. *Arch. Dermatol.*, **128**, 1201–1206

Potard, G., Laugel, C., Baillet, A., Schaefer, H. & Marty, J.P. (1999) Quantitative HPLC analysis of sunscreens and caffeine during in vitro percutaneous penetration studies. *Int. J. Pharmacol.*, **189**, 249–260

van Praag, M.C.G., Out-Luyting, C., Claas, F.H.J., Vermeer, B.-J. & Mommaas, A.M. (1991) Effect of topical sunscreens on the UV-radiation-induced suppression of the alloactivating capacity in human skin in vivo. *J. Invest. Dermatol.*, **97**, 629–633

van Praag, M.C.G., Roza, L., Boom, B.W., Out-Luijting, C., Bergen Henegouwen, J.B.A., Vermeer, B.J. & Mommaas, A.M. (1993) Determination of the photoprotective efficacy of a topical sunscreen against UVB-induced DNA damage in human epidermis. *J. Photochem. Photobiol. B*, **19**, 129–134

Pratt, K. & Borland, R. (1994) Predictors of sun protection among adolescents at the beach. *Aust. Psychol.*, **29**, 135–139

Pruim, B., Wright, L. & Green, A. (1999) Do people who apply sunscreens, re-apply them? *Australas. J. Dermatol.*, **40**, 79–82

Punnonen, K., Puntala, A. & Ahotupa, M. (1991) Effects of ultraviolet A and B irradiation on lipid peroxidation and activity of the antioxidant enzymes in keratinocytes in culture. *Photodermatol. Photoimmunol. Photomed.*, **8**, 3–6

Putnam, G.L. & Yanagisako, K.L. (1982) Skin cancer comic book: Evaluation of a public educational vehicle. *Cancer Detect. Prev.*, **5**, 349–356

Quinn, A.G., Diffey, B.L., Craig, P.S. & Farr, P.M. (1994) Definition of the minimal erythema dose used for diagnostic phototesting. *Br. J. Dermatol.*, **131**, 56–56

Raabe, O.G., Book, S.A. & Parks, N.J. (1980) Bone cancer from radium: Canine dose response explains data from mice and humans. *Science*, **208**, 61–64

Rademaker, M., Wyllie, K., Collins, M. & Wetton, N. (1996) Primary school children's perceptions of the effects of sun on skin. *Australas. J. Dermatol.*, **37**, 30–36

Reding, D.J., Fischer, V., Gunderson, P. & Lappe, K. (1995) Skin cancer prevention: A peer education model. *Wisconsin Med. J.*, **94**, 77–81

Reed, J.C. (1994) Bcl-2 and the regulation of programmed cell death. *J. Cell Biol.*, **124**, 1–6

Reeve, V.E. (1997) The relationship between sunscreen protection from erythema, photoimmunosuppression and photocarcinogenesis in the hairless mouse. In: Gasparro, F.P., ed., *Sunscreen Photobiology: Molecular, Cellular and Physiological Aspects*, Berlin, Springer-Verlag/Landes Bioscience, pp. 157–176

Reeve, V.E., Greenoak, G.E., Gallagher, C.H., Canfield, P.J. & Wilkinson, F.J. (1985) Effect of immunosuppressive agents and sunscreens on UV carcinogenesis in the hairless mouse. *Aust. J. Exp. Biol. Med. Sci.*, **63**, 655–665

Reeve, V.E., Bosnic, M. & Boehm-Wilcox, C. (1990) Effect of ultraviolet (UV) radiation and UVB-absorbing sunscreen ingredients on 7,12-dimethylbenz(a)anthracene-initiated skin tumorigenesis in hairless mice. *Photodermatol. Photoimmunol. Photomed.*, **7**, 222–227

Reeve, V.E., Bosnic, M., Boehm-Wilcox, C. & Ley, R.D. (1991) Differential protection by two sunscreens from UV radiation-induced immunosuppression. *J. Invest. Dermatol.*, **97**, 624–628

Reeve, V.E., Boehm-Wilcox, C., Bosnic, M. & Reilly, W.G. (1994) Differential photoimmuno-protection by sunscreen ingredients is unrelated to epidermal *cis* urocanic acid formation in hairless mice. *J. Invest. Dermatol.*, **103**, 801–806

Ren, Z.P., Hedrum, A., Pontén, F., Nister, M., Ahmadian, A., Lundeberg, J., Uhlen, M. & Pontén, J. (1996) Human epidermal cancer and accompanying precursors have identical *p53* mutations different from *p53* mutations in adjacent areas of clonally expanded non-neoplastic keratinocytes. *Oncogene*, **12**, 765–773

Reynolds, K.D., Blaum, J.M., Jester, P.M., Weiss, H., Soong, S. & Diclemente, R.J. (1996) Predictors of sun exposure in adolescents in a southeastern US population. *J. Adolescent Health*, **19**, 409–415

Rhodes, L.E. & Diffey, B.L. (1996) Quantitative assessment of sunscreen application technique by *in vivo* fluorescence spectroscopy. *J. Soc. Cosmet. Chem.*, **47**, 109–115

Ricci, C., Vaccari, S., Cavalli, M. & Vincenzi, C. (1997) Contact sensitization to sunscreens. *Am. J. Contact Derm.*, **8**, 165–166

Rivers, J.K. & Gallagher, R.P. (1995) Public education projects in skin cancer. Experience of the Canadian Dermatology Association. *Cancer*, **75** (Suppl.), 661–666

Roberts, L.K. & Beasley, D.G. (1995) Commercial sunscreen lotions prevent ultraviolet-radiation-induced immune suppression of contact hypersensitivity. *J. Invest. Dermatol.*, **105**, 339–344

Roberts, L.K. & Beasley, D.G. (1997a) Sunscreen lotions prevent ultraviolet radiation-induced suppression of antitumor immune responses. *Int. J. Cancer*, **71**, 94–102

Roberts, L.K. & Beasley, D.G. (1997b) Sunscreens prevent local and systemic immunosuppression of contact hypersensitivity in mice exposed to solar-simulated ultraviolet radiation. *J. Photochem. Photobiol. B*, **39**, 121–129

Roberts, L.K., Beasley, D.G., Learn, D.B., Giddens, L.D., Beard, J. & Stanfield, J.W. (1996) Ultraviolet spectral energy differences affect the ability of sunscreen lotions to prevent ultraviolet-radiation-induced immunosuppression. *Photochem. Photobiol.*, **63**, 874–884

Robinson, J.K. (1987) Risk of developing another basal cell carcinoma. A 5-year prospective study. *Cancer*, **60**, 118–120

Robinson, J.K. (1992) Compensation strategies in sun protection behaviors by a population with nonmelanoma skin cancer. *Prev. Med.*, **21**, 754–765

Robinson, J.K. & Rademaker, A.W. (1992) Relative importance of prior basal cell carcinomas, continuing sun exposure, and circulating T lymphocytes on the development of basal cell carcinoma. *J. Invest. Dermatol.*, **99**, 227–231

Robinson, J.K. & Rademaker, A.W. (1995) Skin cancer risk and sun protection learning by helpers of patients with nonmelanoma skin cancer. *Prev. Med.*, **24**, 333–341

Robinson, J.K. & Rademaker, A.W. (1998) Sun protection by families at the beach. *Arch. Pediatr. Adolescent Med.*, **152**, 466–470

Robinson, J.K., Rigel, D.S. & Amonette, R.A. (1997a) Trends in sun exposure knowledge, attitudes and behaviors: 1986 to 1996. *J. Am. Acad. Dermatol.*, **37**, 179–186

Robinson, J.K., Rademaker, A.W., Sylvester, J.A. & Cook, B. (1997b) Summer sun exposure: Knowledge, attitudes, and behaviors of Midwest adolescents. *Prev. Med.*, **26**, 364–372

Robinson, W.A., Lemon, M., Elefanty, A., Harrison-Smith, M., Markham, N. & Norris, D. (1998a) Human acquired naevi are clonal. *Melanoma Res.*, **8**, 499–503

Robinson, J.K., Amonette, R., Wyatt, S.W., Bewerse, B.A., Bergfeld, W.F. & Farris, P.K. (1998b) In: *Sun Safety: Protecting Our Future*, Atlanta, Georgia, Centers for Disease Control and Prevention

Robison, S.H., Odio, M.R., Thompson, E.D., Aardema, M.J. & Kraus, A.L. (1994) Assessment of the *in vivo* genotoxicity of 2-hydoxy-4-methoxybenzophenone. *Environ. Mol. Mutag.*, **23**, 312–317

Robson, J. & Diffey, B.L. (1990) Textiles and sun protection. *Photodermatol. Photoimmunol. Photomed.*, **7**, 32–34

Rodenas, J.M., Delgado-Rodriguez, M., Herranz, M., Tercedor, J. & Serrano, S. (1996) Sun exposure, pigmentary traits, and risk of cutaneous malignant melanoma: A case–control study in a Mediterranean population. *Cancer Causes Control*, **7**, 275–283

Rodriguez, G., Ortiz, R. & Suarez, R. (1993) Patterns in sun exposure and sunscreen use among Puertorican adolescents. *Bol. Assoc. Med. P. R.*, **85**, 21–23

Roffo, A.H. (1934) [Cancer and sun. Carcinomas and sarcomas induced by the action of the sun *in toto*.] *Bull. Assoc. Fr. Étude Cancer*, **23**, 590–616 (in French)

Romero-Graillet, C., Aberdam, E., Clement, M., Ortonne, J.P. & Ballotti, R. (1997) Nitric oxide produced by ultraviolet-irradiated keratinocytes stimulates melanogenesis. *J. Clin. Invest.*, **99**, 635–642

Rooney, J.F., Bryson, Y., Mannix, M.L., Dillon, M., Wohlenberg, C.R., Banks, S., Wallington, C.J., Notkins, A.L. & Straus, S.E. (1991) Prevention of ultraviolet-light-induced herpes labialis by sunscreen. *Lancet*, **338**, 1419–1422

Ros, A.M. & Wennersten, G. (1986) Current aspects of polymorphous light eruptions in Sweden. *Photodermatology*, **3**, 298–302

Rosenman, K.D., Gardiner, J., Swanson, G.M., Mullan, P. & Zhu, Z. (1995) Use of skin-cancer prevention strategies among farmers and their spouses. *Am. J. Prev. Med.*, **11**, 342–347

Rosenstein, B.S., Phelps, R.G., Weinstock, M.A., Bernstein, J.L., Gordon, M.L., Rudikoff, D., Kantor, I., Shelton, R. & Lebwohl, M.G. (1999) *p53* mutations in basal cell carcinomas arising in routine users of sunscreens. *Photochem. Photobiol.*, **70**, 798–806

Rosenthal, F.S., Lew, R.A., Rouleau, L.J. & Thomson, M. (1990) Ultraviolet exposure to children from sunlight: A study using personal dosimetry. *Photodermatol. Photoimmunol. Photomed.*, **7**, 77–81

Rosenthal, F.S., West, S.K., Munoz, B., Emmett, E.A., Strickland, P.T. & Taylor, H.R. (1991) Ocular and facial skin exposure to ultraviolet radiation in sunlight: A personal exposure model with application to a worker population. *Health Phys.*, **61**, 77–86

Ross, S.A. & Sanchez, J.L. (1990) Recreational sun exposure in Puerto Rico: Trends and cancer risk awareness. *J. Am. Acad. Dermatol.*, **23**, 1090–1092

Rossi, J.S., Blais, L.M. & Weinstock, M.A. (1994) The Rhode Island Sun Smart Project: Skin cancer prevention reaches the beaches. *Am. J. Public Health*, **84**, 672–674

Roy, C., Gies, H.P. & Toomey, S. (1996) Monitoring UV-B at the Earth's surface. *Cancer Forum*, **20**, 173–179

Sage, E. (1993) Distribution and repair of photolesions in DNA: Genetic consequences and the role of sequence context. *Photochem. Photobiol.*, **57**, 163–174

Sage, E., Lamolet, B., Brulay, E., Moustacchi, E., Châteauneuf, A. & Drobetsky, E.A. (1996) Mutagenic specificity of solar UV light in nucleotide excision repair-deficient rodent cells. *Proc. Natl Acad. Sci. USA*, **93**, 176–180

Sagebiel, R.W. (1993) Melanocytic nevi in histologic association with primary cutaneous melanoma of superficial spreading and nodular types: Effect of tumor thickness. *J. Invest. Dermatol.*, **100**, 322S–325S

Sakane, T., Steinberg, A.D. & Green, I. (1978) Failure of autologous mixed lymphocyte reactions between T and non-T cells in patients with systemic lupus erythematosus. *Proc. Natl Acad. Sci. USA*, **75**, 3464–3468

Sambuco, C.P., Forbes, P.D., Davies, R.E. & Urbach, F. (1984) An animal model to determine sunscreen protectiveness against both vascular injury and epidermal cell damage. *J. Am. Acad. Dermatol.*, **10**, 737–743

Sambuco, C.P., Davies, R.E., Forbes, P.D. & Hoberman, A.M. (1991) Photocarcinogenesis and consumer product testing: Technical aspects. *Toxicol. Meth.*, **1**, 75–83

Sauermann, G., Mann, T. & Wochnowski, M. (1997) UV protection by sunscreens. In: Altmeyer, P., Hoffmann, K. & Stücker, M., eds, *Skin Cancer and UV Radiation*, Berlin, Springer-Verlag, pp. 296–313

Sayre, R.M. & Dowdy, J.C. (1999) Photostability testing of avobenzone. *Cosmet. Toiletries*, **114**, 85–91

Sayre, R.M., Agin, P.P., LeVee, G. & Marlowe, E. (1979) A comparison of *in vivo* and *in vitro* testing of sunscreening formulas. *Photochem. Photobiol.*, **29**, 559–566

Sayre, R.M., Agin, P.P., Desrochers, D.L. & Marlowe, E. (1980) Sunscreen testing methods: *In vitro* predictions of effectiveness. *J. Soc. Cosmet. Chem.*, **31**, 133–143

Schaefer, H. & Redelmeier, T.E. (1996) *Skin Barrier: Principles of Percutaneous Absorption*, Karger, Basel, p. 133

Schaefer, H., Moyal, D. & Fourtanier, A. (2000) State of the art sunscreens for prevention of photodermatoses. *J. Dermatol. Sci.*, **23** (Suppl. 1), S62–S74

Schallreuter, K.U., Wood, J.M., Farwell, D.W., Moore, J. & Edwards, H.G. (1996) Oxybenzone oxidation following solar irradiation of skin: Photoprotection versus antioxidant inactivation. *J. Invest. Dermatol.*, **106**, 583–586

Scharffetter, K., Wlaschek, M., Hogg, A., Bolsen, K., Schothorst, A., Goerz, G., Krieg, T. & Plewig, G. (1991) UVA radiation induces collagenase in human dermal fibroblasts in vitro and in vivo. *Arch. Dermatol. Res.*, **283**, 506–511

Schauder, S. & Ippen, H. (1986) Photoallergic and allergic contact dermatitis from dibenzoyl-methanes. *Photodermatology*, **3**, 140–147

Schauder, S. & Ippen, H. (1997) Contact and photocontact sensitivity to sunscreens. Review of a 15-year experience and of the literature. *Contact Derm.*, **37**, 221–232

von Schirnding, Y., Strauss, N., Mathee, A., Robertson, P. & Blignaut, R. (1991/92) Sunscreen use and environmental awareness among beachgoers in Cape Town, South Africa. *Public Health Rev.*, **19**, 209–217

Schothorst, A.A., Slaper, H., Schouten, R. & Suurmond, D. (1985) UVB doses in maintenance psoriasis phototherapy versus solar UVB exposure. *Photodermatology*, **2**, 213–220

Schulze, R. (1956a) [Some tests and remarks regarding the problem of sunscreens that are found on the market.] *Parfum. Kosmet.*, **37**, 310–316 (in German)

Schulze, R. (1956b) [Some tests and remarks regarding the problem of sunscreens that are found on the market.] *Parfum. Kosmet.*, **37**, 365–372 (in German)

Sclafani, A., Palmisano, L. & Davi, E. (1990) Photocatalytic degradation of phenol by TiO_2 aqueous dispersions: Rutile and anatase activity. *New J. Chem.*, **14**, 265–268

Segan, C.J., Borland, R. & Hill, D.J. (1999) Development and evaluation of a brochure on sun protection and sun exposure for tourists. *Health Educ. J.*, **58**, 177–191

Seité, S., Moyal, D., Verdier, M.-P., Hourseau, C. & Fourtanier, A. (2000a) Accumulated p53 protein and UVA protection levels of sunscreens. *Photodermatol. Photoimmunol. Photomed.*, **16**, 3–9

Séite, S., Colige, A., Piquemal-Vivenot, P., Montastier, C., Fourtanier, A., Lapière, C. & Nusgens, B. (2000b) A full-UV spectrum absorbing daily use cream protects human skin against biological changes occurring in photoaging. *Photodermatol. Photoimmunol. Photomed.* (in press)

Sellers, R.L. & Carpenter, F.G. (1992) An instrument for in-vitro determinations of SPF. *Cosmet. Toiletries*, **107**, 119–123

Serre, I., Cano, J.P., Picot, M.C., Meynadier, J. & Meunier, L. (1997) Immunosuppression induced by acute solar-simulated ultraviolet exposure in humans: Prevention by a sunscreen with a sun protection factor of 15 and high UVA protection. *J. Am. Acad. Dermatol.*, **37**, 187–194

Setlow, R.B. & Carrier, W.L. (1966) Pyrimidine dimers in ultraviolet-irradiated DNA's. *J. Mol. Biol.*, **17**, 237–254

Setlow, R.B., Grist, E., Thompson, K. & Woodhead, A.D. (1993) Wavelengths effective in induction of malignant melanoma. *Proc. Natl Acad. Sci. USA*, **90**, 6666–6670

Seukeran, D.C., Newstead, C.G. & Cunliffe, W.J. (1998) The compliance of renal transplant recipients with advice about sun protection measures. *Br. J. Dermatol.*, **138**, 301–303

Shaath, N.A. (1997a) Evolution of modern sunscreen chemicals. In: Lowe, N.J., Shaath, N.A. & Pathak, M.A., eds, *Sunscreens, Development, Evaluation, and Regulatory Aspects*, 2nd Ed. (Cosmetic Science and Technology Series, Vol. 15), New York, Marcel Dekker, pp. 3–33

Shaath, N.A. (1997b) The chemistry of sunscreens. In: Lowe, N.J., Shaath, N.A. & Pathak, M.A., eds, *Sunscreens, Development, Evaluation, and Regulatory Aspects,* New York, Marcel Dekker, pp. 263–283

Shaath, N.A. (1997c) Quality control of sunscreens. In: Lowe, N.J., Shaath, N.A. & Pathak, M.A., eds, *Sunscreens, Development, Evaluation, and Regulatory Aspects,* New York, Marcel Dekker, pp. 657–675

Shaath, N.A., Griffin, P.M. & Andemicael, G.I. (1997a) Modern analytical techniques in the sunscreen industry. In: Lowe, N.J., Shaath, N.A. & Pathak, M.A., eds, *Sunscreens, Development, Evaluation, and Regulatory Aspects,* New York, Marcel Dekker, pp. 677–707

Shaath, N.A., Griffin, P.M., Andemicael, G.I. & Paloympis, L.E. (1997b) Interpretation and evaluation: Spectroscopic data from sunscreens. In: Lowe, N.J., Shaath, N.A. & Pathak, M.A., eds, *Sunscreens, Development, Evaluation, and Regulatory Aspects,* New York, Marcel Dekker, pp. 709–761

Shih, M.K. & Hu, M.L. (1996) UVA-potentiated damage to calf thymus DNA by Fenton reaction system and protection by para-aminobenzoic acid. *Photochem. Photobiol.*, **63**, 286–291

Silva, R., Almeida, L.M.S. & Brandão, F.M. (1995) Photoallergy to oxybenzone in cosmetic creams. *Contact Derm.*, **32**, 176

Silvestre, J.F., Rodríguez-Serna, M., Miquel, J.F., Gauchía, R. & Aliaga, A. (1996) Allergic contact dermatitis from Euxyl K 400 in a sunscreen cream. *Contact Derm.*, **35**, 315

Skender-Kalnenas, T.M., English D.R. & Heenan P.J. (1995) Benign melanocytic lesions: Risk markers or precursors of cutaneous melanoma? *J. Am. Acad. Dermatol.*, **33**, 1000–1007

Skov, L., Hansen, H., Allen, M., Villadsen, L., Norval, M., Barker, J.N., Simon, J. & Baadsgaard, O. (1998) Contrasting effects of ultraviolet A1 and ultraviolet B exposure on the induction of tumour necrosis factor-a in human skin. *Br. J. Dermatol.*, **138**, 216–220

Slaper, H. (1987) *Skin Cancer and UV Exposure: Investigations on the Estimation of Risks*, PhD Thesis, University of Utrecht

Snyder, D.S. & May, M. (1975) Ability of PABA to protect mammalian skin from ultraviolet light-induced skin tumors and actinic damage. *J. Invest. Dermatol.*, **65**, 543–546

Sollitto, R.B., Kraemer, K.H. & DiGiovanna, J.J. (1997) Normal vitamin D levels can be maintained despite rigorous photoprotection: Six years' experience with xeroderma pigmentosum. *J. Am. Acad. Dermatol.*, **37**, 942–947

Soriani, M., Hejmadi, V. & Tyrrell, R.M. (2000) Modulation of c-jun and c-fos transcription by UVB and UVA radiations in human dermal fibroblasts and epidermoid KB cells. *Photochem. Photobiol.*, **71**, 551–558

Stamper, B. (1990) *Lyotropic Liquid Crystals as Model Vehicles for Chemical Sunscreens*, PhD Thesis, Sunderland Polytechnic

Staples, M., Marks, R. & Giles, G. (1998) Trends in the incidence of non-melanocytic skin cancer (NMSC) treated in Australia 1985–1995: Are primary prevention programs starting to have an effect? *Int. J. Cancer*, **78**, 144–148

Stenberg, C. & Larkö, O. (1985) Sunscreen application and its importance for the sun protection factor. *Arch. Dermatol.*, **121**, 1400–1402

Stender, I.M., Lock-Andersen, J. & Wulf, H.C. (1996a) Sun exposure and sunscreen use among sunbathers in Denmark. *Acta Derm. Venereol. (Stockh.)*, **76**, 31–33

Stender, I.M., Lock-Andersen, J. & Wulf, H.C. (1996b) Sun-protection behaviour and self-assessed burning tendency among sunbathers. *Photodermatol. Photoimmunol. Photomed.*, **12**, 162–165

Stevenson, C. & Davies, R.J.H. (1999) Photosensitization of guanine-specific DNA damage by 2-phenylbenzimidazole and the sunscreen agent 2-phenyl-benzimididazole-5-sulfonic acid. *Chem. Res. Toxicol.*, **12**, 38–45

Stitt, W.Z.D., Scott, G.A., Martin, R.E. & Gaspari, A.A. (1996) Multiple chemical sensitivities, including iatrogenic allergic contact dermatitis, in a patient with chronic actinic dermatitis: Implications for management. *Am. J. Contact Derm.*, **7**, 166–170

Stockdale, M. (1987) A novel assessment of sunscreen product efficacy against UVA. *Int. J. Cosmet. Sci.*, **9**, 85–98

Stokes, R.P. & Diffey, B.L. (1997a) In vitro assay of high SPF sunscreens. *J. Soc. Cosmet. Chem.*, **48**, 289–296

Stokes, R.P & Diffey, B.L. (1997b) How well are sunscreen users protected? *Photodermatol. Photoimmunol. Photomed.*, **13**, 186–188

Stokes, R.P. & Diffey, B.L. (1999a) Water resistance of sunscreen and day-care products. *Br. J. Dermatol.*, **140**, 259–263

Stokes, R.P. & Diffey, B.L. (1999b) *In vitro* assessment of sunscreen photostability: The effect of radiation source, sunscreen application thickness and substrate. *Int. J. Cosmet. Sci.*, **21**, 341–351

Stokes, R.P. & Diffey, B.L. (2000) A novel *ex vivo* technique to assess the sand/rub resistance of sunscreen products. *Int. J. Cosmet. Sci.* (in press)

Stokes, R.P., Diffey, B.L., Dawson, L.C. & Barton S.P. (1998) A novel *in vitro* technique for measuring the water resistance of sunscreens. *Int. J. Cosmet. Sci.*, **20**, 235–240

Strickland, P.T. (1984) Photocarcino-genesis and influence of UV radiation on autoimmune disease in NZB/N mice. *J. Natl Cancer Inst.*, **73**, 537–541

Stroeva, O.G. & Popov, V.B. (1998) Effect of para-aminobenzoic acid on the development of rat embryos when applied to pregnant females. *Ontogenez*, **29**, 444–449

Studzinski, G.P. & Moore, D.C. (1995) Sunlight—Can it prevent as well as cause cancer? *Cancer Res.*, **55**, 4014–4022

Suarez-Varela, M.M., Gonzalez, A.L. & Caraco, E.F. (1996) Non-melanoma skin cancer: A case–control study on risk factors and protective measures. *J. Environ. Pathol. Toxicol. Oncol.*, **15**, 255–261

Sun, J.S., Shieh, K.M., Chiang, H.C., Sheu, S.Y., Hang, Y.S., Lu, F.J. & Tsuang, Y.H. (1999) Scavenging effect of benzophenones on the oxidative stress of skeletal muscle cells. *Free Radicals Biol. Med.*, **26**, 1100–1107

Sutherland, J.C & Griffin, K.P. (1984) *p*-Aminobenzoic acid can sensitise the formation of pyrimidine dimers in DNA: Direct chemical evidence. *Photochem. Photobiol.*, **40**, 391–394

Suzuki, M. (1987) Protective effect of fine-particle titanium dioxide on UVB-induced DNA damage in hairless mouse skin. *Photodermatology*, **4**, 209–211

Szczurko, C., Dompmartin, A., Michel, M., Moreau, A. & Leroy, D. (1994) Photocontact allergy to oxybenzone: Ten years of experience. *Photodermatol. Photoimmunol. Photomed.*, **10**, 144–147

Tan, M.H., Commens, C.A., Burnett, L. & Snitch, P.J. (1996) A pilot study on the percutaneous absorption of microfine titanium dioxide from sunscreens. *Australas. J. Dermatol.*, **37**, 185–187

Taylor, C.R. & Sober, A.J. (1996) Sun exposure and skin disease. *Annu. Rev. Med.*, **47**, 181–191

Tchou, J., Kasai, H., Shibutani, S., Chung, M.-H., Laval, J., Grollman, A.P. & Nishimura, S. (1991) 8-Oxoguanine (8-hydroxyguanine) DNA glycosylase and its substrate specificity. *Proc. Natl Acad. Sci. USA*, **88**, 4690–4694

Thompson, S.C., Jolley, D. & Marks, R. (1993) Reduction of solar keratoses by regular sunscreen use. *New Engl. J. Med.*, **329**, 1147–1151

Thune, P. (1984) Contact and photocontact allergy to sunscreens. *Photodermatology*, **1**, 5–9

Tornaletti, S. & Pfeifer, G.P. (1994) Slow repair of pyrimidine dimers at *p53* mutation hotspots in skin cancer. *Science*, **263**, 1436–1438

Torres, V. & Correia, T. (1991) Contact and photocontact allergy to oxybenzone and mexenone. *Contact Derm.*, **25**, 126–127

Treffel, P. & Gabard, B. (1996) Skin penetration and sun protection factor of ultra-violet filters from two vehicles. *Pharm. Res.*, **13**, 770–774

Treffel, P., Makki, S., Faivre, B., Humbert, P., Blanc, D. & Agache, P. (1991) Citropten and bergapten suction blister fluid concentrations after solar product application in man. *Skin Pharmacol.*, **4**, 100–108

Trevisi, P., Vincenzi, C., Chieregato, C., Guerra, L. & Tosti, A. (1994) Sunscreen sensitization: A three-year study. *Dermatology*, **189**, 55–57

Trueman, R.W. & Schüpbach, M. (1982) An assessment of the potential genotoxicity of four sunscreen agents. *Prog. Clin. Biol. Res.*, **109**, 415–421

Tyrrell, R.M. (1973) Induction of pyrimidine dimers in bacterial DNA by 365 nm radiation. *Photochem. Photobiol.*, **17**, 69–73

Tyrrell, R.M. (1994) The molecular and cellular pathology of solar ultraviolet radiation. *Mol. Aspects Med.*, **15**, 1–77

Tyrrell, R.M. (1996a) Activation of mammalian gene expression by the UV component of sunlight—From models to reality. *Bioessays*, **18**, 139–148

Tyrrell, R.M. (1996b) UV activation of mammalian stress proteins. In: Feige, U., Morimoto, R.I., Yahara, I. & Polla, B.S., eds, *Stress Inducible Cellular Responses*, Basel, Birkhäuser Verlag, pp. 255–272

Tyrrell, R.M. & Pidoux, M. (1986) Endogenous glutathione protects human skin fibroblasts against the cytotoxic action of UVB, UVA and near-visible radiations. *Photochem. Photobiol.*, **44**, 561–564

Tyrrell, R.M. & Pidoux, M. (1988) Correlation between endogenous glutathione content and sensitivity of cultured human skin cells to radiation at defined wavelengths in the solar UV range. *Photochem. Photobiol.*, **47**, 405–412

Tyrrell, R.M., Keyse, S.M. & Moraes, E.C. (1991) Cellular defense against UVA (320-380 nm) and UVB (290-320 nm) radiations. In: Riklis, E., ed., *Photobiology: The Science and Its Applications,* London, Plenum Press, pp. 861–871

Ullrich, S.E. (1986) Suppression of the immune response to allogenic histocompatibility antigens by a single exposure to ultraviolet radiation. *Transplantation*, **42**, 287–291

Ullrich, S.E. (1995) The role of epidermal cytokines in the generation of cutaneous immune reactions and ultraviolet radiation-induced immune suppression. *Photochem. Photobiol.*, **62**, 389–401

Ullrich, S.E., Kim, T.-H., Ananthaswamy, H.N. & Kripke, M.L. (1999) Sunscreen effects on UV-induced immune suppression. *J. Invest. Dermatol.*, **4**, 65–69

Urano, Y., Asano, T., Yoshimoto, K., Iwahana, H., Kubo, Y., Kato, S., Sasaki, S., Takeuchi, N., Uchida, N., Nakanishi, H., Arase, S. & Itakura, M. (1995) Frequent p53 accumulation in the chronically sun-exposed epidermis and clonal expansion of p53 mutant cells in the epidermis adjacent to basal cell carcinoma. *J. Invest. Dermatol.*, **104**, 928–932

Vail-Smith, K. & Felts, W.M. (1993) Sunbathing: College students' knowledge, attitudes, and perception of risks. *J. Am. Coll. Health*, **42**, 21–26

Vangsted, P. (1985) Alterations to eye structures in hairless mice by long-term ultraviolet irradiation. A histopathological study. *Acta Ophthalmol. Copenh.*, **63**, 199–206

van't Veer, L.J., Burgering, B.M.T., Versteeg, R., Boot, A.J.M., Ruiter, D.J., Osanto, S., Schrier, P.I. & Bos, J.L. (1989) N-*ras* mutations in human cutaneous melanoma from sun-exposed body sites. *Mol. Cell. Biol.*, **9**, 3114–3116

Vila, L.M., Mayor, A.M., Valentin, A.H., Rodriguez, S.I., Reyes, M.L., Acosta, E. & Vila, S. (1999) Association of sunlight exposure and photoprotection measures with clinical outcome in systemic lupus erythematosus. *P. R. Health Sci. J.*, **18**, 89–94

Vile, G.F., Basu-Modak, S., Waltner, C. & Tyrrell, R.M. (1994) Heme oxygenase 1 mediates an adaptive response to oxidative stress in human skin fibroblasts. *Proc. Natl Acad. Sci. USA*, **91**, 2607–2610

Vink, A.A., Yarosh, D.B. & Kripke, M.L. (1996) Chromophore for UV-induced immunosuppression: DNA. *Photochem. Photobiol.*, **63**, 383–386

Vink, A.A., Moodycliffe, A.M., Shreedhar, V., Ullrich, S.E., Roza, L., Yarosh, D.B. & Kripke, M.L. (1997) The inhibition of antigen-presenting activity of dendritic cells resulting from UV irradiation of murine skin is restored by *in vitro* photorepair of cyclobutane pyrimidine dimers. *Proc. Natl Acad. Sci. USA*, **94**, 5255–5260

Vitasa, B.C., Taylor, H.R., Strickland, P.T., Rosenthal, F.S., West, S., Abbey, H., Ng, S.K., Munoz, B. & Emmett, E.A. (1990) Association of nonmelanoma skin cancer and actinic keratosis with cumulative solar ultraviolet exposure in Maryland watermen. *Cancer,* **65**, 2811–2817

Walker, S.L. & Young, A.R. (1997) Sunscreens offer the same UVB protection factors for inflammation and immunosuppression in the mouse. *J. Invest. Dermatol.,* **108**, 133–138

Walker, S.L., Morris, J., Chu, A.C. & Young, A.R. (1994) Relationship between the ability of sunscreens containing 2-ethylhexyl-4¢-methoxycinnamate to protect against UVR-induced inflammation, depletion of epidermal Langerhans (Ia⁺) cells and suppression of alloactivating capacity of murine skin *in vivo. J. Photochem. Photobiol. B,* **22**, 29–36

Walter, J.F. (1981) Evaluation of seven sunscreens on hairless mouse skin. *Arch. Dermatol.,* **117**, 547–550

Walter, J.F. & DeQuoy, P.R. (1980) The hairless mouse as a model for evaluating sunscreens. Prevention of ultraviolet B inhibition of epidermal DNA synthesis. *Arch. Dermatol.,* **116**, 419–421

Walters, K.A., Brain, K.R., Howes, D., James, V.J., Kraus, A.L., Teetsel, N.M., Toulon, M., Watkinson, A.C. & Gettings, S.D. (1997) Percutaneous penetration of octyl salicylate from representative sunscreen formulations through human skin *in vitro. Food chem. Toxicol.,* **35**, 1219–1225

Wamer, W.G., Yin, J.-J. & Wei, R.R. (1997) Oxidative damage to nucleic acids photosensitized by titanium dioxide. *Free Radicals Biol. Med.,* **6**, 851–858

Watts, W.S., Byrnes, T. & Hare, J.W. (1993) Skin cancer awareness campaigns: Are men getting the message? *Health Promot. J. Aust.,* **3**, 40–41

Webb, A.R. (1985) *Solar Ultraviolet Radiation and Vitamin D Synthesis in Man,* PhD Thesis, University of Nottingham

Wei, Q., Matanoski, G.M., Farmer, E.R., Hedayati, M.A. & Grossman, L. (1995) DNA repair capacity for ultraviolet light-induced damage is reduced in peripheral lymphocytes from patients with basal cell carcinoma. *J. Invest. Dermatol.,* **104**, 933–936

Wei, Y.D., Rannug, U. & Rannug, A. (1999) UV-induced CYP1A1 gene expression in human cells is mediated by tryptophan. *Chem. Biol. Interactions,* **118**, 127–140

Weinstock, M.A. (1992) Assessment of sun sensitivity by questionnaire: Validity of items and formulation of a prediction rule. *J. Clin. Epidemiol.,* **45**, 547–552

Weinstock, M.A., Rossi, J.S., Redding, C.A. & Maddock, J.E. (1998) Randomized trial of intervention for sun protection among beachgoers (Abstract). *J. Invest. Dermatol.,* **110**, 589

Weinstock, M.A., Stampfer, M.J., Lew, R.A., Willett, W.C. & Sober, A.J. (1992) Case–control study of melanoma and dietary vitamin D: Implications for advocacy of sun protection and sunscreen use. *J. Invest. Dermatol.,* **98**, 809–811

Weiss, R.B. & Duker, N.J. (1987) Endo-nucleolytic incision of UVB-irradiated DNA. *Photochem. Photobiol.,* **45**, 763–768

Wester, R.C., Melendres, J., Sedik, L., Maibach, H. & Riviere, J.E. (1998) Percutaneous absorption of salicylic acid, theophylline, 2,4-dimethylamine, diethyl hexyl phthalic acid, and *p*-aminobenzoic acid in the isolated perfused porcine skin flap compared to man *in vivo. Toxicol. Appl. Pharmacol.,* **151**, 159–165

Westerdahl, J., Olsson, H., Masbäck, A., Ingvar, C. & Jonsson, N. (1995) Is the use of sunscreens a risk factor for malignant melanoma? *Melanoma Res.,* **5**, 59–65

Westerdahl, J., Ingvar, C., Masbäck, A. & Olsson, H. (2000) Sunscreen use and malignant melanoma. *Int. J. Cancer,* **87**, 145–150

Whiteman, D.C., Frost, C.A., Whiteman, C.A. & Green, A.C. (1994) A survey of sunscreen use and sun-protection practices in Darwin. *Aust. J. Public Health,* **18**, 47–50

Whiteman, D.C., Valery, P., McWhirter, W. & Green, A.C. (1997) Risk factors for childhood melanoma in Queensland, Australia. *Int. J. Cancer,* **70**, 26–31

Whitmore, S.E. & Morison, W.L. (1995) Prevention of UVB-induced immunosuppression in humans by a high sun protection factor sunscreen. *Arch. Dermatol.,* **131**, 1128–1133

WHO (1994) *Ultraviolet Radiation* (Environmental Health Criteria 160), Geneva, pp. 25–44

WHO, WMO, UNEP & International Commission on Non-Ionising Radiation Protection (1995) *Global Solar UV Index,* Oberschleissheim, International Commission on Non-Ionising Radiation Protection

Wichstrom, L. (1994) Predictors of Norwegian adolescents' sunbathing and use of sunscreen. *Health Psychol.,* **13**, 412–420

Wilkinson, F. (1998) Solar simulators for sunscreen testing. In: Matthes, R. & Sliney, D., eds, *Measurements of Optical Radiation Hazards,* Oberschleissheim, International Commission on Nonionising Radiation Protection, pp. 653–684

Wittbrodt, J., Adam, D., Malitschek, B., Maueler, W., Raulf, F., Telling, A., Robertson, S.M. & Schartl, A. (1989) Novel putative receptor tyrosine kinase encoded by melanoma-inducing *Tu* locus in *Xiphophorus. Nature,* **341**, 415–421

Wlaschek, M., Bolsen, K., Herrmann, G., Schwarz, A., Wilmroth, F., Heinrich, P.C., Goerz, G. & Scharffetter-Kochanek, K. (1993) UVA-induced autocrine stimulation of fibroblast-derived-collagenase by IL-6: A possible mechanism in dermal photodamage? *J. Invest. Dermatol.,* **101**, 164–168

Wolf, P., Yarosh, D.B. & Kripke, M.L. (1993a) Effects of sunscreens and a DNA excision repair enzyme on ultraviolet radiation-induced inflammation, immune suppression, and cyclobutane pyrimidine dimer formation in mice. *J. Invest. Dermatol.,* **101**, 523–527

Wolf, P., Donawho, C.K. & Kripke, M.L. (1993b) Analysis of the protective effect of different sunscreens on ultra-violet radiation-induced local and systemic suppression of contact hypersensitivity and inflammatory responses in mice. *J. Invest. Dermatol.,* **100**, 254–259

Wolf, P., Donawho, C.K. & Kripke, M.L. (1994) Effect of sunscreens on UV radiation-induced enhancement of melanoma growth in mice. *J. Natl Cancer Inst.,* **86**, 99-105

Wolf, P., Cox, P., Yarosh, D.B. & Kripke, M.L. (1995) Sunscreens and T4N5 liposomes differ in their ability to protect against ultra-violet-induced sunburn cell formation, alterations of dendritic epidermal cells, and local suppression of contact hypersensitivity. *J. Invest. Dermatol.,* **104**, 287–292

Wolf, P., Quehenberger, F., Mülleger, R., Stranz, B. & Kerl, H. (1998) Phenotypic markers, sunlight-related factors and sunscreen use in patients with cutaneous melanoma: An Austrian case–control study. *Melanoma Res.*, **8**, 370–378

Wong, J.C.F., Airey, D.K. & Fleming, R.A. (1996) Annual reduction of solar UV exposure to the facial area of outdoor workers in southeast Queensland by wearing a hat. *Photodermatol. Photoimmunol. Photomed.*, **12**, 131–135

Wulf, H.C., Poulsen, T., Brodthagen, H. & Hou-Jensen, K. (1982) Sunscreens for delay of ultraviolet induction of skin tumors. *J. Am. Acad. Dermatol.*, **7**, 194–202

Wulf, H.C., Stender, I.M. & Lock-Andersen, J. (1997) Sunscreens used at the beach do not protect against eythema: A new definition of SPF is proposed. *Photodermatol. Photoimmunol. Photo-med.*, **13**, 129–132

Wurst, F., Prey, T., Washuttl, J. & Greiter, F. (1978) Studies on the adhesive power of several UV filter substances on sheep's wool before and after UV radiation. *Arztl. Kosmetol.*, **8**, 144–154

Xie, J., Murone, M., Luoh, S.M., Ryan, A., Gu, Q., Zhang, C., Bonifas, J.M., Lam, C.W., Hynes, M., Goddard, A., Rosenthal, A., Epstein, E.H. & de Sauvage, F.J. (1998) Activating *smoothened* mutations in sporadic basal-cell carcinoma. *Nature*, **391**, 90–92

Xiong, Y., Hannon, G.J., Zhang, H., Casso, D., Kobayashi, R. & Beach, D. (1993) p21 is a universal inhibitor of cyclin kinases. *Nature*, **366**, 701–704

Xu, C. & Parsons, P.G. (1999) Cell cycle delay, mitochondrial stress and uptake of hydrophobic cations induced by sunscreens in cultured human cells. *Photochem. Photobiol.*, **69**, 611–616

Xu, G., Snellman, E., Jansen, C.T. & Hemminki, K. (2000) Levels and repair of cyclobutane pyrimidine dimers and 6-4 photoproducts in skin of sporadic basal cell carcinoma patients. *J. Invest. Dermatol.*, **115**, 95–99

Young, A.R., Magnus, I.A., Davies, A.C. & Smith, N.P. (1983) A comparison of the phototumorigenic potential of 8-MOP and 5-MOP in hairless albino mice exposed to solar simulated radiation. *Br. J. Dermatol.*, **108**, 507–518

Young, A.R., Gibbs, N.K. & Magnus, I.A. (1987) Modification of 5-methoxypsoralen phototumorigenesis by UVB sunscreens: A statistical and histologic study in the hairless albino mouse. *J. Invest. Dermatol.*, **89**, 611–617

Young, A.R., Walker, S.L., Kinley, J.S., Plastow, S.R., Averbeck, D., Morliere, P. & Dubertret, L. (1990) Photo-tumorigenesis studies of 5-methoxypsoralen in bergamot oil: Evaluation and modification of risk of human use in an albino mouse skin model. *J. Photochem. Photobiol. B*, **7**, 231–250

Young, A.R., Potten, C.S., Nikaido, O., Parsons, P.G., Boenders, J., Ramsden, J.M. & Chadwick, C.A. (1998a) Human melanocytes and keratinocytes exposed to UVB or UVA in vivo show comparable levels of thymine dimers. *J. Invest. Dermatol.*, **111**, 936–940

Young, A.R., Chadwick, C.A., Harrison, G.I., Nikaido, O., Ramsden, J. & Potten, C.S. (1998b) The similarity of action spectra for thymine dimers in human epidermis and erythema suggests that DNA is the chromophore for erythema. *J. Invest. Dermatol.*, **111**, 982–988

Young A.R., Sheehan J.M., Chadwick CA. & Potten C.S. (2000) Protection by UVA and UVB sunscreens against *in situ* dipyrimidine photolesions in human epidermis is comparable to protection against sunburn. *J. Invest. Dermatol.*, **115**, 37–41

Zanetti, R., Rosso, S., Martinez, C., Navarro, C., Schraub, S., Sancho-Garnier, H., Franceschi, S., Gafa, L., Perea, E., Tormo, M.J., Laurent, R., Schrameck, C., Cristofolini, M., Tumino, R. & Wechsler, J. (1996) The multicentre south European study 'Helios'. I: Skin characteristics and sunburns in basal cell and squamous cell carcinomas of the skin. *Br. J. Cancer*, **73**, 1440–1446

Zhan, Q., Carrier, F. & Fornace, A.J., Jr (1993) Induction of cellular p53 activity by DNA-damaging agents and growth arrest. *Mol. Cell. Biol.*, **13**, 4242–4250

Zhang, X., Rosenstein, B.S., Wang, Y., Lebwohl, M., Mitchell, D.M. & Wei, H. (1997) Induction of 8-oxo-7,8-dihydro-2'-deoxyguanosine by ultraviolet radiation in calf thymus DNA and HeLa cells. *Photochem. Photobiol.*, **65**, 119–124

Zhang, X.-M., Nakagawa, M., Kawai, K. & Kawai, K. (1998) Erythema-multiforme-like eruption following photoallergic contact dermatitis from oxybenzone. *Contact Derm.*, **38**, 43–44

Ziegler, A., Leffell, D.J., Kunala, S., Sharma, H.W., Gailani, M., Simon, J.A., Halperin, A.J., Baden, H.P., Shapiro, P.E., Bale, A.E. & Brash, D.E. (1993) Mutation hotspots due to sunlight in the p53 gene of nonmelanoma skin cancers. *Proc. Natl Acad. Sci. USA*, **90**, 4216–4220

Ziegler, A., Jonason, A.S., Lefell, D.J., Simon, J.A., Sharma, H.W., Kimmelmann, J., Remington, L., Jacks, T. & Brash, D.E. (1994) Sunburn and *p53* in the onset of skin cancer. *Nature*, **372**, 773–776

Ziegler, A., Jonason, A., Simon, J., Leffell, D. & Brash, D.E. (1996) Tumor suppressor gene mutations and photocarcinogenesis. *Photochem. Photobiol.*, **63**, 432–435

Zinman, R., Schwartz, S., Gordon, K., Fitzpatrick, E. & Camfield, C. (1995) Predictors of sunscreen use in childhood. *Arch. Pediatr. Adolescent Med.*, **149**, 804–807

Zitser, B.S., Shah, A.N., Adams, M.L. & St Clair, J. (1996) A survey of sunbathing practices on three Connecticut State beaches. *Connecticut Med.*, **60**, 591–594

Appendix 1
Chemical UVR Absorbers

The names given in bold and used throughout this handbook are those of the International Nomenclature of Cosmetic Ingredients.

ORGANIC CHEMICAL ABSORBERS

UVB absorbers

Cinnamates

Cinoxate
Empirical formula:
$C_{14}H_{18}O_4$

Chemical names:
2-Ethoxyethyl-*para*-methoxycinnamate; 2-propenoic acid, 3-(4-methoxyphenyl)-2-ethoxyethyl ester; 2-ethoxyethyl-4-methoxycinnamate

Trade names:
Giv Tan F; Phiasol

DEA-methoxycinnamate
Empirical formula:
$C_{14}H_{21}NO_5$

Chemical names:
Diethanolamine salt of *para*-methoxyhydroxycinnamate; 2-propenoic acid, 3-(4-methoxyphenyl)-, compd with 2,2'-iminobis(ethanol)

Trade name:
Nipasorb D

Diisopropyl methyl cinnamate
Empirical formula:
$C_{16}H_{22}O_2$

Chemical names:
2-Propenoic acid, 3-[2,4-bis(1-methylethyl)phenyl]-methyl ester; 2,5-diisopropyl methyl cinnamate

Ethylhexyl methoxycinnamate
Empirical formula:
$C_{18}H_{26}O_3$

Chemical names:
2-Ethylhexyl-4-methoxycinnamate; 2-ethyl-hexyl-*para*-methoxycinnamate; *para*-methoxycinnamic acid, 2-ethylhexyl ester; 3-(4-methoxyphenyl)-2-propenoic acid, 2-ethylhexyl ester; octinoxate; octyl methoxycinnamate; 2-propenoic acid, 3-(4-methoxyphenyl)-2-ethylhexyl ester

Trade names:
AEC Octyl Methoxycinnamate; Escalol 557; Eusolex 2292; Heliosol 3; Jeescreen OMC; Katoscreen OMC; Neo Heliopan, Type AV; Parsol MCX; Solarum OMC; Uvinul MC 80

Ethyl methoxycinnamate
Empirical formula:
$C_{12}H_{14}O_3$

Chemical names:
para-Methoxycinnamic acid, ethyl ester; 3-(4-methoxyphenyl)-2-propenoic acid, ethyl ester

Glyceryl ethylhexanoate dimethoxycinnamate
Chemical names:
Glyceryl octanoate dimethoxycinnamate; 2-propenoic acid, 3-(4-methoxyphenyl)-, diester with 1,3-dihydroxy-2-(2-ethyl-1-oxohexyl)oxypropane

Isoamyl-*para*-methoxycinnamate
Empirical formula:
$C_{15}H_{20}O_3$

Chemical names:
Amyl-4-methoxycinnamate; isopentyl-4-methoxycinnamate; isopentyl-*para*-methoxy-cinnamate; 3-(4-methoxyphenyl)-2-propenoic acid, isopentyl ester

Trade names:
Neo Heliopan type E 1000; Solarum AMC

para-Aminobenzoic acids (PABAs)

Amyl dimethyl PABA
Empirical formula:
$C_{14}H_{21}NO_2$

Chemical names:
Amyl *para*-N,N-dimethylaminobenzoate

Trade names:
Escalol 506; Padimate A

Ethyl dihydroxypropyl PABA
Empirical formula:
$C_{15}H_{23}NO_4$

Chemical names:
Benzoic acid, 4-[bis(2-hydroxypropyl)-amino]ethyl ester (mixed isomers); ethyl-4-bis(2-hydroxypropyl)aminobenzoate, mixed isomers; ethyl dihydroxypropyl para-aminobenzoate, mixed isomers; N-propoxylated-ethyl-4-aminobenzoate (mixed isomers)

Trade name:
Amerscreen P

Ethylhexyl dimethyl PABA
Empirical formula:
$C_{17}H_{27}NO_2$

Chemical names:
Benzoic acid, 4-(dimethylamino)-, 2-ethylhexyl ester; benzoic acid, 4-(dimethyl-amino)-, octyl ester; 4-(dimethyl-amino)benzoic acid, 2-ethyl-hexyl ester; 2-ethylhexyl-4-(dimethylamino)benzoate; 2-ethylhexyl para-dimethylamino benzoate; octyldimethyl PABA; octyl dimethyl para-aminobenzoate

Trade names:
Arlatone UVB; Escalol 507; Eusolex 6007; Katoscreen ODMP; Padimate O; Sunarome PLUS; Uvasorb DMO

Ethyl PABA
Empirical formula:
$C_9H_{11}NO_2$

Chemical names:
Anesthesin; ethyl para-aminobenzoate

Glyceryl PABA
Empirical formula:
$C_{10}H_{13}NO_4$

Chemical names:
1-(4-Aminobenzoate)-1,2,3-propanetriol; 4-aminobenzoic acid glyceryl ester; glyceryl-para-aminobenzoate; glycerol 1-(4-aminobenzoate); PABA monoglyceride; propanetriol 1-(4-aminobenzoate)

Trade name:
Escalol 106

PABA
Empirical formula:
$C_7H_7NO_2$

Chemical names:
Acid (PABA); aminobenzoic acid; 4-aminobenzoic acid; para-aminobenzoic acid; aniline-4-carboxylic acid; benzoic acid, 4-amino-; para-carboxyaniline; para-carboxyphenylamine

Trade names:
Amben; Pabacidum; Pabanol

PEG-25 PABA
Empirical formula:
$C_{59}H_{111}NO_{27}$

Chemical names:
4-Bis(polyethoxy)-4-aminobenzoic acid polyethoxyethyl ester; ethoxylated ethyl-para-aminobenzoic acid; ethoxylated ethyl-4-aminobenzoate

Trade names:
Lusantan 25; Uvinul P-25

Salicylates

Dipropylene glycol salicylate
Empirical formula:
$C_{13}H_{18}O_4$

Chemical names:
2-Hydroxybenzoic acid dipropylene glycol ester; 2-(2-hydroxypropyl)-1-methyl-ethyl salicylate

Ethylene glycol salicylate
Empirical formula:
$C_9H_{10}O_5$

Chemical names:
2-Hydroxybenzoic acid ethylene glycol ester; 1,2-ethanediol salicylate

Ethylhexyl salicylate
Empirical formula:
$C_{15}H_{22}O_3$

Chemical names:
Benzoic acid, 2-hydroxy-2-ethylhexyl ester; 2-ethylhexyl 2-hydroxybenzoate; 2-ethylhexyl salicylate; salicylic acid, 2-ethylhexyl ester; octisalate; octyl salicylate

Trade names:
Dermoblock (OS); Escalol 587; Eusolex OS; Hallbrite 0S; Heliosol 2; Katoscreen OS; Neo Heliopan, Type OS; Neotan L; Solarum OS; Sonnelan UV; Sunarome WMO; Trivent OS; Uvinul O-18

Homosalate
Empirical formula:
$C_{16}H_{22}O_3$

Chemical names:
Benzoic acid, 2-hydroxy- 3,3,5-trimethyl-cyclohexyl ester; cyclohexanol, 3,3,5-trimethyl salicylate; homomenthyl salicylate; metahomomenthyl salicylate; 3,3,5-trimethylcyclohexyl 2-hydroxybenzoate; 3,3,5-trimethyl cyclohexyl salicylate

Trade names:
Eusolex HMS; Filtrosol A; Heliopan; Uniderm HOMSAL

Isopropylbenzyl salicylate
Empirical formula:
$C_{16}H_{16}O_3$

Chemical names:
4-Isopropylbenzyl salicylate; 2-hydroxy-benzoic acid 4-isopropylbenzyl ester

Trade name:
Megasol

Methyl salicylate
Empirical formula:
$C_8H_8O_3$

Chemical names:
Benzoic acid, 2-hydroxy-, methyl ester; betula oil; ortho-hydroxybenzoic acid, methyl ester; 2-(methoxycarbonyl)phenol; methyl ortho-hydroxybenzoate; methyl 2-hydroxybenzoate; oil of wintergreen; salicylic acid, methyl ester; teaberry oil

Phenyl salicylate
Empirical formula:
$C_{13}H_{10}O_3$

Chemical name:
2-Hydroxybenzoic acid phenyl ester

Trade names:
Salol; UVSAM-2142

TEA salicylate
Empirical formula:
$C_{13}H_{21}O_6N$

Chemical names:
Benzoic acid, 2-hydroxy-, compd with 2,2',2''–nitrilotris[ethanol] (1:1); 2-hydroxybenzoic acid, compd with 2,2',2''-nitrilotris[ethanol] (1:1); triethanolamine salicylate; trolamine salicylate

Trade names:
Katoscreen TES; Neo Heliopan, Type TS; Neotan W; Sunarome G; Sunarome W

Camphor derivatives

3-Benzylidene camphor
Empirical formula:
$C_{17}H_{19}O$

Chemical names:
3-Benzylidenebornan-2-one; 1,7,7-trimethyl-3-(phenylmethylene)bicyclo-[2.2.1]heptan-2-one

Trade names:
Mexoryl SD; Ultracyd; Ultren BK

Benzylidene camphor sulfonic acid
Empirical formula:
$C_{17}H_{19}O_4$

Chemical names:
α-(2-Oxoborn-3-ylidene)-toluene-4-sulfonic acid; 3-(4'-sulfobenzylidene) camphor

Trade name:
Mexoryl SL

Camphor benzalkonium methosulfate
Chemical names:
Methyl-N,N,N-trimethyl-4-[(4,7,7-trimethyl-3-oxobicyclo[2.2.1]hept-2-ylidine)-methyl]anilinum sulfate; 3-(4'-trimethylammonium benzylidene)-1-bornan-2-one methyl sulfate; N,N,N-tri-methyl-4-(2-oxoborn-3-ylidene methyl)-anilinium methyl sulfate

Trade name:
Mexoryl SO

4-Methylbenzylidene camphor
Empirical formula:
$C_{18}H_{22}O$

Chemical names:
3-(4-Methylbenzylidene)bornan-2-one; 3-(4'-methylbenzylidene)-1 camphor; 1,7,7-trimethyl-3-(para-methylphenylmethylene)-bicyclo[2.2.1]-heptane-2-one

Trade names:
Eusolex 6300; Neo Heliopan, Type MBC; Parsol 5000; Solarum MBC; Uvinul MBC 95

Polyacrylamidomethyl benzylidene camphor
Chemical name:
Polymer of N-(2 and 4)-[(2-oxoborn-3-ylidone)methyl]-benzyl]-acrylamide

Trade name:
Mexoryl SW

Miscellaneous

Diethylhexylbutamido triazone
Chemical names:
Benzoic acid, 4,4'-[(-6-{[(1,1-dimethylethyl)-aminocarbonyl]-phenylamino}-1,3,5-triazine-2,4-diyl)-diimino]bis-, bis (2-ethylhexyl) ether; dioctylbutamido triazone

Trade name:
Uvasorb HEB

Ethylhexyl triazone
Empirical formula:
$C_{48}H_{66}N_6O_6$

Chemical names:
Octyl triazone; 2,4,6-trianilino-(para-carbo-2'-ethylhexyl-1'-oxy)-1,3,5 triazine

Trade name:
Uvinul T-150

5-Methyl-2-phenylbenzoxazole
Empirical formula:
$C_{13}H_{11}N_3O$

Chemical names:
2-(2H-Benzotriol-2-yl)-para-cresol; 2-(2'-hydroxy-5'-methylphenyl)benzotriazole

Trade name:
Tinuvin P

Octocrylene
Empirical formula:
$C_{24}H_{27}NO_2$

Chemical names:
2-Cyano-3,3-diphenyl acrylic acid, 2-ethylhexyl ester; 2-ethylhexyl 2-cyano-3,3-diphenylacrylate; 2-ethylhexyl 2-cyano-3,3-diphenyl-2-propenoate; 2-ethylhexyl 2-cyano-3-phenylcinnamate; 2-propenoic acid, 2-cyano-3,3-diphenyl-, 2-ethylhexyl ether

Trade names:
Escalol 597; Eusolex OCR; Neo Heliopan, Type 303; Parsol 340; Solarum OCR; UV Absorber 3; Uvinul N-539T

Phenylbenzimidazole sulfonic acid
Empirical formula:
$C_{13}H_{10}N_2O_3S$

Chemical names:
2-Phenylbenzimidazol-5-sulfonic acid; 2-phenyl-5-sulfobenzimidazole

Trade names:
Ensulizole; Eusolex 232; Neo Heliopan, Type Hydro; Novantisol; Parsol HS

Urocanic acid

Empirical formula:

$C_6H_7N_2O_2$

Chemical name:
3-(Imidazol-4-yl)acrylic acid

UVA absorbers

Benzophenones

Benzophenone-1

Empirical formula:
$C_{13}H_{10}O_3$

Chemical names:
Benzoresorcinol; 2,4-dihydroxybenzophenone

Trade names:
ASL-23; Syntase 100; Uvasorb 20H/G; Uvinul 400; UVSAM-214

Benzophenone-2

Empirical formula:
$C_{13}H_{10}O_5$

Chemical names:
Bis(2,4-dihydroxyphenyl) methanone; 2,2',4,4'-tetrahydroxybenzophenone

Trade name:
Uvinul D-50

Benzophenone-3

Empirical formula:
$C_{14}H_{12}O_3$

Chemical names:
2-Benzyl-5-methoxyphenol; 2-hydroxy-4-methoxybenzophenone; (2-hydroxy-4-methoxyphenyl)phenylmethanone; methanone (2-hydroxy-4-methoxyphenyl)phenyl; oxybenzone

Trade names:
ASL 24; Cyasorb UV-9; Escalol 567; Eusolex 4360; EUSORB 228; Jeescreen

Benzophenone 3; Katoscreen B-3; Marsorb 24; Neo Heliopan, Type BB; Protaphenone-3; Solarum B ZP3; Spectra-Sorb UV-9; Syntase 62; Uvasorb MeT/C; Uvinul M-40; Uvistat 24

Benzophenone-4

Empirical formula:
$C_{14}H_{12}O_6S$

Chemical names:
Benzenesulfonic acid, 5-benzoyl-4-hydroxy-2-methoxy-; 5-benzoyl-hydroxy-2-methoxybenzene-sulfonic acid; 5-benzoyl-4-hydroxy-2-methoxybenzene sulfonic acid; 2-hydroxy-4-methoxybenzophenone-5- sulfonic acid; 1-phenol-4-sulfonic acid, 2-benzoyl-5-methoxy-; sulisobenzone

Trade names:
Aduvex 112; Escalol 577; Jeescreen Benzophenone 4; Protaphenone-4; Syntase 230; Uval; Uvasorb S5; Uvinul MS-40; Uvistat 112

Benzophenone-5

Empirical formula:
$C_{14}H_{12}O_6S.Na$

Chemical names:
Benzenesulfonic acid, 5-benzoyl-4-hydroxy-2-methoxy-, monosodium salt; sodium 2-hydroxy-4-methoxy-5-sulfobenzophenone; benzophenone-4 sodium salt

Trade name:
ASL-24S

Benzophenone-6

Empirical formula:
$C_{15}H_{14}O_5$

Chemical names:
Bis(2-hydroxy-4-methoxyphenyl) methanone; 2,2'-dihydroxy-4,4'-dimethoxybenzophenone

Trade name:
Uvinul D-49

Benzophenone-8

Empirical formula:
$C_{14}H_{12}O_4$

Chemical names:
2,2'-Dihydroxy-4-methoxybenzophenone; dioxybenzone; (2-hydroxy-4-methoxyphenyl)(2-hydroxy-phenyl)-methanone; methanone, (2-hydroxy-4-methoxyphenyl)(2-hydroxyphenyl)-

Trade name:
Spectra-Sorb UV-24

Benzophenone-9

Empirical formula:
$C_{15}H_{12}O_{11}S_2.2Na$

Chemical names:
Disodium-3,3'-carbonylbis[4-hydroxy-6-methoxybenzenesulfonate]; sodium 2,2'-dihydroxy-4,4'-dimethoxy-5-sulfobenzophenone

Trade name:
Uvinul DS-49

Benzophenone-10

Empirical formula:
$C_{15}H_{14}O_3$

Chemical names:
2-Hydroxy-4-methoxy-4'-methylbenzophenone; (2-hydroxy-4-methoxyphenyl)-(4-methylphenyl)-methanone

Trade names:
Aduvex 2211; Mexenone; Uvistat 2211

Camphor derivatives

Terephthalylidene dicamphor sulfonic acid

Empirical formula:
$C_{28}H_{34}O_8S_2$

Chemical names:
3,3'-(1,4-Phenylenedimethylene)bis(7,7-dimethyl-2-oxo-bicyclo[2.2.1]hept-1-yl-methanesulfonic) acid

Trade names:
Ecamsule; Mexoryl SX

Dibenzoylmethanes

Butyl methoxydibenzoylmethane
Empirical formula:
$C_{20}H_{22}O_3$

Chemical names:
Avobenzone; 4-*tert*-butyl-4'-methoxydiben-zoylmethane; 1-(4-*tert*-butylphenyl-3-(4-methoxyphenyl)propane-1,3-dione; 1-[4-(1,1-dimethylethyl)phenyl]-3-(4-methoxy-phenyl)-1,3-propanedione; 1,3-propane-dione, 2-butyl-2-methoxy-1,3-diphenyl-; 1,3-propanedione, 1-[4-(1,1-dimethyl-ethyl)phenyl]-3-(4-methoxyphenyl)

Trade names:
Eusolex 9020; Neo Heliopan, Type MA; Parsol 1789; Parsol A; Solarum BMBM; Solarum MA

Anthranilates

Menthyl anthranilate
Empirical formula:
$C_{17}H_{25}NO_2$

Chemical names:
Cyclohexanol, 5-methyl-2-(1-methyl-ethyl)-2-aminobenzoate; menthyl-*ortho*-aminobenzoate; meradimate

Trade names:
Neo Heliopan MA; Trivent MA

Miscellaneous

Bisymidazylate
Chemical name:
2,2'-Bis(1,4-phenylene)-1*H*-benzimida-zole-4,6-disulfonic acid, monosodium salt

UVA and UVB absorbers

Miscellaneous

Anisotriazine
Chemical name:
2,4-Bis[4-(2-ethylhexyloxy)-2-hydroxyl]-phenyl-6-(4-methoxyphenyl)-tetramethyl-butyl)-phenol (1,3,5)-triazine

Drometrizole trisiloxane
Chemical name:
Phenol, 2-(2*H*-benzotriazol-2-yl)-4-methyl-6-{2-methyl-3-[1,3,3,3-tetramethyl-1-(tri-methylsilyl)oxy]disil-oxanyl}propyl

Trade name:
Mexoryl XL

Methylene bisbenzotriazolyl tetra-methylbutylphenol
Chemical names:
2,2'-Methylene-bis-6-(2*H*-benzotriazol-2-yl)-4-(1,1,3,3-tetramethylbutyl)phenol

INORGANIC CHEMICAL ABSORBERS

Titanium dioxide
Empirical formula:
TiO_2

Chemical names:
Amorphous titanium dioxide; micro parti-cle titanium dioxide; pigment white 6; titanium dioxide sol; titanium oxide

Trade names:
A310 Tudor Aspen; Atlas White Titanium Dioxide 09985; C47-5175 Cosmetic White; CI 77891; Kowet Titanium Dioxide 09970; Kronos 1025; KRONOS 2071-U; Micro T; Micro Titanium Dioxide MT-500B; Micro Titanium Dioxide MT-150W; MTD-25; NanoGard AQ; Nano TZ; Oxyde de Titane Organophile W 877; Oxyde de Titane Standard; P25; Sicovit White E 171; SI-UF20-Z; SI-UFTR-Z; Spherititan; TiO2 C9228 Blend; TiO2 D13; Ti-Sphere AA-1515; Ti-Sphere AA-1512-LL; Titanium Dioxide P 25; Titanium Dioxide 10-34-PC-0082; Titanium Dioxide 10-34-PC-0748; Titanium Dioxide, USP, CTFA, Bacteria Controlled; UF-20; UFTR; Uniwhite AO; Uniwhite KO; UV-Titan

Zinc oxide
Empirical formula:
ZnO

Chemical names:
Low temperature burned zinc oxide; pig-ment white 4; zinc white

Trade names:
CI 77947; Finex-25; MZO-25; NanoGard Zinc Oxide; Nano-TZ; Nanox; Nano-Zinc SL; Oxyde de Zinc Micropure; Unichem ZO; USP 1; USP-2; Z-Cote; Zinc Oxide Neutral H&R (PN 104 702); Zinc Oxide USP 66

Appendix 2
Definition of genetic test codes

End-point[a]	Code	Definition
Non-mammalian systems		
Prokaryotic systems		
G	SA0	*Salmonella typhimurium* TA100, reverse mutation
G	SA2	*Salmonella typhimurium* TA102, reverse mutation
G	SA5	*Salmonella typhimurium* TA1535, reverse mutation
G	SA7	*Salmonella typhimurium* TA1537, reverse mutation
G	SA8	*Salmonella typhimurium* TA1538, reverse mutation
G	SA9	*Salmonella typhimurium* TA98, reverse mutation
G	ECW	*Escherichia coli* WP2 *uvr*A, reverse mutation
G	EC2	*Escherichia coli* WP2, reverse mutation
Lower eukaryotic systems		
D	SSD	*Saccharomyces* species, DNA repair-deficient strains, differential toxicity
R	SCG	*Saccharomyces cerevisiae*, gene conversion
G	SCR	*Saccharomyces cerevisiae*, reverse mutation
Insect systems		
G	DMM	*Drosophila melanogaster,* somatic mutation
G	DMX	*Drosophila melanogaster,* sex-linked recessive lethal mutations
Mammalian systems		
Animal cells in vitro		
G	G5T	Gene mutation, mouse lymphoma L5178Y cells, *Tk* locus
G	G51	Gene mutation, mouse lymphoma L5178Y cells, all other loci
S	SIC	Sister chromatid exchange, Chinese hamster cells *in vitro*
C	CIC	Chromosomal aberrations, Chinese hamster cells *in vitro*
Human cells in vitro		
D	DIH	DNA strand breaks, cross-links or related damage, human cells *in vitro*
Animals in vivo		
M	MVR	Micronucleus formation, rats *in vivo*
C	CBA	Chromosomal aberrations, animal bone-marrow cells *in vivo*

[a] End-points are grouped within each phylogenetic category as follows: C, chromosomal aberrations; D, DNA damage; G, gene mutation; M, micronuclei; R, mitotic recombination or gene conversion; S, sister chromatid exchange

Glossary

Actinic radiation

Electromagnetic radiation capable of initiating photochemical reactions; ultraviolet B and C radiation (see below)

Contact hypersensitivity

T-cell-mediated immune response evoked by topically applied antigen

Chromophore

Atomic grouping, which, when introduced into an organic substance, affects its absorption spectrum (and causes it to change colour)

Delayed-type hypersensitivity

T-cell-mediated immune response evoked by internally administered antigen (e.g. injected into the skin)

Derived sun protection factor

Evaluated from the spectral transmission values $(T(\lambda)]$ of a sunscreen applied to a substrate, expressed mathematically as:

$$\sum_{290}^{400} E(\lambda)\varepsilon(\lambda)\Delta\lambda \left/ \sum_{290}^{400} E(\lambda)\varepsilon(\lambda)T(\lambda)\Delta\lambda \right.$$

where $E(\lambda)$ is the spectral irradiance of terrestrial ultraviolet radiation under defined conditions, $e(\lambda)$ is the reference erythema action spectrum of the Commission Internationale de l'Eclairage (McKinlay & Diffey, 1987) and $\Delta\lambda$ is the wavelength increment (e.g. 5 nm)

Effective irradiance

Hypothetical irradiance of monochromatic radiation with a wavelength at which the action spectrum of the relevant photobiological effect is equal to unity

Hairless mouse

An immune-competent mouse lacking hair by virtue of homozygosity at the *Hr* locus

Langerhans cell

An epidermal dendritic antigen-presenting cell

Minimal erythema dose

The minimal erythema dose (MED) is the lowest exposure to radiant ultraviolet radiation that produces a threshold erythemal response 8–24 h after exposure. There is no consensus concerning this response; both just-perceptible reddening of the skin and erythema with sharp margins are used as end-points. There is also no consensus concerning the quantity of exposure that elicits a threshold erythemal response (Urbach & Forbes, 1998).

Photoageing

Progressive deterioration of skin structure caused by long-term exposure to sunlight

Photoproduct	Result of a structural change due to absorption of radiation energy
Protection factor	The protection factor of a sunscreen is the ratio of the exposure to any type of ultraviolet source required to produce a defined biological response (e.g. immunosuppresion) on skin that is protected with a sunscreen and unprotected (see also sun protection factor)
Radiant exposure	Radiant energy delivered to a given area (J/m^2)
Solar-simulated radiation	Radiation from an artificial source (e.g. optically filtered arc lamp) that approximates the terrestial solar spectrum
Solar zenith angle	Angle between the point in the sky directly overhead (the zenith) and the sun; the solar zenith is the 90° complement of 'degrees from horizontal axis'.
Standard erythema dose	The standard erythema dose (SED) is equivalent to an erythemal weighted dose of 100 J/m^2 (Commission Internationale de l'Eclairage, 1988). Minimal erythema on unacclimatized skin would be expected to require a SED of 1.5–6. In order to avoid confusion between the minimal erythema dose (MED) and the SED for particular skin types, a numerical value of 100 J/m^2 was chosen. The SED supersedes arcane units such as the Robertson-Berger unit and the instrumental MED and is the recommended unit for expressing erythemally effective radiant exposure.
Sun protection factor	Ratio of the least amount of ultraviolet energy required to produced minimal erythema on sunscreen-protected skin to the amount of energy required to produce the same erythema on unprotected skin. Applies strictly to human skin exposure *in vivo* to a simulated source of sunlight by defined optical filtering of xenon arc lamps. Protected skin is that to which a 2-mg/cm^2 layer of sunscreen has been applied.
Sunscreen	Formulation of active organic or inorganic chemical absorbers which has undergone testing and is available to the public.
Ultraviolet A	Electromagnetic radiation of wavelength 315–400 nm
Ultraviolet B	Electromagnetic radiation of wavelength 280–315 nm
Ultraviolet C	Electromagnetic radiation of wavelength 100–280 nm
Ultraviolet radiation	Electromagnetic radiation of wavelength 100–400 nm

Sources of figures

1 IARC
2 G. Mollon, IARC
3 IARC
4 A. McKinlay & B. Diffey (1987)
5 Working Group
6 Working Group
7 Working Group
8 IARC
9 Working Group
10 IARC
11 L'Oréal Recherche, Centre Charles Zviak, 92583 Clichy, France
12 Loyola University, Dermatology Department, Chicago, USA
13 Working Group
14 Working Group
15 B. Diffey (1999)
16 B. Diffey & H. Giess (1998)
17 Office of National Statistics (1988), London
18 IARC
19 B. Diffey (1998)
20 L'Oréal Recherche, Centre Charles Zviak, 92583 Clichy, France

21 IARC
22 IARC
23 27ème Dimension, 6 rue Emile Pathé, 78400 Chatou, France
24 Anti-Cancer Council of Victoria, Australia
25 Loyola University, Dermatology Department, Chicago, USA
26 G. Mollon, IARC
27 Loyola University, Dermatology Department, Chicago, USA
28 Loyola University, Dermatology Department, Chicago, USA
29 Loyola University, Dermatology Department, Chicago, USA
30 Loyola University, Dermatology Department, Chicago, USA
31 IARC
32 L'Oréal Recherche, Centre Charles Zviak, 92583 Clichy, France
33 *Journal of Investigative Dermatology*
34 L'Oréal Recherche, Centre Charles Zviak, 92583 Clichy, France

35 IARC
36 IARC
37 L'Oréal Recherche, Centre Charles Zviak, 92583 Clichy, France
38 L'Oréal Recherche, Centre Charles Zviak, 92583 Clichy, France
39 Professor R.StC. Barnetson, University of Sydney, Australia
40 L'Oréal Recherche, Centre Charles Zviak, 92583 Clichy, France
41 L'Oréal Recherche, Centre Charles Zviak, 92583 Clichy, France
42 Loyola University, Dermatology Department, Chicago, USA
43 IARC

Working Procedures for the *IARC Handbooks of Cancer Prevention*

The prevention of cancer is one of the key objectives of the International Agency for Research on Cancer (IARC). This may be achieved by avoiding exposures to known cancer-causing agents, by increasing host defences through immunization or chemoprevention or by modifying lifestyle. The aim of the series of *IARC Handbooks of Cancer Prevention* is to evaluate scientific information on agents and interventions that may reduce the incidence of or mortality from cancer.

Scope

Cancer-preventive strategies embrace chemical, immunological, dietary and behavioural interventions that may retard, block or reverse carcinogenic processes or reduce underlying risk factors. The term 'chemoprevention' is used to refer to interventions with pharmaceuticals, vitamins, minerals and other chemicals to reduce cancer incidence. The *IARC Handbooks* address the efficacy, safety and mechanisms of cancer-preventive strategies and the adequacy of the available data, including those on timing, dose, duration and indications for use.

Preventive strategies can be applied across a continuum of: (1) the general population; (2) subgroups with particular predisposing host or environmental risk factors, including genetic susceptibility to cancer; (3) persons with precancerous lesions; and (4) cancer patients at risk for second primary tumours. Use of the same strategies or agents in the treatment of cancer patients to control the growth, metastasis and recurrence of tumours is considered to be patient management, not

prevention, although data from clinical trials may be relevant when making a *Handbooks* evaluation.

Objective

The objective of the *Handbooks* programme is the preparation of critical reviews and evaluations of evidence for cancer-prevention and other relevant properties of a wide range of potential cancer-preventive agents and strategies by international working groups of experts. The resulting *Handbooks* may also indicate when additional research is needed.

The *Handbooks* may assist national and international authorities in devising programmes of health promotion and cancer prevention and in making benefit–risk assessments. The evaluations of IARC working groups are scientific judgements about the available evidence for cancer-preventive efficacy and safety. No recommendation is given with regard to national and international regulation or legislation, which are the responsibility of individual governments and/or other international authorities. No recommendations for specific research trials are made.

Working Groups

Reviews and evaluations are formulated by international working groups of experts convened by the IARC. The tasks of each group are: (1) to ascertain that all appropriate data have been collected; (2) to select the data relevant for the evaluation on the basis of scientific merit; (3) to prepare accurate summaries of the data to enable the reader to follow the reasoning of the Working Group; (4) to evaluate the signifi-

cance of the available data from human studies and experimental models on cancer-preventive activity, and other beneficial effects and also on adverse effects; and (5) to evaluate data relevant to the understanding of the mechanisms of preventive activity.

Approximately 13 months before a working group meets, the topics of the *Handbook* are announced, and participants are selected by IARC staff in consultation with other experts. Subsequently, relevant clinical, experimental and human data are collected by the IARC from all available sources of published information. Representatives of producer or consumer associations may assist in the preparation of sections on production and use, as appropriate.

Working Group participants who contributed to the considerations and evaluations within a particular *Handbook* are listed, with their addresses, at the beginning of each publication. Each participant serves as an individual scientist and not as a representative of any organization, government or industry. In addition, scientists nominated by national and international agencies, industrial associations and consumer and/or environmental organizations may be invited as observers. IARC staff involved in the preparation of the *Handbooks* are listed.

About eight months before the meeting, the material collected is sent to meeting participants to prepare sections for the first drafts of the *Handbooks*. These are then compiled by IARC staff and sent, before the meeting, to all participants of the Working Group for review. There is an opportunity to return the compiled specialized sections of the draft to the experts, inviting preliminary comments, before the complete first-draft document is distributed to all members of the Working Group.

Data for *Handbooks*

The *Handbooks* do not necessarily cite all of the literature on the agent or strategy being evaluated. Only those data considered by the Working Group to be relevant to making the evaluation are included. In principle, meeting abstracts and other reports that do not provide sufficient detail upon which to base an assessment of their quality are not considered.

With regard to data from toxicological, epidemiological and experimental studies and from clinical trials, only reports that have been published or accepted for publication in the openly available scientific literature are reviewed by the Working Group. In certain instances, government agency reports that have undergone peer review and are widely available are considered. Exceptions may be made on an ad-hoc basis to include unpublished reports that are in their final form and publicly available, if their inclusion is considered pertinent to making a final evaluation. In the sections on chemical and physical properties, on production, on use, on analysis and on human exposure, unpublished sources of information may be used.

The available studies are summarized by the Working Group. In general, numerical findings are indicated as they appear in the original report; units are converted when necessary for easier comparison. The Working Goup may conduct additional analyses of the published data and use them in their assessment of the evidence. Important aspects of a study, directly impinging on its interpretation, are brought to the attention of the reader.

Criteria for selection of topics for evaluation

Agents, classes of agents and interventions to be evaluated in the *Handbooks* are selected on the basis of one or more of the following criteria.

- The available evidence suggests potential for significantly reducing the incidence of cancers.
- There is a substantial body of human, experimental, clinical and/or mechanistic data suitable for evaluation.
- The agent is in widespread use and of putative protective value, but of uncertain efficacy and safety.
- The agent shows exceptional promise in experimental studies but has not been used in humans.
- The agent is available for further studies of human use.

Evaluation of cancer-preventive agents

A wide range of findings must be taken into account before a particular agent can be recognized as preventing cancer, and a systematized approach to data presentation has been adopted for *Handbooks* evaluations.

Characteristics of the agent or intervention

Chemical identity and other definitive information (such as genus and species of plants) are given as appropriate. Data relevant to identification, occurrence and biological activity are included. Technical products of chemicals are given, including trade names, relevant specifications and information on composition and impurities.

Preventive interventions can be broad, community-based interventions, or interventions targeted to individuals (counselling, behavioural alterations, chemoprevention).

Human exposure

Occurrence

Information on the occurrence of an agent in the environment is obtained from monitoring and surveillance in occupational environments, air, water, soil, foods and animal and human tissues. When available, data on the generation, persistence and bioaccumulation of the agent are included. For interventions, data on prevalence are supplied.

Production and use

The dates of first synthesis and of first commercial production of a chemical are provided, with the dates of first reported occurrence. In addition, methods of synthesis used in past and present commercial production and methods of production that may give rise to various impurities are described. For interventions, the dates of first mention of their use are given.

Data on the production, international trade and uses and applications of agents are obtained for representative regions. In the case of drugs, mention of their therapeutic applications does not necessarily represent current practice, nor does it imply judgement as to their therapeutic efficacy.

If an agent is used as a prescribed or over-the-counter pharmaceutical product, the health status, age, sex and medical condition of the person receiving the product are described. For non-pharmaceutical agents, particularly those taken because of cultural traditions, the characteristics of use or exposure and the relevant populations are given. In all cases, quantitative data, such as dose–response relationships, are considered to be of special importance.

Metabolism of and metabolic responses to the agent or intervention

In evaluating the potential utility of a suspected cancer-preventive agent or strategy, a number of different properties, in addition to direct effects upon cancer incidence, are described and weighed. Furthermore, as many of the data leading to an evaluation are expected to come from studies in experimental animals, information that facilitates interspecies extrapolation is particularly important; this includes metabolic, kinetic and genetic data. Whenever possible, quantitative data, including information on dose, duration and potency, are considered.

Information is given on absorption, distribution (including placental transfer), metabolism and excretion in humans and experimental animals. Kinetics within the target species may affect the interpretation and extrapolation of dose–response relationships, such as blood concentrations, protein binding, tissue concentrations, plasma half-lives and elimination rates. Comparative information on the relationship between use or exposure and the dose that reaches the target site may be of particular importance for extrapolation between species. Studies that indicate the metabolic pathways and fate of an agent in humans and experimental animals are summarized, and data on humans and experimental animals are compared when possible. Observations are made on interindividual variations and relevant metabolic polymorphisms. Data indicating long-term accumulation in human tissues are included. Physiologically based pharmacokinetic models and their parameter values are relevant and are included whenever they are available. Information on the fate of the compound within tissues and cells (transport, role of cellular receptors, compartmentalization, binding to macromolecules) is given.

The metabolic consequences of interventions are described.

Genotyping will be used increasingly, not only to identify subpopulations at increased or decreased risk for cancers but also to characterize variation in the biotransformation of and responses to cancer-preventive agents.

This subsection can include effects of the compound on gene expression, enzyme induction or inhibition, or pro-oxidant status, when such data are not described elsewhere. It covers data obtained in humans and experimental animals, with particular attention to effects of long-term use and exposure.

Cancer-preventive effects
Human studies
Types of study considered
Human data are derived from experimental and non-experimental study designs and are focused on cancer, precancer or intermediate biological end-points. The experimental designs include randomized controlled trials and short-term experimental studies; non-experimental designs include cohort, case–control and cross-sectional studies.

Cohort and case–control studies relate individual use of, or exposure to, the agent or invervention under study to the occurrence of cancer in individuals and provide an estimate of relative risk (ratio of incidence or mortality in those exposed to incidence or mortality in those not exposed) as the main measure of association. Cohort and case–control studies follow an observational approach, in which the use of, or exposure to, the agent is not controlled by the investigator.

Intervention studies are experimental in design — that is, the use of, or exposure to, the agent or intervention is assigned by the investigator. The intervention study or clinical trial is the design that can provide the strongest and most direct evidence of a protective or preventive effect; however, for practical and ethical reasons, such studies are limited to observation of the effects among specifically defined study subjects of interventions of 10 years or fewer, which is relatively short when compared with the overall lifespan.

Intervention studies may be undertaken in individuals or communities and may or may not involve randomization to use or exposure. The differences between these designs is important in relation to analytical methods and interpretation of findings.

In addition, information can be obtained from reports of correlation (ecological) studies and case series; however, limitations inherent in these approaches usually mean that such studies carry limited weight in the evaluation of a preventive effect.

Quality of studies considered
The *Handbooks* are not intended to summarize all published studies. The Working Group considers the following aspects: (1) the relevance of the study; (2) the appropriateness of the design and analysis to the question being asked; (3) the adequacy and completeness of the presentation of the data; and (4) the degree to which chance, bias and confounding may have affected the results.

Studies that are judged to be inadequate or irrelevant to the evaluation are generally omitted. They may be mentioned briefly, particularly when the information is considered to be a useful supplement to that in other reports or when it provides the only data available. Their inclusion does not imply acceptance of the adequacy of the study design, nor of the analysis and interpretation of the results, and their limitations are outlined.

Assessment of the cancer-preventive effect at different doses and durations
The Working Group gives special attention to quantitative assessment of the preventive effect of the agent under study, by assessing data from studies at different doses. The Working Group also addresses issues of timing and duration of use or exposure. Such quantitative assessment is important to clarify the circumstances under which a preventive effect can be achieved, as well as the dose at which a toxic effect has been shown.

Criteria for a cancer-preventive effect
After summarizing and assessing the individual studies, the Working Group makes a judgement concerning the evidence that the agent or intervention in question prevents cancer in humans. In making their judgement, the Working Group considers several criteria for each relevant cancer site.

Evidence of protection derived from intervention studies of good quality is particularly informative. Evidence of a substantial and significant reduction in risk, including a 'dose'–response relationship, is more likely to indicate a real effect. Nevertheless, a small effect, or an effect without a dose–response relationship, does not imply lack of real benefit and may be important for public health if the cancer is common.

Evidence is frequently available from different types of study and is evaluated as a whole. Findings that are replicated in several studies of the same design or using different approaches are more likely to provide evidence of a true protective effect than isolated observations from single studies.

The Working Group evaluates possible explanations for inconsistencies across studies, including differences in use of, or exposure to, the agent, differences in the underlying risk of cancer and metabolism and genetic differences in the population.

The results of studies judged to be of high quality are given more weight. Note is taken of both the applicability of preventive action to several cancers and of possible differences in activity, including contradictory findings, across cancer sites.

Data from human studies (as well as from experimental models) that suggest plausible mechanisms for a cancer-preventive effect are important in assessing the overall evidence.

The Working Group may also determine whether, on aggregate, the evidence from human studies is consistent with a lack of preventive effect.

Experimental models

Experimental animals

Animal models are an important component of research into cancer prevention. They provide a means of identifying effective compounds, of carrying out fundamental investigations into their mechanisms of action, of determining how they can be used optimally, of evaluating toxicity and, ultimately, of providing an information base for developing intervention trials in humans. Models that permit evaluation of the effects of cancer-preventive agents on the occurrence of cancer in most major organ sites are available. Major groups of animal models include: those in which cancer is produced by the administration of chemical or physical carcinogens; those involving genetically engineered animals; and those in which tumours develop spontaneously. Most cancer-preventive agents investigated in such studies can be placed into one of three categories: compounds that prevent molecules from reaching or reacting with critical target sites (blocking agents); compounds that decrease the sensitivity of target tissues to carcinogenic stimuli; and compounds that prevent evolution of the neoplastic process (suppressing agents). There is increasing interest in the use of combinations of agents as a means of improving efficacy and minimizing toxicity. Animal models are useful in evaluating such combinations. The development of optimal strategies for human intervention trials can be facilitated by the use of animal models that mimic the neoplastic process in humans.

Specific factors to be considered in such experiments are: (1) the temporal requirements of administration of the cancer-preventive agents; (2) dose–response effects; (3) the site-specificity of cancer-preventive activity; and (4) the number and structural diversity of carcinogens whose activity can be reduced by the agent being evaluated.

An important variable in the evaluation of the cancer-preventive response is the time and the duration of administration of the agent or intervention in relation to any carcinogenic treatment, or in transgenic or other experimental models in which no carcinogen is administered. Furthermore, concurrent administration of a cancer-preventive agent or implementation of an intervention may result in a decreased incidence of tumours in a given organ and an increase in another organ of the same animal. Thus, in these experiments it is important that multiple organs be examined.

For all these studies, the nature and extent of impurities or contaminants present in the cancer-preventive agent or agents being evaluated are given when available. For experimental studies of mixtures, consideration is given to the possibility of changes in the physicochemical properties of the test substance during collection, storage, extraction, concentration and delivery. Chemical and toxicological interactions of the components of mixtures may result in nonlinear dose–response relationships.

As certain components of commonly used diets of experimental animals are themselves known to have cancer-preventive activity, particular consideration should be given to the interaction between the diet and the apparent effect of the agent or intervention being studied. Likewise, restriction of diet may be important. The appropriateness of the diet given relative to the composition of human diets may be commented on by the Working Group.

Qualitative aspects An assessment of the experimental prevention of cancer involves several considerations of qualitative importance, including: (1) the experimental conditions under which the test was performed (route and schedule of exposure, species, strain, sex and age of animals studied, duration of the exposure, and duration of the study); (2) the consistency of the results, for example across species and target organ(s); (3) the stage or stages of the neoplastic process, from preneoplastic lesions and benign tumours to malignant neoplasms, studied and (4) the possible role of modifying factors.

Considerations of importance to the Working Group in the interpretation and evaluation of a particular study include: (1) how clearly the agent was defined and, in the case of mixtures, how adequately the sample composition was reported; (2) the composition of the diet and the stability of the agent in the diet; (3) whether the source, strain and quality of the animals was reported; (4) whether the dose and schedule of treatment with the known carcinogen were appropriate in assays of combined treatment; (5) whether the doses of the cancer-preventive agent were adequately monitored; (6) whether the agent(s) was absorbed, as shown by blood concentrations; (7) whether the survival of treated animals was similar to that of controls; (8) whether the body and organ weights of treated animals were similar to those of controls; (9) whether there were adequate numbers of animals, of appropriate age, per group; (10) whether animals of each sex were used, if appropriate;

(11) whether animals were allocated randomly to groups; (12) whether appropriate respective controls were used; (13) whether the duration of the experiment was adequate; (14) whether there was adequate statistical analysis; and (15) whether the data were adequately reported. If available, recent data on the incidence of specific tumours in historical controls, as well as in concurrent controls, are taken into account in the evaluation of tumour response.

Quantitative aspects The probability that tumours will occur may depend on the species, sex, strain and age of the animals, the dose of carcinogen (if any), the dose of the agent and the route and duration of exposure. A decreased incidence and/or decreased multiplicity of neoplasms in adequately designed studies provides evidence of a cancer-preventive effect. A dose-related decrease in incidence and/or multiplicity further strengthens this association.

Statistical analysis Major factors considered in the statistical analysis by the Working Group include the adequacy of the data for each treatment group: (1) the initial and final effective numbers of animals studied and the survival rate; (2) body weights; and (3) tumour incidence and multiplicity. The statistical methods used should be clearly stated and should be the generally accepted techniques refined for this purpose. In particular, the statistical methods should be appropriate for the characteristics of the expected data distribution and should account for interactions in multifactorial studies. Consideration is given as to whether the appropriate adjustment was made for differences in survival.

Intermediate biomarkers
Other types of study include experiments in which the end-point is not cancer but a defined preneoplastic lesion or tumour-related, intermediate biomarker.

The observation of effects on the occurrence of lesions presumed to be preneoplastic or the emergence of benign or malignant tumours may aid in assessing the mode of action of the presumed cancer-preventive agent or intervention. Particular attention is given to assessing the reversibility of these lesions and their predictive value in relation to cancer development.

In-vitro models
Cell systems *in vitro* contribute to the early identification of potential cancer-preventive agents and to elucidation of mechanisms of cancer prevention. A number of assays in prokaryotic and eukaryotic systems are used for this purpose. Evaluation of the results of such assays includes consideration of: (1) the nature of the cell type used; (2) whether primary cell cultures or cell lines (tumorigenic or nontumorigenic) were studied; (3) the appropriateness of controls; (4) whether toxic effects were considered in the outcome; (5) whether the data were appropriately summated and analysed; (6) whether appropriate quality controls were used; (7) whether appropriate concentration ranges were used; (8) whether adequate numbers of independent measurements were made per group; and (9) the relevance of the end-points, including inhibition of mutagenesis, morphological transformation, anchorage-independent growth, cell–cell communication, calcium tolerance and differentiation.

Mechanisms of cancer prevention
Data on mechanisms can be derived from both human studies and experimental models. For a rational implementation of cancer-preventive measures, it is essential not only to assess protective end-points but also to understand the mechanisms by which the agents or interventions exert their anticarcinogenic action. Information on the mechanisms of cancer-preventive activity can be inferred from relationships between chemical structure and biological activity, from analysis of interactions between agents and specific molecular targets, from studies of specific end-points *in vitro*, from studies of the inhibition of tumorigenesis *in vivo,* from the effects of modulating intermediate biomarkers, and from human studies. Therefore, the Working Group takes account of data on mechanisms in making the final evaluation of cancer prevention.

Several classifications of mechanisms have been proposed, as have several systems for evaluating them. Cancer-preventive agents may act at several distinct levels. Their action may be: (1) extracellular, for example, inhibiting the uptake or endogenous formation of carcinogens, or forming complexes with, diluting and/or deactivating carcinogens; (2) intracellular, for example, trapping carcinogens in non-target cells, modifying transmembrane transport, modulating metabolism, blocking reactive molecules, inhibiting cell replication or modulating gene expression or DNA metabolism; or (3) at the level of the cell, tissue or organism, for example, affecting cell differentiation, intercellular communication, proteases, signal transduction, growth factors, cell adhesion molecules, angiogenesis, interactions with the extracellular matrix, hormonal status and the immune system.

Many cancer-preventive agents and interventions are known or suspected to act by several mechanisms, which may operate in a coordinated manner and allow them a broader spectrum of anticarcinogenic activity. Therefore, multiple mechanisms of action are taken into account in the evaluation of cancer-prevention.

Beneficial interactions, generally resulting from exposure to inhibitors that work through complementary mechanisms, are exploited in combined cancer-prevention. Because organisms are naturally exposed not only to mixtures of carcinogenic agents but also to mixtures of protective agents, it is also important to understand the mechanisms of interactions between inhibitors.

Other beneficial effects
An expanded description is given, when appropriate, of the efficacy of the agent in the maintenance of a normal healthy state and the treatment of particular diseases.

Information on the mechanisms involved in these activities is described. Reviews, rather than individual studies, may be cited as references.

The physiological functions of agents such as vitamins and micronutrients can be described briefly, with reference to reviews. Data on the therapeutic effects of drugs approved for clinical use are summarized.

Toxic effects

Toxic effects are of particular importance in the case of agents or interventions that may be used widely over long periods in healthy populations. Data are given on acute and chronic toxic effects, such as organ toxicity, increased cell proliferation, immunotoxicity and adverse endocrine effects. Some agents or interventions may have both carcinogenic and anticarcinogenic activities. If the agent has been evaluated within the *IARC Monographs on the Evaluation of Carcinogenic Risks to Humans*, that evaluation is accepted, unless significant new data have appeared that may lead the Working Group to reconsider the evidence. If the agent occurs naturally or has been in clinical use previously, the doses and durations used in cancer-prevention trials are compared with intakes from the diet, in the case of vitamins, and previous clinical exposure, in the case of drugs already approved for human use. When extensive data are available, only summaries are presented; if adequate reviews are available, reference may be made to these. If there are no relevant reviews, the evaluation is made on the basis of the same criteria as are applied to epidemiological studies of cancer. Differences in response as a consequence of species, sex, age and genetic variability are presented when the information is available.

Data demonstrating the presence or absence of adverse effects in humans are included; equally, lack of data on specific adverse effects is stated clearly.

Information is given on carcinogenicity, immunotoxicity, neurotoxicity, cardio-toxicity, haematological effects and toxicity to other target organs. Specific case reports in humans and any previous clinical data are noted. Other biochemical effects thought to be relevant to adverse effects are mentioned.

Effects on fertility, teratogenicity, fetotoxicity and embryotoxicity are also described. Information on nonmammalian systems and in-vitro systems is presented only if it has clear mechanistic significance.

The results of studies of genetic and related effects in mammalian and nonmammalian systems *in vivo* and *in vitro* are summarized. Information on whether DNA damage occurs via direct interaction with the agent or via indirect mechanisms (e.g. generation of free radicals) is included, as is information on other genetic effects such as mutation, recombination, chromosomal damage, aneuploidy, cell immortalization and transformation, and effects on cell–cell communication. The presence and toxicological significance of cellular receptors for the cancer-preventive agent are described.

Structure–activity relationships that may be relevant to the evaluation of the toxicity of an agent are included.

Summary of data

In this section, the relevant human and experimental data are summarized. Inadequate studies are generally not included but are identified in the preceding text.

Recommendations for research

During the evaluation process, it is likely that opportunities for further research will be identified. These are clearly stated, with the understanding that the areas are recommended for future investigation. It is made clear that these research opportunities are identified in general terms on the basis of the data currently available.

Evaluation

Evaluations of the strength of the evidence for cancer-preventive activity and carcinogenic effects from studies in humans and experimental models are made, using standard terms. These terms may also be applied to other beneficial and adverse effects, when indicated. When appropriate, reference is made to specific organs and populations.

It is recognized that the criteria for these evaluation categories, described below, cannot encompass all factors that may be relevant to an evaluation of cancer-preventive activity. In considering all the relevant scientific data, the Working Group may assign the agent or intervention to a higher or lower category than a strict interpretation of these criteria would indicate.

Cancer-preventive activity

The evaluation categories refer to the strength of the evidence that an agent or intervention prevents cancer. The evaluations may change as new information becomes available.

Evaluations are inevitably limited to the cancer sites, conditions and levels of exposure and length of observation covered by the available studies. An evaluation of degree of evidence, whether for an agent or an intervention, is limited to the materials tested, as defined physically, chemically or biologically, or to the intensity or frequency of an intervention. When agents are considered by the Working Group to be sufficiently closely related, they may be grouped for the purpose of a single evaluation of degree of evidence.

Information on mechanisms of action is taken into account when evaluating the strength of evidence in humans and in experimental animals, as well as in assessing the consistency of results between studies in humans and experimental models.

Cancer-preventive activity in humans

The evidence relevant to cancer prevention in humans is classified into one of the following categories.

- *Sufficient evidence of cancer-preventive activity*
  The Working Group considers that a causal relationship has been established between use of the agent or intervention and the prevention of human cancer in studies in which chance, bias and confounding could be ruled out with reasonable confidence.

- *Limited evidence of cancer-preventive activity*
  The data suggest a reduced risk for cancer with use of the agent or intervention but are limited for making a definitive evaluation either because chance, bias or confounding could not be ruled out with reasonable confidence or because the data are restricted to intermediary biomarkers of uncertain validity in the putative pathway to cancer.

- *Inadequate evidence of cancer-preventive activity*
  The available studies are of insufficient quality, consistency or statistical power to permit a conclusion regarding a cancer-preventive effect of the agent or intervention, or no data on the prevention of cancer in humans are available.

- *Evidence suggesting lack of cancer-preventive activity*
  Several adequate studies of use of or exposure to the agent or intervention are mutually consistent in not showing a preventive effect.

The strength of the evidence for any carcinogenic effect is assessed in parallel.

Both cancer-preventive activity and carcinogenic effects are identified and, when appropriate, tabulated by organ site. The evaluation also cites the population subgroups concerned, specifying age, sex, genetic or environmental predisposing risk factors and the relevance of precancerous lesions.

Cancer-preventive activity in experimental animals

Evidence for cancer prevention in experimental animals is classified into one of the following categories.

- *Sufficient evidence of cancer-preventive activity*
  The Working Group considers that a causal relationship has been established between the agent or intervention and a decreased incidence and/or multiplicity of neoplasms.

- *Limited evidence of cancer-preventive activity*
  The data suggest a cancer-preventive effect but are limited for making a definitive evaluation because, for example, the evidence of cancer prevention is restricted to a single experiment, the agent or intervention decreases the incidence and/or multiplicity only of benign neoplasms or lesions of uncertain neoplastic potential or there is conflicting evidence.

- *Inadequate evidence of cancer-preventive activity*
  The studies cannot be interpreted as showing either the presence or absence of a preventive effect because of major or quantitative limitations (unresolved questions regarding the adequacy of the design, conduct or interpretation of the study), or no data on cancer prevention in experimental animals are available.

- *Evidence suggesting lack of cancer-preventive activity*
  Adequate evidence from conclusive studies in several models shows that, within the limits of the tests used, the agent or intervention does not prevent cancer.

Overall evaluation

Finally, the body of evidence is considered as a whole, and summary statements are made that encompass the effects of the agent or intervention in humans with regard to cancer-preventive activity and other beneficial effects or adverse effects, as appropriate.

Available in the same series:

IARC Handbooks of Cancer Prevention:

Volume 1	Non-Steroidal Anti-inflammatory Drugs (NSAIDs)
Volume 2	Carotenoids
Volume 3	Vitamin A
Volume 4	Retinoids

These books can be ordered from:

IARC*Press*
150 Cours Albert Thomas
69372 Lyon cedex 08, France
Fax: +33 4 72 73 83 02
E-mail: press@iarc.fr

Oxford University Press
Walton Street
Oxford, UK OX2 6DP
Fax: + 44 1865 267782